D1715919

Self-Care Theory in Nursing

in Nursing

Selected Papers of
Dorothea Orem

Katherine McLaughlin Renpenning, MSN, holds a Bachelors of Science from the University of Saskatchewan and a Masters from the University of British Columbia. She is president and chief nursing consultant of MCL Educational Services, Inc., and McLaughlin Associates. She has held a variety of positions in nursing education and nursing service and consulted extensively in relation to self-care deficit nursing theory in research, practice, and education. Ms. Renpenning was coauthor of *Nursing Administration in the 21st Century: A Self-Care Theory Approach*, published by Sage Publishing, and has worked with Dorothea Orem since 1983.

Susan Gebhardt Taylor, PhD, RN, FAAN, is Professor Emerita, Sinclair School of Nursing, University of Missouri-Columbia. Her Bachelor degree is from Alverno College, Milwaukee, Wisconsin, and her graduate degrees are from The Catholic University of America, Washington, DC. She is the recipient of awards, including Alumnae of the year from Alverno College, Missouri Tribute to Nurses Nurse Educator, Kemper Fellow for Teaching Excellence, and MU Alumni Association Faculty Award. Dr. Taylor has worked with Dorothea Orem since 1976, collaborating on writing, consultations, and presenting work related to self-care deficit nursing theory.

Self-Care Theory in Nursing

Selected Papers of
Dorothea Orem

Katherine McLaughlin Renpenning, MSN
Susan G. Taylor, RN, PhD, FAAN
Editors

 Springer Publishing Company

Springer Publishing Company, Inc.
536 Broadway
New York, NY 10012-3955

Acquisitions Editor: Ruth Chasek
Production Editor: Sara Yoo
Cover design by Joanne Honigman

03 04 05 06 07/5 4 3 2 1

Library of Congress Cataloging-in-Publication Data

Self-care theory in nursing / Katherine McLaughlin Renpenning, Susan G. Taylor, editors.
    p. cm.
    Includes bibliographical references and index.
    ISBN 0-8261-1725-2
    1. Nursing—Philosophy. 2. Self-care, Health—Study and teaching.
  3. Patient education—Study and teaching. 4. Nurse and patient.
  5. Nursing—Study and teaching. I. Renpenning, Kathie McLaughlin.
  II. Taylor, Susan G.
  RT84.5 .S456 2003
  610.73'01—dc21   2002036655

Printed in the United States of America by Maple-Vail Book Manufacturing Group.

To Dorothea Orem
for the wisdom and foresight she manifests in the papers
and for working with us through the years
to enhance the scholarliness of nursing

Contents

PART II: INTERNATIONAL PERSPECTIVES ON OREM'S WORK

Contributors

Dorothea Orem, MSNEd, FAAN
Savannah, GA

Other Contributors

Gerd Bekel, Soz Wiss RN FIG
Cloppenburg, Germany

Esther C. Gallegos, PhD
Universidad Autonoma De Nuevo
   Leon
Monterrey, N.L.
Mexico

Somchit Hanucharurnkul, PhD,
   RN
Ramathibodi Hospital
Bangkok, Thailand

Yuwadee Luecha, EdD, RN
Ramathibodi Hospital
Bangkok, Thailand

Wantana Maneesriwongul, DScN,
   RN
Ramathibodi Hospital
Bangkok, Thailand

Jariya Wittaya-sooporn, DNS, RN
Ramathibodi Hospital
Bangkok, Thailand

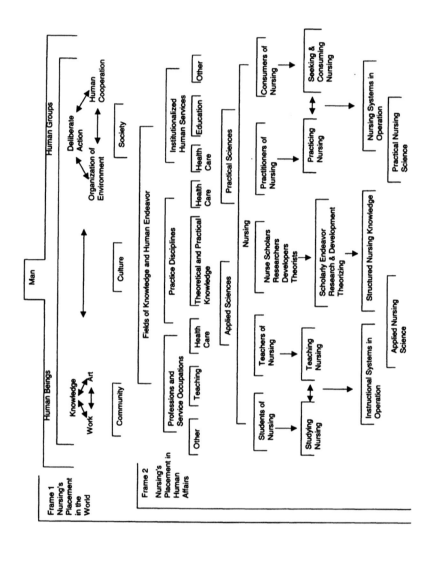

FIGURE P.1 Nursing's placement in the world of humankind and in human affairs.
Nursing Development Conference Group (1979). *Concept Formalization in Nursing* (2nd ed.), p. 22.

A Note From Dorothea Orem

The writings selected for publication by the editors represent three areas of professional responsibility that have been of interest and concern to me during my years in nursing. The papers reveal some results of my search for understanding of the nursing sciences, nursing education, and nursing practice, including formalized and expressed insights about their nature, structure, content, and relations. The papers are historical in the sense that they reflect time-specific conditions, events, and issues in nursing about which nurses had questions and sought answers.

My work confirmed for me that the three above-named areas of responsibility of the nursing profession, while distinct from one another but also related, must be investigated and developed separately. Investigation in one area, often proceeding in the same time frame with investigation in another area, led to verified insights about the nature of each and the relationships between them. For example, the identification and formalization of the proper object of nursing in society and the subsequent modeling of the self-care deficit theory of nursing (nursing science area) led to conceptualizations and the formalizations of the end product of nursing practice, namely systems of nursing care, to the expression of the human results to be sought through nursing, and to the form, structure, and content areas of nursing practice (nursing practice area).

In 1973, while preparing a paper on the processes of developing conceptual frameworks for nursing practice and nursing education, I experienced a need for an answer to the question: Where does nursing fit in the world of humankind and human affairs? Figure P.1 is an illustration of the outcome of my deliberations. Accepting that nursing, like all areas of human endeavor, has its origins and existence in the tendencies, interests, and capabilities of individual men and women working alone or in groups, I located nursing within a broad frame of human affairs that I named "fields of knowledge and human endeavor." I identified three subframes that would subsume nursing, namely, professions and service occupations, practice disciplines, and institutionalized human services. Nursing practice and nursing education are located in the subframe of institutionalized human services and nursing science in the subframe of practice disciplines. Nursing practice is located within the broader category of health services. In my subsequent work I found the results of this exercise of formally locating nursing in the world of human affairs a continuing guide in boundary setting. The fit of nursing in the world in which we live is an essential understanding for all nurses who seek to fulfill their professional responsibilities for nursing. I did not do in-depth work to formally develop the subframe "professions and service occupations." However, it was necessary for me to be knowing about and use knowledge from this area to make some developments in the area of nursing education, including its relations to the nursing practice area.

The writings in this book are for the most part general in their orientation. They are pieces of a larger picture. Together with *Nursing: Concepts of Practice* and *Concept Formalization in Nursing: Process and Product*, they have afforded some direction to practitioners of nursing, educators and teachers of nursing, and nursing researchers who work at the operational level to ensure that nursing and nursing education, as they are provided in their communities, are in accord with the needs and concerns of persons served.

I thank the editors for their interest in my work and for the efforts they have expended in developing this publication. Susan Taylor and Kathie Renpenning have made major contributions to the continuing effort to bring nursing true status as a profession in our society.

Dorothea Orem

Foreword

This publication of the collected papers of Dorothea E. Orem is a significant and valuable contribution to the nursing literature. These writings give insight into the development and range of thinking about nursing over the years. Orem's conceptualizations have provided a mental model essential to the development of nursing as a discipline of knowledge—a practical science with applied sciences and the foundational nursing sciences. As Mary B. Collins, an experienced clinical nurse, once said, "It gives me the words to express what I *know* to be nursing."

Through six editions of her book, *Nursing: Concepts of Practice*, and two editions of *Concept Formalization in Nursing: Process and Product* by the Nursing Development Conference Group, of which Orem was the leader, key contributor, and editor, Orem has provided the theoretical structure upon which to develop and expand nursing knowledge. She has clarified nursing's particular contribution to health care and given direction for its future development.

Dorothea Orem has a unique ability to listen to a group of nurses expressing their concerns and ideas about nursing and to analyze and conceptualize the essence of meaning in what is being said. Through this process she frequently formulates an abstract model to illustrate the relationships among the concepts.

Dorothea Orem has always been gracious and considerate about others' ideas and exemplifies a scholarly approach to whatever subject is under consideration. She always functions as an integral part of the group, never dominating, but sharing with others in a collaborative working relationship. She quietly encourages input from nurses, facilitating in developing their ideas, helping them gain insights and stimulating them to take a similar scholarly approach to nursing.

Notable about Orem is not only her depth of thought but also her continuing growth over the years in developing her conceptualizations, as evidenced in this collection of papers and the six editions of her book. In the most recent edition of *Nursing: Concepts of Practice*, Orem not only added to the structure of her nursing theories but laid the groundwork for areas needing further development in the practical science of and the foundational sciences of nursing.

For more than thirty years, Orem's concepts, based on the self-care deficit theory of nursing, have given direction to many nurses, inspiring them to seek better ways to develop and express the knowledge base of nursing. She has been a consultant to many groups of nurses in education, practice, and nursing administration, both nationally and internationally. She also has made a significant contribution in developing a theory of nursing administration. From the late 1960s to the present, numerous regional and international conferences and institutes based on her conceptualizations have taken place. In honor of her contributions to nursing, Orem has received recognition from many sources, including Sigma Theta Tau, the National League for Nursing, the Distinguished Alumni Award from The Catholic University of America, and three honorary doctorates.

The International Orem Society for Nursing Science and Nursing Scholarship was established in 1990 for the purpose of advancing nursing science and nursing scholarship through the use of Dorothea E. Orem's conceptualizations in nursing education, practice, and research. The Society seeks to establish a worldwide network for interaction among nursing scholars and sponsors conferences and promotes scholarly activities designed to encourage the advancement of nursing science.

Much research has been done based on the self-care deficit nursing theory, beyond serving as the basis for master's theses and doctoral dissertations. A few examples of its use are: the early development by Horn and Swain (1977) at the University of Michigan on *Criterion Measures of Nursing Care*; the W. K. Kellogg Foundation grant to Alcorn State University for development of family-centered adolescent health promotion centers in rural Mississippi; the establishment of the Center for Experimentation and Development in Nursing at The Johns Hopkins Hospital during the late 1960s and early 1970s, whose projects for developing nursing practice were based on Orem's concepts; and a grant for a post-doctoral program at Wayne State University for scholars to work with the theory. Moreover, the self-care deficit nursing theory has been used to develop nursing practice in many service agencies, such as hospitals, home health care, and community health agencies. It is the basis for nursing practice and education in Thailand and is being used in other countries around the world.

In education, it has been the basis of nursing courses and curricula in baccalaureate and community college nursing programs.

Orem served as a consultant for many of these agencies, helping them to develop creative and innovative approaches to achieve desired outcomes. Some of this work has been published. Her model has provided impetus for the development of exemplary programs in nursing practice, in the teaching of nursing and nursing curricula, as well as in nursing research.

As two members of the former Nursing Development Conference Group who early on had the benefit and privilege of working with Orem and applying her ideas in both practice and education, we have found her mental model for nursing to be insightful, logical, and representative of the reality of nursing. Working with Orem's conceptualizations has been both exciting and challenging in our professional lives. Orem has provided the structure for the ongoing and future development of nursing as a practical science and as a practice discipline.

Sarah E. Allison, RN, MSN, EdD
Cora S. Balmat, RN, MSN, PhD
Members of the Nursing Development Conference Group

REFERENCE

Horn, B. J., & Sevain, M. A. (1977). Development of Criterion Measures of Nursing Care: Volumes I and II. Prepared for National Center for Health Services Research. Hyattsville, MD.

Introduction

HOW THIS BOOK CAME ABOUT

We, the editors of this book, both have a long association with Dorothea Orem—Susan Taylor since 1976 and Kathie Renpenning since 1983. Collaboration between the two of us began in 1983 at the instigation of Orem and continues to this day through theory development activities, writing and publishing, and giving presentations in North America, South America, Asia, and Europe. As we have worked with Orem and learned of her theoretical and conceptual work, we also got to know her personally and were privileged to have access to her working papers and presentations. There is great value in these materials and we wanted to share them with the nursing community.

The papers that are included in this book are representative of Orem's thinking throughout the years. Most of the papers were developed for presentation. In a few instances notes that Orem had made in preparation for presentations, writings, or classes are included. The materials are presented in chronological order to illuminate the development of Orem's ideas about nursing theory, education, and practice over time. At the end of the book there are papers by nurses in other countries which highlight the status of Orem's theory internationally.

Papers that had been typed were scanned into the computer and edited for accuracy. Handwritten papers were edited for readability, abbreviations converted into words, transcribed by a professional typist, and edited by one of us. Some format changes were made for readability and publication style such as the format of references, lists, and publications. The original papers were not written in a particular style. However, whenever possible APA was used in editing.

As with any historical document, these papers need to be read with consideration of the historic and cultural context in which they were written or presented. For example, it should be noted that in the early years, the use of *man* or the pronoun *he* was acceptable when referring to the individual. Because of where Orem was working, the early focus is on hospital nursing, while in later years many settings were represented.

THE ROOTS OF DEVELOPMENT OF SELF-CARE DEFICIT NURSING THEORY

In 1945, after working as a nurse in the operating room, emergency room, private duty, pediatrics, and adult medical/surgical nursing and teaching at The Catholic University of America (CUA), Orem accepted a position as Director of Nursing Service and Director of Nursing Education at Providence Hospital in Detroit. In a personal communication (11/20/97) she recounted an experience she had when she was director of the school.

> We had a good program, good students. We were having a curriculum committee meeting, and a question was asked; it was a substantive question. I had no glimmer of an answer to it. I knew there was something missing. I was director of the school. We had a good faculty. It was a question that raised questions in my mind. What's the answer? I don't know. I knew that I should, but, if you don't have a conceptualization of nursing there are certain things that you can't answer. You're oriented to doing this and doing that and doing the other.

The lack of a substantive, structured body of nursing knowledge surfaced again when she was working in Indiana. She went to Indiana in 1949, with the Indiana State Board of Health, Hospital Division, to help in upgrading of nursing services in general hospitals. She worked closely with Ann Poorman Donovan, conducting studies of organizational structure of nursing services and variations in types of patients and length of stay. She described this period.

> Some of the things we came up with included the demands placed on nurses by length of stay of patients, by the scheduling of admission and discharges, by how activities were planned throughout the day in nursing units . . . nurses had difficulty representing their needs to hospital administrators. They didn't know how to talk about nursing, they didn't know how to represent what they needed. The same would be true in communicating with boards of trustees and with physicians. But one of the things I found in talking with physicians was that if

you talk nursing, they understood. They weren't anti-nursing, they just needed somebody to represent things properly to them. (personal communication, 11/20/97)

Orem reports that it was at the end of writing a report on the study of administrative positions that she felt the need to write a chapter on hospital nursing services and then a chapter on the art of nursing that included her first definition of nursing.

I actually had to construct it. I think one of the important things was that I had some conceptualization of how a science develops because of my background in biology, including the sequence of courses through bachelor's and master's programs in biology. At least, I had some understanding of scientific knowledge. I knew that it didn't exist in nursing, but to develop nursing science, that wasn't in my mind. I was concerned with expressing what nursing is. (personal communication, 11/20/97)

The first two chapters reflect the results of her thinking at this time. Although the study from which these chapters are extracted was done in the 1950s they are included here for the definition of nursing with the first specification of self-care limitations of persons as the object of nursing and the clear statements of the inherent distinctions between nursing and medicine. During this time in nursing there was beginning to be a focus on planning nursing care. Orem became aware that the "point of departure for planning care had to be the patient's, not the nurses', tasks." The emphasis on planning nursing care led Orem to ask, "What is the basis for planning? What are you planning? To me, there wasn't anything" (personal communication, 11/20/97).

Following her work in Indiana, Orem returned to Washington, D.C., and took a position with the Office of Education, Vocational Section of the Technical Division, where there was an ongoing project to upgrade practical nurse training. It was at this time that the more formal work of structuring began including authoring *Guides for Developing Curricula for the Education of Practical Nurses* (Orem, 1959).

In my thinking that started at that time, I came to the conclusion that the question that had to be answered was "Why do people need nursing?" I didn't go back to the work I had done in Indiana. I didn't look at nursing references but I asked myself the question. I can still remember the situation in which I had the insight to answer the question "Why do people need nursing?" The knowledge was within me. I was able to use that knowledge in answering the question. I remember sitting, how I was sitting at the desk when I did ask and answer that question. It is a specific memory. From that time onward, the knowledge I had about nursing began to structure itself. It wasn't anything I did deliberately, but the pieces started to come together. (personal communication, 11/20/97)

NURSING THEORY AND NURSING EDUCATION

Orem returned to the CUA School of Nursing in 1959 to teach graduate students and direct them in their research. During the next twenty years the development of self-care deficit nursing theory, theory-based curriculum building, and the design of nursing practice from a nursing theory perspective occurred synergistically as can be seen particularly in chapters 3–16. These chapters reflect Orem's interaction with educators and practitioners. In addition to being active in curriculum development at CUA Orem was active as a curriculum consultant for schools of nursing developing nursing theory based curricula. The interactions with faculty at CUA and three other schools (Morris Harvey College, Charleston, West Virginia, the newly developing nursing program at the University of Southern Mississippi, Hattiesburg, Mississippi, and the Georgetown University School of Nursing, Washington, D.C.) were particularly meaningful in the development of self-care deficit nursing theory. Publications and papers describing this work contain much information of interest to nursing educators and historians. These materials are outside the scope of this book, as they were developed by people working with Orem and not Orem herself. In 1974, the accrediting body of the National League for Nursing (NLN) revised the standards for accreditation to include the requirement that nursing curricula have a theoretical basis (NLN, 1972). This was a stimulus for continuing theory development.

There are identifiable themes in the chapters on education. In the early ones, Orem is dealing with the then current issue of levels of nursing education programs and the need for maintaining standards that would be helpful to both the profession and society. This was a period when there was a nursing personnel shortage and increasing complexity in practice. This led to the development of the nursing technician programs in the junior and community colleges as well as an increase in the number of baccalaureate programs for nurses in colleges and universities, and master's clinical specialization. The ideas expressed in these papers remain meaningful in the contemporary health care milieu, as ways of dealing with the current issues of nursing shortages and the essential and legitimate roles of professional nursing are debated. The later papers reflect the influence of theory development on Orem's understanding of curriculum development and the need for theoretical understanding of the object of nursing. She spoke and wrote to the need for knowing the object of nursing and using structured knowledge to build curricula. She maintained her belief that the intellectual work of nursing is most appropriately the work of the professionally educated nurse.

NURSING THEORY AND NURSING PRACTICE

Coincidentally with the curriculum work, the Nursing Development Conference Group (NDCG), which grew out of the CUA Nursing Models Committee, was formalized in 1968. This group was made up of eleven nurses from a variety of backgrounds in education and practice who were concerned about the lack of an organizing framework for nursing. This group set about working with Orem and the embryonic self-care deficit nursing theory to continue the work of formulating the theory. One of the "laboratories" for analyzing nursing and designing of nursing practice was The Center for Experimentation and Development of Nursing at The Johns Hopkins Hospital. Orem was an active consultant to this center and personnel from the center were members of the NDCG. The results of the deliberations of Orem and the NDCG were published in two editions of *Concept Formalization: Process and Product* (NDCG, 1973 and 1979). The scholarly activity and productivity of this group under the leadership of Orem is illustrated in chapter 16.

With the publication of the first edition of *Nursing: Concepts of Practice* (Orem 1971) information about self-care deficit nursing theory became widely disseminated and Orem came to be much in demand as a speaker and consultant in relation to the theory itself and in relation to nursing practice and education issues. In chapters 17–31 the development of the theory can be seen and the specific contribution of the theory to advancing nursing education and nursing practice can be appreciated.

Orem frequently refers to self-care deficit nursing theory as a theory of nursing practice. The theory emerged in part as Orem sought answers to the question "Why does a person need a nurse?" Answering the question has resulted in the lifelong work of theorizing about nursing and making "explicit the elements and relationships that give form and meaning to nursing as a field of practice and a field of knowledge" (Orem, 2001, p. 489). In the first chapter in this book Orem lays out the essential requirements for the practice of nursing. Although this was written in 1955 it still has meaning today. This early work has been influential in Orem's thinking as self-care deficit nursing theory has evolved.

Orem's facility for listening to nurses; observing and analyzing practice situations; breaking down and analyzing systems, individual acts, and sequences of actions; and categorizing and structuring the disparate pieces of information, as well as her ability to bring out the scholar in practicing nurses resulted in the Nursing Development Conference Group's contributing to laying out the substantive structure of the variables of concern to nursing (NDCG, 1973, 1979). This also resulted in making explicit and sharing insights about the relationships among those variables. This was a significant milestone in the development of nursing as a practice discipline. The theories and knowledge bases of other disciplines would remain important to nursing but the issues and questions of concern to nurses and their answers could now be framed and explored from the perspective of nursing rather than from that of another discipline.

Development of nursing as a discipline is dependent in part on structuring the knowledge base of nursing practice so that nurses can share with each other what they have learned through their many and varied experiences. This requires a language that enables nurses to describe experiences and to articulate what they have learned from those experiences. Without this specific language nurses rely on the language of other disciplines which incompletely describe nursing's focus of concern. In chapters 7, 8, and 9 the value of identifying the variables of concern to nursing and the provision of a nursing language to the processes of nursing are illustrated. As a point of interest, these workshops occurred prior to the publication of *Nursing: Concepts of Practice* and *Concept Formalization: Process and Product*. In these chapters the utility of self-care deficit nursing theory in guiding and making specific data collection, designing, and planning systems of nursing assistance is presented.

Early in her career Orem recognized the interrelationships among organizational structure, nursing practice, and the development of nursing knowledge. She frequently writes and speaks about the need for nurses and persons responsible for delivery of health care and nursing services to recognize and address the articulation of nursing systems with other organizational systems, and the need for nurses to recognize their responsibility and to have a strong voice in the development of health care delivery systems. Chapters 16, 19, 24, 25, and 31 are concerned with nursing administration and delivering nursing services on an agency-wide basis. Orem emphasized that in delivering such services it is necessary to think beyond those provided by individual nurses to individual patients and to focus on designing and delivering services to groups of persons and populations.

FUTURE WORK

In 1993 Orem wrote a paper titled "Work to be done" (see chapter 34). The work to be done includes further development of self-care deficit nursing theory, but more importantly, it involves the further development of the practical science of nursing and the structuring of nursing knowledge. This is the work of nurse scholars, researchers, practitioners and educators. Recognizing the need for continuing development of self-care deficit nursing theory, students of the theory have formed the International Orem Society for Nursing Science and Scholarship. This group has held conferences in the United State, Belgium, and Thailand, and is currently planning a conference to be held in Germany. At the conference in Belgium a development group established by Orem reported on the work they were doing. Orem did not attend the conference but she introduced the work of the development group via video. In the introduction (chapter 36) she outlined the process of theory development as it has been pertinent to self-care deficit nursing theory. This paper provides one set of directions for future action.

Susan G. Taylor, RN, PhD, FAAN
Professor Emerita
Sinclair School of Nursing, University of Missouri-Columbia

Katherine McLaughlin Renpenning
President, Chief Nursing Consultant, MCL Educational Services, Inc.

PART *I*

Orem's Writings

CHAPTER 1

Essential Requirements for the Practice of Nursing: An Analysis

The application of the art of nursing to specific persons in need of nursing assistance constitutes the practice of the art. Nursing, like all arts, has a range of practice that extends from the simple to the complex and at all times has undeveloped, partially developed, as well as unknown areas of practice. Since nursing is an art that renders a personal service to patients and physicians, it is necessarily practiced in those situations. The requirements for the effective practice of the art of nursing are derived from the art itself, from its modes or forms of practice, from the situations where patients reside and where physicians give medical care, and from the practitioners of nursing. There is need to understand these requirements, since the practitioner of nursing does not have responsibility for, and often has no control over, the specific situations in which she practices her art. The nurse goes where she is needed by patients and by physicians.

The essential requirements for the effective practice of nursing fall into three groups: relationships, qualifications of practitioners, and situational requirements. The specific requirements that constitute each group are listed as follows.

ESSENTIAL REQUIREMENTS FOR THE PRACTICE OF NURSING

Relationships

1. A personal relationship between the nurse and her patient, like the relationship between friends, with the nurse in the role of the more

This paper was originally presented as a report prepared for the Division of Hospital and Institutional Services of the Indiana State Board of Health in October, 1956.

objective, the able-bodied, the unselfish, and the skilled practitioner of nursing

2. A personal relationship between the nurse and the patient's physician, like the relationship between partners in an enterprise
3. A personal relationship between the nurse and the relatives, friends, and associates of her patient like the relationship of members of a family who are concerned with the well-being of one who is in need, the patient
4. A personal relationship between the nurse and all other persons who participate in the care of the patient, like the relationship of business associates

Qualifications of Practitioners

1. Ability to understand the kinds of relationships necessary in the practice of the nursing art and the capacity to evolve reasonably satisfactory relationships as required in various types of situations under ordinary and extraordinary conditions of actions
2. Ability to determine and evaluate the nursing care needs of patients, the ability to plan for meeting these needs in an effective and reasonable manner, and the skills to effectively meet the care needs of patients under changing conditions of action
3. Ability to determine, evaluate, and plan for the needs of the physician for nursing assistance in various types of situations under ordinary and extraordinary conditions of action, and the skills to effectively meet these needs

Situational Requirements

1. Conditions of action that permit for the evolving of essential relationships with the patient, the physician, the relatives, friends, and associates of the patient, and other persons who participate in the care of the patient as required
2. Conditions of action that provide the time and the contacts necessary for determining, evaluating, and planning for the nursing care needs of the patient

3. Conditions of action that provide the time and the contacts necessary for determining, evaluating, and planning for the needs of the physician relative to nursing assistance
4. Conditions of equipment, supplies, and facilities in accord with the nursing care needs of patients, the nursing assistance needs of physicians, and the specific forms of application of the nursing art
5. Conditions of work and employment that permit the practitioner of nursing to apply her art in accord with its nature and with the specific requirements just listed, and that provide for the personal welfare and the just remuneration of the practitioners

These requirements may be considered as standards of nursing practice that are essential in any situation where nurses practice their art. The degree to which these standards are met is a criterion of nursing effectiveness in specific situations and in particular institutions and agencies. Structuring procedures that thwart rather than provide for these requirements are detrimental to the patient, the physician, the nurse, and the institution or agency where nursing is practiced. Continued failure to meet the requirements for the practice of the art of nursing results in the substitution of numerous technical services, and the patient has no nurse to act with and for him in his dependency.

CHAPTER 2

The Art of Nursing in Hospital Nursing Service: An Analysis

Thus far, nursing has been discussed as one of the functional entities of a hospital. It is necessarily understood that nursing, like medicine and other health disciplines, does not derive its reason for existence or its essential characteristics from the hospital. The substantial elements of nursing are always the same whether nursing be practiced in the patient's home, in a hospital, a clinic, or in the physician's office. The place where nursing is practiced modifies its application but does not change its substantial character. For this reason a brief analysis of the art of nursing is presented.

NURSING DEFINED

Nursing is an art through which the practitioner of nursing gives specialized assistance to persons with disabilities of such a character that more than ordinary assistance is necessary to meet daily needs for self-care and to intelligently participate in the medical care they are receiving from the physician. The art of nursing is practiced by doing for the person with the disability, by *helping him to do for himself* and/or by *helping him to learn how to do for himself.* Nursing is also practiced by helping a capable person from the patient's family or a friend of the patient to learn how *to do for* the patient. Nursing the patient is thus a practical and a didactic art.

Nursing as an art also includes the special assistance that the practitioner of nursing gives directly to the physician. The nurse prepares situations

This paper was originally presented as a report prepared for the Division of Hospital and Institutional Services of the Indiana State Board of Health in October, 1956.

of action in which the physician will perform medical care measures for a patient; she maintains selected conditions of action while he performs the measures with which she may assist him in the care of the patient, and with the handling of equipment and supplies as he performs the measure; she may assist him with the care of the patient immediately following the performance of the measure; and she may perform or direct the performance of measures to care for the equipment and supplies used and the facility where the measure was performed. What the nurse does is what the physician would otherwise have to do for himself. The nurse frees the physician in situations of action that extend to many details so that his efforts may be directed to decision making and to the actual performance of the measure. The nurse makes many decisions in light of the physician's directives and the known requirements for the performance of the measure. The nurse does not make decisions that relate to the medical reason for the measure, to the measure itself, or to its outcome.

The nurse in the practice of her art is personally responsible for her actions as they relate to the patient and to the physician. This extends to the carrying out of the physician's directives for medications and treatments for a patient, as well as the physician's directives about assisting him with medical care measures. This means that the nurse's understandings and skills must be adequate for making judgments and decisions about (1) what needs to be done, (2) the correctness of the things she has been requested to do by the physician, (3) her ability to act, and (4) her right to act. The physician always retains responsibility for his actual directives to the nurse; the nurse is responsible for the action she takes in light of them.

The art of nursing does not include in its practice the performance of measures which, by nature and by standards of medical practice, are the rightful worries of the physician. Nurses may acquire the understandings and skills to intelligently perform selected measures of medical care. When they perform such measures in accord with physicians' directives, they are not practicing nursing but are acting in place of the physician. The physician, of necessity, retains responsibility not only for the directive given but also for the actions of the nurse who carries out his directive, for she is performing a medical and not a nursing act.

NURSING THE PATIENT

The nurse applies her art to patients with disabilities that have resulted in physical, intellectual, or psychological dependency upon another for daily self-care, including intelligent patient participation in medical care. The physician directs the medical care of the patient, including that which the patient must do for himself, or the nurse must do for him, or help him do, or instruct him so that he will learn to do. Medical care is directed specifically to the disabilities of the patient, their causes, and their effects. Nursing care is directed to helping the patient meet his continuous requirements for self-care during the twenty-four hours of the day in light of his disability, his specific dependencies, his physician's directives for medical care, and his needs arising from his personality, habits, and status in life.

The forms of application of the art of nursing to a patient are three, as previously mentioned: caring for the patient, helping the patient to care for himself, and instructing the patient and/or another to acquire the knowledge and the skills necessary to give the required care. The specific forms or modes of application of the nursing art to the patient are determined by the character, degree, and extent of the patient's dependencies. The unconscious patient is totally dependent and must be *cared for*. The patient with uncontrolled diabetes mellitus, with circulatory impairment of the lower extremities, may need nursing care in all three forms, since he has some degree of physical dependency, may lack the knowledge and skills to participate in his own care, and may feel personally inadequate to cope with the situation. Other patients may require nursing only in the form of helping them learn to care for themselves. The form of application of the nursing art will, of necessity, change as patients progress and dependencies are eliminated.

Thus, the art of nursing in application to the patient has two general goals: to meet or to help the patient meet, during the twenty-four hours of the day, his continuous needs for self-care and self-participation in the medical care directed by his physician, and to help the patient when his condition so permits to become self-directing in his personal care and able to carry out his physician's directives for participation in medical care. The specific application of the art of nursing to a patient will help the patient meet, with the required assistance of the physician and others, the following:

1. His specific ordinary demands for self-care and daily living related to
   a. daily care of the body
   b. eating and the taking of fluids
   c. elimination from bladder, bowels, and skin

    d. needs for privacy, rest, and sleep

    e. needs for a safe and comfortable physical environment

    f. needs for diversion, recreation, intellectual activity, and physical activity

    g. contacts with family, friends, and associates

    h. the spiritual practices of his religion

2. The extraordinary requirements for self-care and daily living that result directly from the disabilities present, their causes, their effects, and the medical care being received

    a. specific modifications of self-care and daily living

    b. relief and prevention of stress from physical causes such as discomfort and pain; from emotional causes such as fear, apprehension, and guilt; from social causes such as lack of normal family solicitude, over-solicitude, and specific social and economic family difficulties; and from spiritual difficulties

3. Participation in the medical care of the patient during the twenty-four hours of the day as directed by the patient's physician

    a. the fulfillment of orders for specific medications and treatments

    b. the continuous determination of the condition of the patient, his response to medications and treatments, and the presence or absence of signs and symptoms relevant to the patient's pathological state and his medical care

    c. securing the assistance of the patient's physician, as required, in emergencies

    d. assisting the patient to meet the directives of his physician in regard to aspects of his medical care in which other physicians and persons from other health disciplines participate; for example, ensuring that the patient is prepared for ordered x-ray examinations, that his appointment is in order and that he keeps his appointment

    e. assisting the patient either through his physician or directly, if so advised by the physician, to secure specific assistance that the patient needs from social workers, family assistance groups, or spiritual ministers and others

4. Giving the patient's physician, each day, or more often as required, specific information about the following:

    a. the general condition of the patient during the twenty-four hours of the day and his abilities and difficulties in meeting the ordinary requirements of daily living

   b. the specific condition of the patient as it relates to his disability, its cause, effects, and medical care during the twenty-four hours of the day, including response to medications, treatments, and so on

   c. the presence of stress or of factors that may result in it

   d. the patient's desires and feelings, suppressed or expressed, which the physician may find of value in his medical care of the patient

   e. the patient's response to specific measures of care applied by other persons in accord with the physician's directives.

That which the nurse does to accomplish the above and the manner or form in which she does each specific activity involved should be derived from a careful analysis of the nursing needs of each patient. To be of value to the nurse and to the patient, such an analysis must relate to those aspects of the person's life and his disability that give rise to specific needs for nursing care, and it must be reasonably exhaustive.

DISABILITIES OF PATIENTS AND RESULTANT NURSING CARE REQUIREMENTS

The General Nature of Disabilities

Because the nurse's relationship to a patient has its origin in the patient's dependencies, and dependencies result from disabilities, it is necessary to understand the types of disabilities to which people are subject as well as the effects of disabilities. A disability is the absence or partial absence of a power, a capacity, or an ability normal or usual to a person. Since the powers of a person are physical, mental, emotional, spiritual, and psychosocial, disabilities will relate to these powers. The following is a suggested classification of disabilities according to their general character

1. Disabilities of internal physiological functioning
2. Disabilities of musculoskeletal functioning
3. Disabilities of sight, hearing, speech, muscular sense, equilibrium, touch, smell, and taste
4. Disabilities of intellection
5. Disabilities of self-control in regard to behavior

6. Disabilities of self-direction in regard to personal action
7. Disabilities of emotional control
8. Disabilities of emotional tone and response
9. Disabilities of psychosocial adequacy to meet life's demands upon the individual as a member of society

A major disability results from grave pathological retardation, loss, or from extreme limitation of the normal exercise of those powers of the person that are essential to complete and natural functioning. Limited disabilities result from temporary or permanent interference with the exercise of powers essential to complete and natural functioning but are amenable to control or to substitution therapy. Major disabilities are ones in which the person has

1. Loss or congenital absence of parts, organs, and tissues of the body essential to complete and natural functioning
2. Loss or congenital absence of natural structural relationships between parts, organs, and tissues of the body essential to complete and natural functioning
3. Extensive functional failure of existing parts, organs, and tissues of the body
4. Apparent absence or extreme or moderate limitation of powers of intellection, self-control and self-direction
5. Apparent absence or extreme or moderate limitation of the power to be objective

Limited disabilities are ones in which the person has

1. A moderate or minor limitation of function of existing, parts, organs, and tissues of the body
2. A minor limitation of the powers of intellection, self-control, and self-direction
3. A minor limitation of the power to be objective

Causes of Disabilities

Disabilities to which man is subject have many specific and many precipitating causes. The specific causes of disabilities are within the subject matter of medicine. A discussion of specific causes is not possible here. The nurse, however, is concerned with causes of disabilities insofar as they specifically affect the nursing care of the patient. The following is a listing of general, not specific, causes of disabilities.

1. Trauma to parts, organs, and tissues of the body from external sources
2. Trauma to parts, organs, and tissues of the body from sources within the patient
3. Lack or limitation of experiences and practices through which the person develops his existing powers of intellection, self-control, and self-direction
4. Lack or limitation of experiences and practices through which the person develops his existing powers of objectivity

Effects of Disabilities

The presence of a disability is first recognized through its specific effects by the patient, the physician, the nurse, or by other persons caring for or in contact with the patient. Effects of disabilities are always in the nature of a temporary or permanent impairment or an actual loss of function. The effects of disabilities are naturally related to types of disabilities as listed previously. Classification of the effects of disabilities is not an easy matter. What is cause and what is effect is of the very essence of medicine and is often of grave concern to the physician in the making of a diagnosis and in prescribing treatment. The same is true for the physiologist and the psychologist. The following is a suggested grouping of the effects of disabilities in general, not specific, terms.

1. Complete or partial failure of the normal physiological activity of specific internal organs and tissues or of any combination of tissues and organs of the body
2. Complete or partial failure of the normal physiological activities related to the external movement of the person
3. Complete or partial failure of the person to maintain a normal body chemistry, a normal rate of metabolism, a normal amount of body fat, and a normal energy reserve
4. Complete or partial failure of the normal physiological activity of the organs of sense

5. Complete or partial failure of the intellectual operations and the operations of the will of the person
6. Complete or partial failure of the operations necessary for psychological integration and wholeness and for leading a wholesome life in society

The patient lives the twenty-four hours of each day with the specific effects of his disabilities and their combined general effect. The effects of disabilities may necessitate modifications of the patient's habits of self-care and living; they may produce demands for special types of care to support impaired functioning; and they may require specific medical treatment. The nurse helps the patient meet the demands placed upon him by the specific and general effects of his disabilities when he needs such assistance. Patients with disabilities with effects confined to localized areas of the body may need nursing care that is primarily concerned with helping them to intelligently carry out their physician's directives and to learn to modify their own self-care as necessary. The person who is self-directing in relation to his self-care and the ordinary aspects of daily living and is able to participate effectively in his medical care is not in need of the special help of nurses, even though he may need things brought to him or other non-medical assistance.

Nursing Care Requirements of Patients

A careful analysis of the needs of each patient for nursing assistance is fundamental to the application of the art of nursing in specific situations. The results of such an analysis should lead to conclusions about

1. The existence of specific needs of the patient for the assistance of a nurse
2. The character, extent, and intensity of the patient's needs for nursing assistance
3. The major and minor measures of nursing care necessary to meet the nursing needs of the patient for the twenty-four hours of the day
4. The form of application of each major and minor measure of nursing care
5. The qualifications of nurse practitioners and nurse assistants to meet the needs of the patient, and the specific periods of the day

when the patient will need nurses and assistants with these
qualifications

The main areas of such an analysis are listed below.

1. The major personal characteristics of the patient in terms of
    a. age
    b. sex
    c. social state
    d. cultural state
    e. mentality
    f. personality
    g. habits of self-care
    h. habits of daily living
2. The major or limited disabilities of the patient for which he is
    receiving medical and related care
    a. the character, extent, and cause of each disability as known
        to the physician
    b. the effects of these disabilities as known to the physician, the
        patient, and persons who have been caring for the patient
    c. the general nature of the medical care the patient has been
        and is receiving from his physician
    d. the physician's specific directives for care of the patient related
        directly to the cause and the effects of the disability, as well
        as all directives for specific diagnostic, treatment, rehabilita-
        tion, and preventive measures to be performed for or by the
        patient
    e. how the patient and his family have been meeting the patient's
        needs arising from the disability
3. The major or limited disabilities of the patient that are not the
    main objective of present medical care but that complicate present
    care
    a. the character, extent, cause, and effects of each disability as
        known to the physician and the patient
    b. the relationships of these disabilities to present care and to
        the well-being of the patient
    c. the manner in which the patient has met or is meeting the
        general and specific results of these disabilities
    d. the physician's directives in regard to these disabilities

It can be readily understood that such an analysis and the reaching of conclusions in light of the results can be adequately done only by a physician who fully understands the nursing aspects of care of a patient, or by a nurse practitioner qualified to practice the full range of the nursing art. A careful and reasonably exhaustive analysis of the care requirements of a patient is basic to nursing care worthy of the name. An able and experienced nurse practitioner who is constantly with a patient makes such an analysis without going through a formalized process. It is done rather instinctively and the process itself often does not come to consciousness.

In situations where it is necessary to provide and plan for the nursing care of many patients, a formalized analysis is essential if the nursing needs of patients are to be known and met.

NURSING AS IT RELATES TO THE PHYSICIAN

The art of nursing as practiced in relation to the patient is a direct service to the patient. At the same time a service is rendered to the physician if the nursing care is of such nature and quality that it contributes to the well-being and progress of the patient, effectively applies measures of care ordered and advised by the physician, and keeps the physician informed of the general and specific condition of the patient and the patient's responses to care and his needs. The art of nursing as previously defined has an area of practice that serves the physician directly. This direct service relates to the physician's own performance of medical care measures. Nursing service to the physician is directed to accomplish the following.

1. The preparation of situations of action in which the physician will perform one or more medical care measures for a patient; this preparation includes the detailed activities necessary
   a. to ensure that required environmental conditions exist and can be maintained within the facility where the measure will be performed
   b. to ensure that the required equipment and supplies are present in a state of readiness for use
   c. to ensure that the physician's directives in regard to special needs are carried out
   d. to ensure that the patient is ready and present for the performance of the measure

2. The maintenance of required conditions of action while the physician performs the measure

3. Assisting the physician with the handling and the care of equipment and supplies as he performs the measure, and with the handling, preparation, and dispatching of specimens taken from the patient

4. Assisting with the details of caring for the patient before, during, and after the performance of the care measure

5. The aftercare of situations where physicians have performed medical care measures

This aftercare includes activities necessary to ensure that the facility is clean and safe for reuse and to ensure that the equipment and supplies are cared for or disposed of in accord with the use they have had.

The physician requires nursing service relative to the above matters in selected situations. The factors within a situation that give rise to a special need on a part of a physician for nursing service arise from (1) the measure itself, (2) the patient, (3) the physician and his work, or (4) from various combinations of the first three items. The physician needs nursing service in the performance of measures of care that are in themselves detailed and require detailed preparation and aftercare. He may need nursing assistance when he applies even moderately detailed measures of care to patients who are gravely ill physically, emotionally, or mentally, or when he and/ or the patient would be more at ease with a nurse present. He may need nursing assistance when his work involves performing numerous medical care measures for many patients in relatively short periods of time.

Nursing assistance to the physician is a personal service in which the nurse follows the directives, the known requirements, and the major personal needs of the physician in rendering assistance relative to the physician's performance of a medical care measure for individual patients.

The Nurse Acts for the Physician

When the nurse performs a measure of care that is within the category of medical practice, she is not serving in the role of a nurse. As she performs such a measure as directed by the physician, the nurse acts as a medical and not as a nurse assistant to the physician. Nurses, and in some instances technical assistants, may acquire the specific skills necessary to effectively perform selected medical care measures that the physician may deem necessary to assign to them. Only measures that possess all of the following characteristics should be so assigned.

1. The measure requires primarily mechanical skill with a minimum of adaptation to individual patients, and requires a relatively limited body of knowledge for its safe and accurate performance
2. The measure is such that it must be applied immediately when the need for it arises in the patient, or else must be applied so frequently that it would be a hardship, if not an impossibility, for the physician to be with the patient each time it is required
3. The measure is such that the life of the patient is not endangered by the measure itself, or, conversely, the patient will die if the measure is not immediately carried out
4. The measure is such that it may be effectively performed by carrying out a set procedure, step by step, with a minimum of adaptation required because of the individuality of the patient or his clinical situation

Nurses should perform such medical care measures only when qualified, able, and when so directed by the physician, and in an institutional situation only with the agreement of their immediate supervisor.

Measures that physicians tend to delegate are those that are repetitive and of a relatively fixed character. Such medical care measures eventually become integral parts of the practice of nursing but still remain integral parts of the practice of medicine. The taking of temperatures and blood pressure of patients are examples of medical care measures that are now integral parts of nursing practice as well as medical practice. The giving of medications and fluids intravenously is an example of a medical care measure that is in a state of transition between medical practice and nursing practice.

CHAPTER 3

Nursing Education, 1966–1967

A s nursing moves toward professional status in the United States, the problems of nursing practice and nursing education become not only more numerous but also more complex. In part nursing problems are rooted in the health needs of society and the rapid changes in the scientific foundation for health care, but they also are the result of the ways in which nursing education and practice have developed in our country. The focus of this paper is a description of roles for which nurses are prepared through particular forms of nursing education.

FORMS OF INITIAL EDUCATION FOR NURSING

The traditional form of education for nursing in our country developed within the institutional setting of the hospital. This form of education for nursing (the hospital-controlled diploma program) has undergone considerable change and presently exists alongside other forms of preservice or initial nursing education. To understand problems that confront nurses today, both from the perspective of practice and of education, it is necessary to have and to be able to apply two very different concepts of nursing: (1) the concept of nursing as a health service to people, something that nurses do in their assisting or helping roles in society, and (2) the concept of nursing as an area of subject matter, a body of knowledge that can be continuously developed and extended through the efforts of nurse practitioners, scholars, and researchers. Nurses and nurse educators would do well to give attention to both concepts and to identify the implications

---

This paper was first presented at the Nursing Services Conference of the American Red Cross, Eastern Area, in Alexandria, VA, June 2, 1966.

18

inherent in each to the eternal problem of providing nursing in society. Citizens of every community and all nurses have roles in finding solutions to this problem, but professionally educated nurses have a prime role in setting directions for its solution.

Today, attention is focused on making changes in initial educational preparation for nursing practice, changes that medicine, engineering, and agriculture started to make in the century prior to this one. But at the same time, nurses and citizens of our communities continue to be confronted with the social responsibility for getting people nursed. It seems to me that, in some way or other, old modes of nursing practice (or what we accept as nursing) must be put aside and new forms or revitalized older forms instituted. Modes or forms of nursing are not the focus of this paper but its topic is a closely related one—the roles of nurses prepared in various existing types of educational programs preparatory for nursing practice. It is my premise that what nurses can do to extend or improve nursing as a health service in society is set to a large degree by their initial education for nursing.

The development of nursing education in our country took place primarily within the framework of the hospital. In the early period of hospital development the nurse and the physician formed the health team and also performed the duties of present-day highly specialized paramedical workers. In the developmental period of hospital service in the United States there was specialization but in a different form than it prevails today. For example, I had an aunt who was a nurse, a pharmacist, and an x-ray technician and was recognized as effective in these three very different roles within the health field.

For many years nursing was a stable field of practice. Because of lack of rapid change in the foundational sciences and in medical science and technology, new developments in health care could be easily taken into the not-too-broad scope of nursing practice. The vocational or vocational-technical type education of the hospital school seemed to be adequate to meet society's need and it was so accepted by nurse leaders. What was never made explicit in the hospital diploma programs was that it was a vocational or vocational-type education. There were efforts to bring nursing education into educational institutions, but for the most part they were nonproductive. Nurse leaders continued to label this vocational or vocational-technical type of education as preparatory for functioning as a professional nurse in society.

The system of vocational and vocational-technical education that developed in hospital-controlled nursing schools left the country without a corps of professionally educated nurses. It placed the burdens of control of nursing practice and the development of nursing as an organized body of knowledge upon the shoulders of the hospital educated nurse—burdens for which she was ill prepared by education. If we look back in nursing history, however, we can note that the nurses who gave enlightened leadership to nursing were often women with a liberally or scientifically directed education that was acquired prior to entrance into a nursing school.

Following World War II, there was the phenomenal increase in the number of practical nurses and in the number of auxiliary personnel that many nurses practicing or teaching today experienced. Today we are experiencing the rapid growth of associate degree programs in nursing, and the closing or modification of the traditional three-year hospital school programs, and we are confronted with the recommendation that the preservice nursing education programs be limited to two types: the baccalaureate program controlled by senior colleges and universities and the associate degree program controlled by junior or senior colleges. It is not the purpose of this paper to extol any one program or to speak against any type of existing program. The plea is that we as nurses examine each type objectively so that we can understand that the social roles for which nurses are prepared are fashioned by their preservice education for nursing.

In the United States, three types of education for the occupations have been developed and presently prevail: professional, technical, and vocational. Today a fourth type is being recognized: vocational-technical. This seems to be a form that combines some features of both the technical and the traditional vocational approach to education preparatory for the occupations. In nursing education there are, today, preservice programs that are representative of these four types of approaches to occupational education. Graduates of these programs are all afforded the title of *nurse* by society, and in one type only—the vocational—are the title and functioning of the nurse qualified or limited by law. In the early days of the associate degree program movement in nursing education there was use of the term *nurse technician* to identify the graduate of this program; this term seems to be used less and less frequently. In 1967, the hospital or independent school program of two to three years duration, the associate degree program, and the baccalaureate program each made graduate nurses eligible to sit for the same examination to become registered nurses with an unlimited license to practice *professional nursing* as defined by state laws. It should be noted that according to program objectives and curriculums, the first two types or programs are specifically designed to prepare nurses for the limited practice of nursing. Thus nurses and nurse educators, at least by inaction, seem willing to have nurses licensed to function at a level for which they have not been prepared.

Today, if not in 1930 and earlier, nurses must admit that the foundation for nursing practice received in diploma programs and in associate degree programs does not provide a base for the full, unrestricted practice of professional nursing.

THE PROFESSIONALLY EDUCATED NURSE

The provision of professional education for nursing has been accepted by the universities and senior colleges of our country. As with any emerging profession there are problems, but progress is being made and there is some movement away from the vocational approach to teaching nursing that today still characterizes to some degree all types of initial programs of nursing education. The roles of the professionally educated nurse are for the sake of the profession and thus for the services to society for which the profession exists. It is my conviction that nursing cannot be developed on a scientific basis in any country of the world without a corps of professionally educated nurses. Many of the ills from which nursing and nursing education suffer today are caused by this lack. As long as a country denies itself this group of workers and negates a need for them, nursing in that country can never rest on a sound base and move as a social force for the good of the society.

The roles of the professionally educated nurse as I see them are as follows: (1) to render nursing assistance to persons in situations where creativity and flexibility in the application of scientific principles must be utilized in selecting and applying ways to assist them in achieving health results through continuing therapeutic self-care. The creative use of nursing technologies and the creation of new nursing technologies are essential parts of this role. This nurse must be able to think scientifically and be able to bring theory to bear in observing the reality of nursing situations for which nursing technologies are unformalized and in devising and applying ways to use nursing to aid in the accomplishment of health results; (2) to validate nursing technologies and to make them part of the body of knowledge that is nursing; (3) to extend the frontiers of nursing practice; (4) to develop the applied nursing sciences; and (5) to transmit to others formalized knowledge basic to nursing practice through writing and teaching.

Today, the baccalaureate program in nursing exists to provide a foundation that should enable the graduate to become a professional practitioner of nursing. She is not a professional practitioner upon graduation—she has a foundation for becoming one. She also has a foundation for professional specialization in nursing through graduate study in the university. Professional specialization requires a narrowing down of nursing focus, and the study of one aspect of the subject matter of nursing and its practice in depth. This includes the study of the applied sciences and the technologies of the specialty area, the acquisition of skills needed in the practice of the specialty, and beginning skills in extending the body of nursing knowledge and the practice of the specialty.

The pattern for professional education for nursing should adhere in a creative fashion to the patterns set for such education in the United States. This pattern includes a liberal arts and humanities component, a foundational science component; a nursing component, that ideally would have three parts: (1) applied nursing science, (2) the practical science of nursing (including the major nursing technologies), and (3) a nursing experience component. Ideally, the professionally educated nurse would have depth of preparation in several of the foundational sciences to facilitate development of scientific habits of thought. She would have less than depth preparation in a number of sciences. And, importantly, she would know in a general way the methods of derivation of the applied nursing sciences and the practical science of nursing.

Nurses who are graduated from the programs leading to the baccalaureate degree with a solid nursing major should become the expert generalized practitioners of professional nursing. It is these nurses who should, through graduate education in nursing, become the professional clinical nurse specialists and the scholars and researchers in nursing—the makers of nursing science. Sometimes we forget that science is not nature but the results of some hard-working, painstaking person's conceptualization and study of natural or behavioral phenomena. Too, the professionally educated nurse must collaborate with other professional health workers, with volunteers, with the public, and especially with other professional nurses or with technically or vocationally educated nurses, who may be her partners in providing nursing to individuals. The professional nurse will not turn to or accept from persons outside of the nursing profession answers to questions that are purely nursing problems. She bears responsibility before society for nursing and for its practice.

VOCATIONALLY AND TECHNICALLY PREPARED WORKERS

In an occupation where there is a professional level of practice as well as technically and vocationally prepared workers, the roles and rationales for the preparation of these workers must be identified. The role of the practical nurse has been and still is a major issue in nursing. We are now confronted with a similar problem relative to associate degree program graduates. Unless nurses resolve it, nursing will fail in its social mission. Technically and vocationally prepared nurses are a corps of nurses whose nursing roles should be limited by their education, including their continuing and extension education and related experiences. The tasks or the cluster of jobs these nurses are prepared to perform must be identified, and curriculums must be geared to prepare students for the effective and efficient practice of nursing within the limitations set. The limits of practice should be set before curriculums are developed. In technical and vocational education there must be a close liaison among employing institutions, educational institutions, and the profession. As nursing practice changes, so should vocational and technical nursing education programs. Ideally the corps of professionally educated nurses will be directing the change by feeding new and validated nursing technologies into nursing practice and by developing the scientific foundations underlying them. Educational programs for the vocational and technically educated nurse are merged in the plan for nursing education developed by the American Nurses Association.

One group of general educators have suggested the following as the level of intellectual functioning demanded of the nurse with reference to associate degree programs: (1) apply the principle of rational systems to solve practical problems, (2) integrate a variety of instructions furnished in written, oral, and diagrammatic or schedule form, and (3) deal with a variety of concrete variables. The nursing of some persons requires intellectual functions beyond this level. Variables may not be concrete; they may be quite abstract and so tied with the concrete that much scientific knowledge must be brought to bear even to identify the variables, much less to work with them.

Situations of mental illness, rehabilitation situations, and situations of illness where vital organs are involved are but a few examples. The vocationally and/or the vocationally-technically educated nurse from associate degree programs in nursing have important nursing roles but they can never be substituted for the professional nurse.

What the less-than-professionally educated nurse of the future should be educated to with respect to nursing must be identified in terms of the populations of our hospitals and the clientele of our community health agencies. We should recognize that a worker who has a depth of knowledge for a limited area of functioning can be more effective than a worker with limited knowledge spread over a large area of functioning. Should we not think of what are the nursing needs of society before there is a rapid and related unrestricted growth in the associate degree program? Some nurses in this audience have experienced the rapid growth of the hospital degree program, the practical nurse program, and now will be living through the same thing with the associate degree program.

My plea tonight is that all professionally licensed nurses in this audience, regardless of the type of preservice program in which they received their initial education for nursing, become active in setting standards for and controlling the practice of professional nursing. But let us see that a part of our responsibility is the setting straight of the future. Let us ensure that the education of the nurse who is licensed as a professional nurse be prepared for professional responsibility and let us not place professional responsibility upon the shoulders of non-professionally educated nurses.

CHAPTER *4*

Inservice Education and Nursing Practice

The topic, inservice education and nursing practice, poses the questions: What is inservice education? and How does inservice education relate to nursing practice? Two assumptions are made to serve as guides in exploration of the topic.

1. Inservice education is education for licensed nurses who are functioning in settings where nursing is practiced; this education is provided or sponsored by an agency or institution through which nursing as well as other health services are provided. The nurses are thus organizational members of the sponsoring agency or institution; they are *in service*.
2. The education offered is related to nursing as it is or as it should be practiced within the agency or institution.

Since nurses are the legitimate practitioners of scientifically derived and scientifically practiced nursing within agencies and institutions, the topic of inservice education and nursing practice can be developed from both an institutional point of view and from the point of view of the nurse and nursing practice. Consideration is given to institutional factors and nursing factors that are relevant to inservice education for nurses; suggestions then are made about a nursing focus to guide inservice education within agencies and institutions with nurse members.

This chapter was previously published in *Forces Affecting Nursing Practice: The Proceedings of the Continuing Education Series* conducted under the auspices of the Workshops Office of the Catholic University of America, March 7–May 2, 1968, ed. D. D. Petrowski & M. T. Partheymuller. Washington, DC: The Catholic University of America.

THE NURSE AS A MEMBER OF AN ORGANIZATION

Hospitals, short-term and long-term nursing homes, extended care facilities, community health agencies, health centers, and clinics are types of institutions or units of institutions within which nursing is practiced. Nurses who are organizational members of these institutions practice nursing in structured settings; they have expectations of themselves as well as of other members of the organization who fill positions different from their own.

A concept of an institution is a necessary aid in visualizing the nurse as a member of a community health agency or a hospital.

> Institutions are structures of mutual expectations attached to roles that define what each of its members shall expect from others and from himself. . . . The members of a human institution are related by three main modes of interaction—co-operation, conflict and competition. All three are necessary to maintain that dynamic balance that is the condition of survival. [Vickers, 1957, pp. 3–4]

The concept of an institution provides a base for examining the nurse as a member of an organization in order to see the demands that this membership places upon her. Nurses should be seen as interacting not only with patients but with one another and with organizational members from other health services, especially medicine.

Nurses and other persons who give health services may be said to be functioning in operational roles since they contribute to bringing about the institution's end product: health service to individuals, families, and communities. There is another group of organizational members who are directly concerned with maintaining "that dynamic balance that is the condition of survival" (Vickers) for each health care institution, namely those with executive or administrative roles.

Executives or administrators interact among themselves and with persons with operational roles at that level of organization where the institutional system brings persons with these roles together. Administrators at this level should seek information to establish what mutual expectations are held by institutional members as well as the degrees of cooperation, conflict, and competition among institutional members.

At this point, inservice education can be seen as an instrument or tool that can be utilized to formalize or clarify mutual expectations and thus establish a basis for cooperation, or to resolve conflict by objective study of issues and solving of problems, or to provide a basis for healthy competition in goal accomplishment.

The complexity of interactions and expectations should not be underestimated. Figures 4.1 and 4.2, which are oversimplified examples of areas of interaction of administrators and different types of operational members and a patient care situation respectively, attempt to illustrate some of the complexities of being an organizational member. The institutional problem of having members with valid and reliable expectations is a grave one; this problem must be solved on a continuing basis. In the four-person situation shown in Figure 4.2, it can be seen that a patient-care situation can be described not only in terms of roles and role expectations, but also in terms of requirements for communication among members of the health care team and between members of the team and the patient. If the time dimension is added to indicate that service is provided on a twenty-four hour basis, the picture becomes even more complex, because more than one organizational member who is able and qualified to assume the various roles will be needed. If organizational roles are split and tasks divided among a number of persons, the problem of role expectations increases in complexity; when the dimension of change in the patient's condition is added, complexity may be increased or decreased. Improvement and stability of the patient's condition lead to a decrease in complexity, and worsening and instability increase the demand for interactions and for relevant communications.

The roles nurses have in various types of health care situations can be viewed as determining their responsibilities for maintaining the dynamic balance of health teams. Since other team members also have similar responsibilities, the need for an institutional mechanism for bringing nurses together with other health team members should be evident. Team conferences are of course a part of team operation. However, joint study and exploration of health care and service problems presented by different types of cases could be an effective way for preparing nurses as well as others for efficient and effective functioning in rendering health services in specific situations. Joint study of cases by nurses and other organizational members who give health care is a fruitful form of inservice education.

SOME DEVELOPMENTS IN INSERVICE EDUCATION

An annotated bibliography prepared at Teachers College in 1944 provides some background information about inservice education in relation to nursing practice (Rogers, 1944). The annotated materials, which cover the

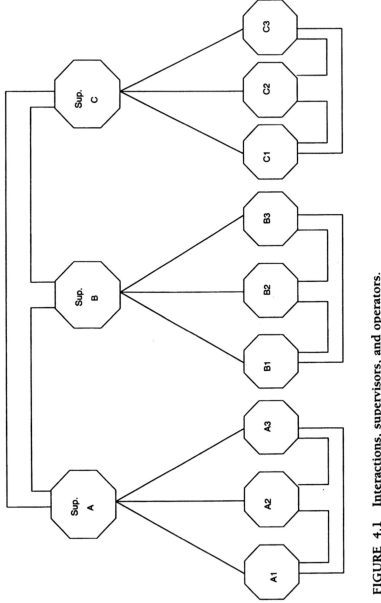

FIGURE 4.1 Interactions, supervisors, and operators.

—— Interaction

Sup. A, B, C: Supervisors with different health care and supervising roles

A, B, C: Operators with different health care roles

Sets of Expectations: (with A, B, and C representing different health care personnel in a health care situation).

1. Patient's expectations of his own roles as related to A, B, and C
   Patient's expectations of A, B, & C
2. A's expectations of himself and of B and C
   A's expectations of the patient as related to himself and to B and C
3. B's expectations of himself and of A and C
   B's expectations of the patient as related to himself and to A and C
4. C's expectations of himself and of A and B
   C's expectations of the patient as related to himself and to A and C

FIGURE 4.2 A health care situation—roles, interactions, and expectations.

period from 1926 to 1943, show that the state of development of nursing in society was reflected in what was being done or suggested as appropriate for inservice education. Some extractions are presented by decades.

The Period 1920 to 1930

In this period, the reasons for and the instruments of inservice education were highlighted. Reasons included the following.

1. Education is necessary for continuous progressive growth in order that appropriate levels of skills may be maintained while in service.
2. Education increases a growing person's responsibility for living.
3. Staff education is educating a constituency—attitudes, objectives, and educational media are necessary.
4. Education is for self-improvement, including organizational expedients for self-improvement.
5. Inservice training for nurses can enlarge the usefulness of nursing as a profession, that is, promote the well-being of the nation.

6. Staff education enables nurses to teach more effectively.
7. Topics used in staff education should be selected to make general-duty nursing more attractive and to promote growth of the nurse in service.

Some of the means and areas of education mentioned during this period were

1. Supervision as a medium for staff education
2. Staff conferences
3. Need for technical and general education
4. Staff education as a mutual benefit—nurses learn from each other
5. Staff education requires programming

The Period 1931 to 1940

The period 1931 to 1940 gave emphasis to means and reasons for inservice education with some reference to education of the nurse as related to administration and to specific clinical cases. Some extracts from the annotations are presented to demonstrate similarities to as well as evidence of change from the earlier decade covered in the bibliography.

Reasons for staff education reflect those of the earlier period. The needs of the institution were referred to in one annotation.

1. Post-graduate and staff education is related to professional growth.
2. Staff education is a tentative program for developing full time workers on the job.
3. Inservice education needed for the staff nurse.
4. Informal staff education is needed for staff nurses and head nurses.
5. Staff education comprehends the needs of the institution and the patients it serves, as well as the total personnel engaged in rendering the service.
6. Staff education is for the purpose of improving nursing practice.
7. Staff education is to meet needs for growth in service.

Changes from the earlier decade were most evident in the instruments for and the focus of staff education.

1. Opportunities for inservice staff education for the general staff nurse include participation in the administrative program of the nursing department.
2. Staff seminars can meet needs for continuing education in a psychiatric hospital.
3. Staff program was for the study of pneumonia and for the study of nursing problems.
4. Content of staff education should be related to clarification of techniques and establishment of uniformity in procedures.
5. Content of inservice should be based on what nurses want.
6. There should be conferences for staff nurses.
7. The staff is responsible for the success of an inservice program.

The Period 1941 to 1943

The last period covered in the bibliography included the years 1941 to 1943. There was some evidence of the formalization of inservice programs within institutions and a recognition of some aspects of operation and control of inservice programs.

1. Staff education for an all-graduate staff, for educating nurses for specialties, and for effective clinical teaching
2. Inclusion of theoretical instruction and practical experience for the graduate staff nurse to promote integration of nursing care of cancer patients into all existing nursing services
3. Staff education viewed as a well-organized integrated program comprehending the needs of the institution, patients, and total personnel, and as enlarging the understanding and appreciation of workers
4. Provision of inservice training for new staff members without increasing the number of supervisors by using senior staff nurses to assist in the inservice training program
5. Techniques necessary for determining the needs of a group for staff education

SUMMARY

An analysis of annotations from a bibliography for inservice education from 1920 to 1943 revealed evidence that inservice education was viewed as (1) institution sponsored, (2) designed for nurses so that by improving themselves, nursing and institutional goals could be achieved more effectively, (3) related to patients requiring nursing and to nursing problems, (4) requiring programming and resources, (5) involving costs, and (6) dependent upon staff support and staff involvement.

The period covered in the bibliography saw the gradual emergence of the *staff nurse* as an operational member of health care institutions, especially hospitals; staff nurses gradually replaced nursing students who were both *in training* and *in service*. Health care institutions had not been subjected to the demands for rapid change that followed the Second World War. There was recognition, however, of a need for the staff nurse to be provided with inservice education by the employing institution. But developments in the health field in general, and in nursing in particular, demand new guidelines for inservice education for nursing practice.

SOME GUIDELINES FOR INSERVICE EDUCATION

Two guidelines are suggested as aids in relating inservice education to nursing practice. The first is more general than the second. As a first guideline, it is proposed that institutional members with different roles as well as with different educational and experiential backgrounds have different requirements for inservice education. Professionally educated organizational members should have different inservice education from that provided for members prepared in technical or vocation-technical type educational programs. Professionally educated persons should also be expected to select what they need and be responsible and contributing participants in inservice education. Ordinarily, members not prepared through professionally qualifying education are not expected to be as self-directing as the professional with respect to identification of educational needs. The work of nurses prepared in vocational or semi-professional preservice educational programs is specified by the clusters of tasks they perform under the supervision of professionally educated members of the organization. In general, it can be assumed that the scope of an institution's responsibility for organized inservice education programs and projects is determined (1) by the way in which institutional positions and roles are defined, (2) by the number of members holding these positions, and (3) by the educational preparation and the experiences of these members.

Within the framework of this guideline, inservice education is confined to formally programmed education. It thus excludes learning concomitant with an institutional member's day-to-day performance of his roles in interaction with other organizational members; it also excludes teaching and learning as they are related to supervision. Supervision is that guidance, direction, and overseeing of work that every institution owes to each of its members: for example, the day-to-day supervision of a practical nurse or a nurse who completed a program of preservice education for nursing in a junior college by an experienced, professionally educated nurse. The kind and amount of supervision provided should be in accord with the present competency of a nurse to perform her role responsibilities.

Failures in supervision are common in nursing; some of these failures, perhaps the majority of them, are due to inadequate role definitions and to invalid expectations about what nurses with various educational and experiential backgrounds can do in nursing patients and in supervising the work of other nurses. No inservice education program can do away with the need for effective supervision, but effective inservice education can decrease the amount of supervision needed and can promote more effective interactions between the nurse who is supervised and the nurse who is supervising.

A role expectation focus is suggested to guide inservice education to improve nursing practice. Outcomes can be visualized in terms of cooperative effort toward the achievement of goals for patients who are under nursing care as well as in programming for the nursing of individual patients and groups of patients. Consideration would be given to attitudes, motives, knowledge, and skills that bear upon interaction, communication, and coordination between nurse and patient, nurse and nurse, and nurse and other health workers and supporting personnel. Figures 4.1 and 4.2 are suggested as guides for use in identification of sets of expectations and requirements for interactions and communication in patient care situations and between nurses engaged in nursing patients and their nurse supervisors.

The second guideline for use in relating inservice education to nursing practice is the development of the first guideline to give a more specific nursing focus to inservice education. This guideline suggests that inservice education for nurses can have as its focus any combination of the following: (1) the nursing process as related to specific types of nursing cases, (2) nursing demands arising from a patient population, (3) results, including the limits of the results that can be achieved through nursing, and (4) the control of the effectiveness and the efficiency of nursing in an institution through specific mixes or combinations of nurses and patients. Since these foci cannot be treated here in detail, two suggestions may serve to give direction to designing and planning for inservice education in relation to demands for nursing practice in institutions. The first suggestion is that the patient population served be studied so that it can be described in its relation to nursing demands, and the second is that nurse members of the institution be placed in categories according to their education, experience, and licensure to practice nursing.

A study of the *patient population* served by a health care institution can yield data from which types of demands for nursing can be inferred. Consistency or lack of consistency of characteristics of the population, changes in the reasons for needs for health care and nursing, changes in size of the population, and the duration of requirements for nursing can be determined from patient data that is readily available in many health care institutions. Information about changes in the technologies of health care and trends in utilization of health services is also of importance in designing and planning for inservice education for nurses.

Patient data as compiled for hospitals in the *Professional Activity Study* is one example of readily available information about patient populations from which some inferences about nursing requirements can be made (Commission on Professional and Hospital Activity, 1966). For example, for a six-month period in 1966, one metropolitan hospital in one of the Middle Atlantic States in a population of 6,082 patients had 625 patients with diseases of organs of the digestive system. Table 4.1 shows the distribution of this patient group by final diagnosis, total days in hospital, age, and the frequency of operative therapy.

It is necessary for nurses responsible for inservice education in institutions and agencies to have information about patients served and to have some reliable expectations about the characteristics of future demands for service. Without such information and without its utilization, inservice education cannot be related to demands for nursing in specific agencies and institutions.

The placement of nurses who are organizational members of institutions according to education, experience, and licensure is another task to be done by nurses who are responsible for inservice education. For purposes of illustration, three groups or categories are suggested; these groups are developed around the roles of nurses in relation to designing, planning, giving, and controlling nursing care for individual patients and groups of patients.

Group One: Nurses prepared through education and experience, qualified by licensure, and able to engage in the initial and continuing assessment

TABLE 4.1 Hospitalized Patients With Diagnosed Diseases of the Digestive System for a Six-Month Period, 1966

Patients by Final Diagnosis	Total Patients	Total Days	Patients by Age		Operative therapy
			13 and under	65 or older	
Dental	44	145	2	1	42
Mouth and Esophagus	12	98	—	2	7
Stomach and Duodenum	163	2264	2	34	52
Appendicitis	52	513	19	1	51
Other Intestine	206	2268	42	42	72
Liver, Gallbladder, and Pancreas	148	2414	—	37	92

of nursing requirements for the care of patients, to design systems of nursing care for patients, to plan for the institution and control of these systems of care, and to select and supervise nurses to contribute to the process of nursing the patients for whom the systems of care were designed.

Group Two: Nurses licensed to practice nursing in situations that demand nursing judgments requiring utilization by the nurse of scientifically derived knowledge. This group would include all nurses licensed as Registered Nurses; the group of nurses would be divided into subgroups according to education for nursing and the institution's plans relative to each nurse's career in nursing within the institution.

Group Three: Nurses licensed to participate in the nursing of patients under the direction and supervision of a registered nurse or a licensed physician, but who, according to licensure, are not to be placed in nursing situations demanding the use of scientifically derived knowledge in making nursing judgments. This group would include all licensed practical or vocational nurses and would be subdivided according to education and experience.

These three groups and their institutional roles should give direction to the kind of inservice education that would advance the nurses in these groups in nursing practice. Nurses must be related to the population to be nursed. This involves the development of positions and the defining of nurses' roles as they relate to characteristics of a patient population, to other nurses, and to other persons who give health care. Nurses who design systems of nursing care for individual patients define both the roles of the patient and the nurse who will provide nursing assistance. It is thus imperative that all nurses be assisted through inservice education to learn how to develop realistic expectations of themselves, of patients, and other personnel, and to learn their roles in terms of the nursing process as it is applied in the types of situations in which they will be expected to nurse.

CHAPTER 5

Clinical Evaluation

Clinical evaluation is approached within a framework of a course or programs that have a goal of preparing persons to be able to render direct health care service to patients through vocational instruction. In this frame of reference, clinical evaluation should be related to the patient, the student, and the course or program of vocational instruction. It is a component of the *control* function when clinical instruction is considered as a process through which selected changes are to be brought about in students so that they can, in turn, effect certain changes in patients in need of nursing. See Figure 5.1.

The course specifies what the student or the trainee is to become able to do for patients—what services will be given and under what circumstances these services may or may not be given; it also specifies the instructions and guidelines to be given to the student and establishes the evaluation. Patients are living subjects who require services that students are being taught to render; clinical evaluation is a process of ascertaining whether the student is able to render these services effectively, that is, in such a way that the service to the patient accomplishes its designed result or end, and efficiently, so that no undesired or untoward effects result for the patient, the student, or others, including no undue expenditure of energy or loss of materials.

Since clinical evaluation is activity, there must be an agent or a doer. The teacher who gives the vocational instruction should be the agent or the evaluator of the service rendered by the student to the patient since he has developed the objectives of the care and has instructed and guided

This paper consists of notes for presentation at the Introduction and Orientation for Directors, Clinical Specialist Courses, for the Surgeon General, Department of the Army, Walter Reed Hospital, held at the Woodner Hotel, Washington, DC, June 17–21, 1968.

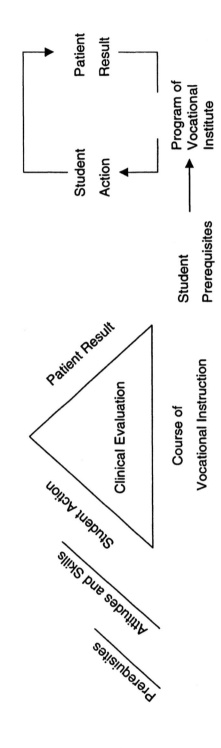

FIGURE 5.1 Framework for clinical evaluation.

the student, but by necessity, the student is also an evaluator of his own acts; he is not only a perceptive, thinking, responsible person, but he is in a position to control what he does as he renders.

The student and the teacher ideally utilize the same specifications: services to patients. Clinical evaluation is thus an essential aspect of rendering health care services to living subjects regardless of who is in the position of agent, as well as an essential aspect of the process of vocational instruction. See Figure 5.2.

These ideas are further developed into a set of assumptions about clinical evaluation.

1. Clinical evaluation has as its focus or object health care services rendered to patients by students receiving vocational instruction.
2. Clinical evaluation is a process of appraising or estimating the value of health care rendered to a patient in terms of the end result sought and achieved and in terms of the presence or absence of undesirable results that were not sought.
3. Clinical evaluation requires
   a. that a student's learning experiences have prepared him to become able to accomplish the result being evaluated
   b. that the teacher and the student are in contact and communication with one another and that the student knows the specifications for the health care to be given and the result to be sought
   c. that the student and teacher be in the presence of the patient and that each be aware of his or her roles in the situation
   d. that the student act to give a defined and limited health care service to a patient toward achievement of a defined result, evaluating and controlling his actions as he proceeds in light of relevant factors and results sought
   e. that the teacher act to weigh what the student accomplishes for the patient against the results sought for the patient and weigh unsought results in terms of their desirability or undesirability.

FOCUS ON THE OBJECT OF CLINICAL EVALUATION

Occupational preparatory courses or programs have the goals of preparing persons for gainful employment within specific occupations. Vocational education has traditionally been based upon the concurrent existence of three conditions in society.

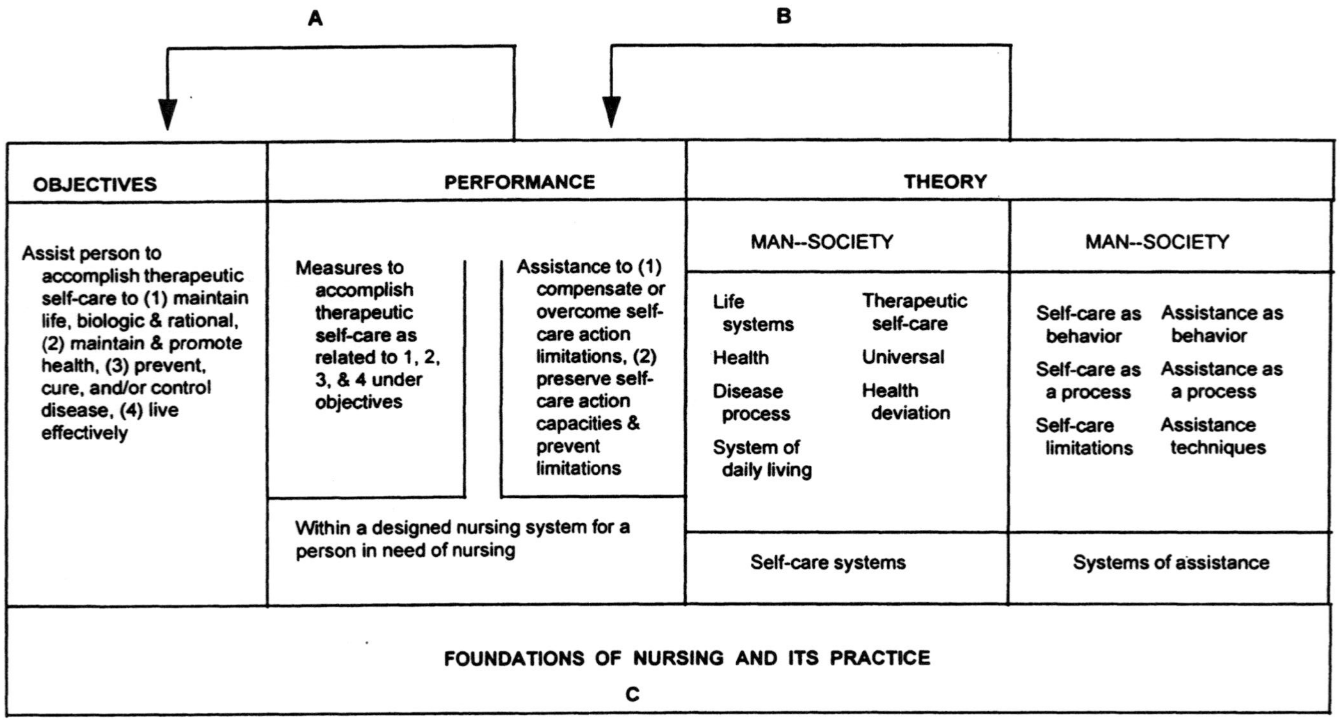

FIGURE 5.2 The focus and the components of vocational instruction in nursing.

A—The focus of the vocational program
B—Necessary for A
C—Necessary for A & B

1. There are defined jobs within various occupations and occupational settings, the effective performance of that will accomplish specified results that contribute to the attainment of some defined and limited purpose
2. The ways to accomplish these results have been established and systematized
3. Workers are needed to perform these jobs

The existence of jobs, the essential work operations required in effective job performance, and the need for workers to fill the jobs all exist prior to vocational courses or programs. It is the descriptive definition of what the job is to accomplish and the tasks or work involved that are the source of the educational objectives of vocational courses or programs. An example from a personal service, the vocation of hairdresser, may aid in understanding an approach to describing results for health vocations. Moyer and Beach (1967) suggest these objectives in relation to the task of hairstyling: "Given scissors, comb, and brush, be able to shape and style a client's hair to her satisfaction, taking into consideration facial contour and hair color and texture, within a half hour. Acceptable performance is achieved when the client is satisfied" (p. 43). This objective describes and sets the specifications for the results to be achieved through the performance of the task of hairstyling. A student would be evaluated by appraising what she accomplished for the client against the specifications set by the objective. This is illustrated in Figure 5.3.

ESTABLISHING THE FOCUS

In the health service occupations, particularly practical or vocational nursing, the defining of jobs and job tasks has been a problem for educators and for health care institutions and agencies. This problem has become increasingly complex and, in some instances, is ignored rather than analyzed in an attempt to find solutions. The literature on practical nursing education that has been published by federal and state agencies presents a number of approaches that have been utilized or suggested: for example, types of nursing cases (the convalescent or the chronically ill); procedures required in giving *care* (the problem is to define care) to a patient or in taking care of his environment or his clothing or preparing his food; criteria for selection of nursing cases appropriate for the practical nurse. The roles

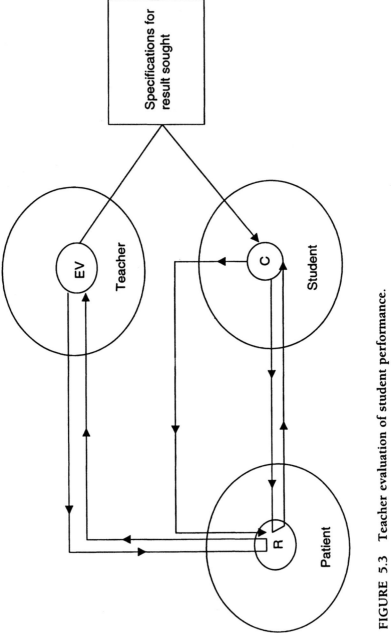

FIGURE 5.3   Teacher evaluation of student performance.

R—Results
C—Control action for health care
EV—Evaluative action control and judgment

42

and functions of the practical nurse are described in state laws as well as in publications of national groups such as the NFLPN (National Federation of Licensed Practical Nurses), the ANA (American Nurses Association), and the NLN (National League for Nursing). Despite these efforts to offer guidelines to both educators and health care agencies, practical nurses continue to be both over- and underutilized, and at times the question can be asked: Do the jobs for which vocational education programs prepare practical nurses actually exist? If the jobs do not exist, what basis is there for a vocational program or for clinical evaluation? However, neither past nor present conditions should deter efforts to attack, again, the problem of the *results* that *practical nurses* or *clinical specialists* in the military service can achieve for patients. Vocational education should not only be accepted but actually utilized in the development of institutional programs for practical nurses or clinical specialists prepared through vocational instruction. But it does seem essential that the instruction to be given be derived from nursing. The following are suggested standards to guide in describing results. These standards are general and would be made specific in terms of the characteristics of the patient population to be served.

1. Results are developed for types of nursing cases
2. The result specifies some condition(s) to be brought about or maintained or some change(s) to be effected in the person served. This condition(s) or change(s) is health related and its effects will be beneficial to the patient in terms of life, health, or effective living
3. The result is to be accomplished by specific sets of tasks that are to be performed by the practical or vocational nurse in order to bring about or maintain the health-related condition or the health-related change in the patient. The patient's role in bringing about or maintaining the condition or in effecting the change is described in relation to the roles of the practical or vocational nurse
4. The roles of the practical or vocational nurse are defined not only in terms of action to bring about results for patients but also in terms of relation to the roles of professional nurses, physicians, and others when giving health care to the patients, and the practical nurse's supervisor.

The vocational instructor who chooses to define results to be achieved in the work situation other than in terms of nursing cases, patients, and patient and nurse roles as related to types of cases ignores the *patient* as the focus of health care services. Furthermore, if what is done by the practical nurse or clinical specialist is not patient oriented, then it is not *clinical*.

ENSURING A PATIENT AND A ROLE FOCUS

How can a vocational program or vocational teachers go about establishing a patient and a role focus for a vocational course or program? Admittedly, the problem is a complex one but not beyond solution. The first requisite is that the health care service's frame of reference be identified and described. As vocational programs in the health services are developing today there seem to be at least four types: nursing, medicine, dentistry, and various paramedic fields, and in some instances there are no doubt combinations of these.

Nursing as a frame of reference for the vocational and practical nurse should provide to the course or program developer, the vocational teacher, and the clinical evaluations of student performance in course or program objectives, sets of tasks to be performed and theory to be applied as the tasks are performed. There are guides toward doing this but there is much that the person involved in vocational instruction must create and bring together. If the vocational instruction is in the field of nursing, it is essential to begin course development, revision, or adjustment with a well-formulated concept of nursing as the organizing principle. When used in conjunction with the three conditions justifying vocational instruction a concept of nursing provides the first set of standards for a course or program developer; keeping in mind that the objectives set for the course or program provide the basis for evaluation of student performance.

Figure 5.2 shows some of the components and relations among components in a program for the vocation of practical nurse. These components are four in number: objectives, performance components, theory, and a component that answers the "What is nursing?" question and "What are the characteristics of its practice in society?" Within the vocational frame of reference: performance is for the sake of the objectives, theory is basic to performance, and a guiding conceptualization of nursing is the component justifying or validating the presence of all other components. It sheds, so to speak, guiding light.

The descriptive definition of nursing, therapeutic self-care, nursing roles, and relations and nursing system, that are implicit in the figure, are taken from *Foundations of Nursing & Its Practice* to be published by McGraw-Hill. These ideas, first presented in *Nurse Case Identification, Selection, and Description* are essential in the taking of a patient result focus in clinical evaluation. Some guides toward doing this include accumulated patient data, criteria for selecting patients for PNs, and guides for looking at patients from a nursing point of view. [*Ed. note*—This was never published. The definitions can be found in any edition of *Nursing: Concepts of Practice.*]

ADDITIONAL NOTES

From the *Wall Street Journal*, December 2, 1966:

> The HEW Dept, The Labor Dept, and the Office of Economic Opportunity—planned to allocate $50 million or more to extra nursing grant—nearly double the 100,000 nursing and sub-professional personnel—technicians and orderlies—normally graduate annually from a variety of Federal-sponsored health programs. Experts say the nation's hospitals need 275,000 more nurses and other employees quickly (20% increase). Labor Dept. Manpower administration expects to enroll 52,000 persons in health organizations (double last year's total).

The ANA—reports three types of Initial Programs for Professional nursing—Diploma, Baccalaureate and Associate degree.

1. Treating nursing students as students and not as nurses creates employment opportunities for registered nurses.
2. The traditional fields of nursing practice as defined by ANA have not been extended in the last ten years. There has, however, been an increasing demand for specialization within the various fields defined by the ANA.

CHAPTER 6

Levels of Nursing Education and Practice

INTRODUCTION

The forms of institutionalized education or schooling preparatory for the practice of nursing in American society is the topic developed in this paper. It is my conviction that the form and the level at which education for nursing is offered, as well as the quality of the education, contributes to defining what nurses are able to do in nursing practice. The subject of levels of education and practice in nursing can be considered from the historical and comparative perspective, or from a combined nursing and educational perspective. The latter approach has been chosen because it serves to bring attention to norms and trends from the field of occupational education and their applicability to nursing education.

LEGITIMATE FORMS OF NURSING EDUCATION

Preliminary attention is given to the question: What programs of nursing education are legitimate in American society? This is an important question, for the answer to it should be seen as an influencing force in the determination of which of the existent programs will continue, which are likely to go out of existence, and, finally, what types of programs are likely to be or should be introduced.

This paper was first presented to the Alumnae Association of the Johns Hopkins Hospital School of Nursing, October 12, 1968.

Acceptable or legitimate programs of nursing education are necessarily identified in terms of what is acceptable to specific social groups. The original question would be more properly stated in these terms: What programs of nursing education are accepted by

1. Organized nurses and organizations that focus on nursing as a health service in society
2. The various states as establishing eligibility for persons to take examinations for licensure or registration as nurses
3. The public considered as the source of recruits to nursing, consumers of nursing, and financial and political support
4. Employing institutions such as hospitals or community health agencies
5. Persons in nursing-related occupations and professions who work with nurses in the rendering of health services in communities

As available information about nursing education is organized around these questions, or as individuals and groups seek answers to them, the characteristics of variety and differences emerge; there emerges also the central theme of change in the status of the nurse educated in hospital-controlled schools. This nurse no longer has the status of the most highly qualified nurse in society and the only type of nurse recognized in society as professional. Today she is one among many, and only by law or by virtue of her own nursing expertise and her concern and consideration for her patients, is she afforded the right to call herself a professional nurse.

In the years that brought the nineteenth century to its close The Johns Hopkins Hospital and its School of Nursing gave form and direction to nursing education with the purpose of offering to society "what is best in nursing" (Robb, 1907). During the past year, the Alumnae Association of The Johns Hopkins Hospital School of Nursing has given attention to the directions that nursing education should take in The Johns Hopkins institutions. In this effort, the Alumnae Association is contributing to the fulfillment of the social responsibility of appraising what is being offered and determining what should be offered so that those who elect to do so and those who can be stimulated to do so can pursue a career in nursing, at least in part, in The Johns Hopkins Institutions. A "career in nursing" (Gerstl, 1967) is used here to mean the filling of a succession of nursing positions in the occupational life cycle of a person as well as the person's movement into and out of nursing.

Modern efforts to introduce change and innovation in nursing education and practice seem to be of two general types: (1) those directed toward incorporation of modern science and technologies relevant to health care and interpersonal relations into nursing education and nursing practice and (2) those directed toward the distribution of the nursing required by a person or by members of a family among a number of different kinds of nurses and assistants to nurses. Nursing educators are confronted not only with needs for modernization of curricula and for keeping curricula up to date in terms of science and technology, but also with the problem of levels of education for nursing. The demand that nursing education be provided at a number of different levels came from various sectors of society and has resulted in at least four different types of nurses when classified by basic education for nursing. Three of these types of nurses are granted the same kind of licensure to practice. The demand that preservice nursing education be offered at no more than two levels has come from organized nurses (American Nurses' Association, 1965).

Decision making relative to continuity and change in nursing education requires information about demands for nursing, educational trends, and current conditions in society that influence both nursing education and nursing practice. To these you have given your attention (Alumnae Association, 1967). But decision making also requires a set of standards that describes what nursing education can and should be in present-day society. These standards would necessarily reflect the increasing volume of available knowledge and the increase in technical and professional specialization that will continue to affect nursing practice in our "complex, specialized and swiftly changing society" (Kneller, 1966, p. 13). Standards should reflect the state of the culture, particularly those segments that are integrated with nursing and with education. The beliefs, the convictions, the hopes, as well as the antagonisms of members of our society must not be disregarded when groups undertake to ensure continuity of nursing education programs or bring about change in them.

Nurses and nurse educators must continue to address themselves to the matter of levels of nursing education and levels of nursing practice. The problems connected with levels of education are complex and analyses of an extensive nature are required if the problems are to be understood, much less solved; relations to nursing practice must be identified clearly.

The remaining sections of this paper are devoted to a consideration of levels of nursing education. The purpose is to make explicit some educational considerations related to levels of nursing education and practice.

TYPES AND LEVELS OF NURSING EDUCATION

Nursing education is of the type referred to as education for the occupations and professions. The most general term we can use is *work preparatory education*, that stands in contrast to liberal and general education; these seek to make a man by drawing on the rich heritage of the race, studying this heritage as an end in itself or as a means for understanding problems in daily living (Brubacher & Rudy, 1958). The place of education for the occupations and professions within the school and college curriculum has been and remains controversial among educationists (King & Brownell, 1966). One trend seems to be clear: that all types of occupational education be offered in combination with liberal or general education or be built upon it, as has been the practice in the professions of law, medicine, and theology. This trend is evident in the vocational high schools and the two-year colleges, as well as in specialized educational institutions and programs. At last there seems to be rather widespread consensus in regard to something that has been recognized since antiquity—the inadequacy of occupationally centered education to move a man toward the fullness of his stature as a man. Some educationists, in fact, continue to use the term *occupational training* rather than *occupational education*, to emphasize that the scope and depth of program offerings are derived from *occupational demands* (King & Brownell, 1966). This label is usually not attached to the professions named above because of their requirement that professional education be built upon a solid base of liberal education.

As nursing education has advanced in its movement toward the achievement of professional status in American society, the baccalaureate degree with a nursing major has become necessary for this status. This educational criterion requires the placement of these programs in senior colleges or universities, institutions that have the power to grant baccalaureate and higher degrees, and liberal or general education has become a necessary component of the professional nursing curriculum. The following list of types of educational components specific to professional education are adapted from McGrath (1962):

1. General education outside the vocational field needed by individuals, regardless of their chosen work, to discharge their civic duties and to live an effective personal life
2. The theoretical foundations basic to professional practice and the subjects necessary to understand these theoretical foundations

3. The general core of instruction in the professional practice and the particular knowledge and technical skills that characterize a profession and distinguish it from others
4. Continuing education, professional and general

The necessity of practical experience in relating theory and practice has been recognized in professional education. The focus is not, however, on "how-to-do-it techniques," but on understanding, that enables the professional man to use techniques under conditions of change (McGrath, 1962).

At the other extreme of work-preparatory education is what has been referred to in the United States as *vocational education*. This type of education focuses on preparation for work that is characterized by demands for the performance of specific tasks. The curriculum offerings of vocational high schools and adult vocational programs were and are primarily of this type. The education of practical nurses, as it took on momentum and developed during the 1940s, was vocational education in this sense. Curricula emphasized the tasks to be done for patients within a system of nursing care and the techniques to be used in the performance of the tasks. The scientific rationales for the tasks and for the techniques were taught sometimes separately, sometimes in application to the techniques. Vocational education in the United States has been and is being offered in the high school, in programs of adult education within vocational schools, and in two-year colleges. Students in vocational education programs may or may not be high school graduates.

Programs of vocational education are short-term, and are offered to prepare people for, or upgrade them in, jobs that actually exist in a community; programs are discontinued when there are no jobs to be filled in the community. Because of our failure to see nursing clearly, and consequently to define clearly the position and roles of practical nurses, we have had and continue to have unfortunate and unsafe practices related to utilization of practical nurses. The vocational level of nurse preparation has moved in a number of programs from the purely vocational partly into the next level of preparation. This movement was in part the basis for the ANA position that practical nurse education be upgraded to merge with the technical level.

In the middle range of the spectrum of work-preparatory education is that type referred to as technical education. The worker prepared through this type of education in both the engineering and the non-engineering technologies (that include the health services) is called a technician. A technician has been defined as "any person who assists with the applied aspects of a trade or a profession" (Blocker, Plummer, & Richardson, 1965, p. 215). Technicians are not ordinarily involved in the development of new theory; they apply existing knowledge to immediate practical problems. Because their theoretical education is substantial, though more limited than that of the professional. Because their general educational background is sound, technicians should have great job flexibility and opportunity for general advancement.

Technical education programs are differentiated according to their offering of higher- and lower-level courses—higher-level referring to courses where there is a greater focus on theory as related to the technology and the sciences foundational to it than on practical skills, the reverse being true in lower-level courses. Today two-year colleges, area vocational schools, and technical institutes offer technical curricula in a variety of engineering and non-engineering technologies. The associate degree is granted upon the completion of technical programs by two-year colleges with such power. In nursing education, programs leading to the associate degree in two-year colleges, as well as programs in hospital-controlled schools of nursing, may be classified as technical whenever they exhibit the characteristics and components just described. In summary, components of a technical education program include (1) general education subjects, (2) the sciences foundational to the technology, and (3) the technology and the derived techniques.

In a consideration of the relation between the level and form of preservice nursing education and resultant capabilities of individual nurses in contributing to the continued existence of nursing in society, more detailed attention is given to levels of work preparatory training or education. For it is the level of education that must be used to give form to a curriculum and subsequently to nursing practice, and it is that level that affects engagement in nursing research and theory development. Three levels of preparation, and consequently of practice, are described. (The descriptions of levels of education were developed from remarks made by Dr. Eamon P. O'Doherty, University of Dublin, Consultant to the Committee for the Development of a Nursing Model, at The School of Nursing, The Catholic University of America, March 16, 1965.)

Level I   The teaching of what to do: Emphasizes the development of certain limited skills and use of techniques necessary for task performance without much conceptualization as to where and how the techniques are derived

Level II   The solving of practical problems in the occupational field or profession so that a certain end product can be produced: Emphasizes information gathering to the extent that it is needed for the end product and emphasizes the use of techniques already validated

Level III   The discovery of problems in the occupational or professional field and discovery of ways to solve them: Emphasizes creative thinking and demands development and validation of techniques

The selection of one level, or of an upward combination of levels, as guiding principles to give direction to course and program development results in the occupationally relevant characteristics of a work preparatory program. These grades or levels of work preparatory education should not be seen as an extension in quantity of knowledge and skills. Movement from one level to another requires qualitative changes, and appropriate environments must be provided if persons are to move from one level to another. I see simplistic approaches to career ladders in nursing as the result of failure to recognize qualitative characteristics that must be developed by students in the upper levels of nursing education.

The types of preservice nursing education programs previously described—practical or vocational, technical, and professional—do not fit neatly into these three levels of education and practice. The closest correspondence is perhaps between the traditional type practical nurse program and Level I. It is recognized, however, that upon examination, the nursing component of some preservice programs in two-year colleges, hospital controlled schools of nursing, and even in four-year colleges and universities may reveal a large number of Level I characteristics.

Present-day technical type preservice nursing education programs are viewed as attempts to combine the Level I and Level II approaches. I suggest that, despite the taking of the problem-solving approach to the selection of nursing actions in clinical nursing situations, the nursing component of technical programs in two-year colleges and in other institutions is more often than not of the Level I Type.

Baccalaureate education is viewed primarily as Level II education, with the possibility of laying a foundation for the nurse to move toward Level III education and practice. What can be accomplished in a combined program of liberal and professional education compressed into a four-year period should be carefully studied. The interests and capabilities of students should be taken into consideration. Perhaps it would be more realistic to develop some nursing programs leading to the baccalaureate degree that emphasize straight Level II education and others that combine Level II education with preparation in the foundations for Level III education.

Graduate education at the master's level would narrow down the technological focus of Level II education through clinical nursing specialization, and would lay a foundation for Level III education in the nursing specialty. Nurses prepared through graduate education at the master's level should be able to perform in an actively and positively therapeutic manner in nursing situations.

Level III education would be conducted at the postmaster's and doctoral levels. This is the level of research proper, and emphasizes the development of qualities that enable the nurse to be creative, inventive, and instructive.

Can nursing education programs be appraised in terms of these levels, and can the levels be helpful to nurses and nurse educators in their effort to bring about constructive change? I believe that they can.

FOUNDATIONS FOR PROGRESS

It is suggested that progressive and developmental movement in nursing education cannot take place until nurses begin to build the foundations for such movement. Three foundations are identified. The *first* foundation would result from nurses' development of the ability to conceptualize nursing in terms of its unique social focus, and to understand and accept nursing as both a health service in society and a body of knowledge, however poorly this body of knowledge is developed at the present time.

The *second* foundation would arise from nurses' overcoming their tendencies to underestimate their roles in the delivery of health services. Nurses must come to see themselves as therapeutic agents with (1) a set of therapeutic skills derived from the technologies foundational to nursing; practice—technologies that represent application of specific sciences toward the accomplishment or the practical results of nursing—and (2) sets of motivations that together lead up to a set of social roles (O'Doherty, 1965).

The building of the *third* foundation for change in nursing education requires the delineation and development of the technologies of nursing practice. Some technologies are in the process of development, but the majority are relatively unformalized and undeveloped. I suggest that the failure of nurses to formally recognize the unique social focus of nursing and to use this focus as the formal base for the organization of nursing-relevant knowledge is in part the cause of the presently unstructured state of nursing knowledge and the lack of structured application of nursing-relevant knowledge. This state is or should be of great concern to nurses, especially to those who constitute faculties of nursing in universities, and to those who are considering the institution of university-based programs. It is my conviction that society must give more support to high quality professional nursing education at the undergraduate and graduate levels if nursing knowledge is to become formalized and validated. For years society has placed the social burdens of the professional person on nurses with Level I type training.

The development, or further development, of the following technologies in their relations to nursing practice is seen as essential to future progress in preservice nursing education at all levels:

1. The technologies or processes through which interpersonal, intergroup, and intragroup relations are brought into existence and maintained as long as such relations are essential for achievement of nursing and nursing-related goals in specific social situations.

2. The technologies of human assistance through which help or service is rendered by one person to another. The reasons for the requirements for help and the matters about which persons need help determine the characteristics of assisting processes. The use of these processes in nursing practice is dependent upon intrapsychic factors in nurse and patient. It is suggested that assisting technologies are of three general types: wholly compensatory, partly compensatory, and developmental. All systems of nursing assistance are seen as coming in part from the application of techniques and procedures derived from one or a combination of these assisting technologies toward the accomplishment of nursing goals.

3. The technologies of individual personal care that is self-administered by adults and administered by them to infants and children. When such care has as its goal positive health, and when it has a base in scientifically derived knowledge, I refer to it as *therapeutic self-care demand*. Some components of therapeutic self-care may be prescribed by the individual's physician.

4. The technologies for appraising, changing, and controlling man's integrated functioning with emphasis on physiologic or psychologic modes of functioning in health and disease. These are the medically derived technologies.

5. The processes that bind persons together in therapeutic relations (relations from which flow positively therapeutic results) that contribute to the maintenance of personal integrity and development, despite disease and disability.
6. The processes for bringing about and controlling the position and movement of persons in their physical environment.
7. The research processes, methods, and techniques necessary for the nursing-relevant development and application of the above technologies, including validation of the techniques and rules for application under conditions encountered in nursing practice.

Much work is required if these foundations are to be developed to the point where they form a substantial body of content from which nursing curricula can be constructed. Nurses hope that universities that have supported past efforts to move nursing education forward will continue their support and that other universities will take up the social cause of nursing. There are nurses throughout the country who are engaged in the development of nursing and nursing education. It is my hope that the efforts of this Association in this regard will be fruitful and provide data from which a new page in nursing history can be written.

CHAPTER 7

The Nursing Process With a Focus on Data Collection

W hen we begin to focus on getting nursing accomplished, we must see nursing as a *whole thing*, as a *system of action* directed toward (1) the achievement of a patient's required therapeutic self-care and (2) the overcoming of his limitations to act for himself in therapeutic self-care. Goals of nursing action may be phrased in these terms as illustrated in Figure 7.1.

A *system* is a collection of interrelated elements characterized by a boundary and a functional unity. It is a set of objects together with relationships between the objects and between their attributes. *Objects* are the parts or components of the system; *attributes* are the properties of the objects; *relationships* are the connections among the objects that tie the system together. We may properly speak of a system of nursing assistance. The elements would be as illustrated in Figure 7.2. But we see a system of nursing action (labeled I) as distinct from a system of medical care (labeled II) and the patient's system of family life (labeled III).

The actions of nurse and patient that produce intra-relations are essential to the system. We want to focus on what the nurse does deliberately to bring about and maintain an effective system of nursing for the patient. This we refer to as the *nursing process*. Every human action deliberately performed, and nursing, in which not one act but a series of actions is performed over time, is conceptualized as having three phases: (1) the phase of planning, (2) the phase of doing, and (3) the phase of seeing or checking.

This paper was first presented at a workshop sponsored by the Catholic University of America, Washington, DC, on July 22, 1969.

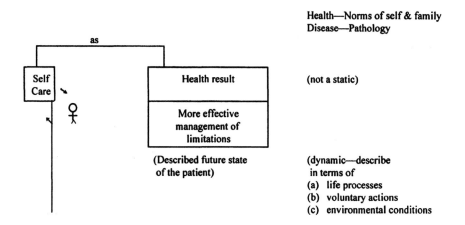

FIGURE 7.1   Goals of nursing action.

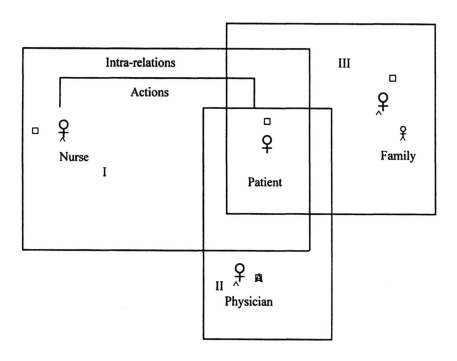

FIGURE 7.2   Elements of a system of nursing assistance.

These phases of human action become extremely important when action systems are complex in the sense that (1) many actions must be performed and related to achieve a simple result and (2) some of the actions need to be performed simultaneously or in some necessary sequential relationship.

What guides do we have in helping us to see and understand elements, attributes, and relationships in complex new action systems? We are not confronted with a problem of one-way causality, for example, if X—then Y. We are confronted with organized complexity; in fact we are confronted with making organized complexity.

As a guide toward making "an organized complexity"—nursing—the steps have been identified by nurses in variety of ways, but all conform to the scheme of Plan, Do, and See.

1. The initial and continuing determination of why a person should be under nursing care, including requirements for nursing assistance to compensate for, or overcome limitations to meet present and future requisites for self-care
2. The designing and design of a system of nursing, assistance, or a series of systems to be used in progression
3. Initial, continuing, and controlling systems of nursing assistance

This process is illustrated in Figure 7.3.

PROPOSITION

Every step of the nursing process requires

1. Data to describe the reality of the nursing situation that actually exists
2. Knowledge from the sciences and technologies needed to understand the factors that describe the situation from a nursing point of view; knowledge is required to
   a. recognize the existence of factors
   b. collect data to describe them
   c. make judgments about their relevance and degree of importance
   d. make decisions about the nursing actions to be taken in light of changes indicated
   e. recognize the evidence of changes

FIGURE 7.3   Nursing as a Process of Plan, Do, and See

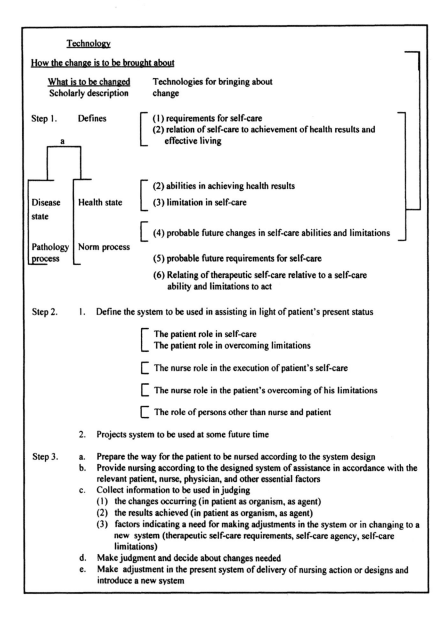

f. judge if the change is desired or undesired
g. judge if the evidence of specific changes together constitute evidence of the result desired

Data collection is in itself a complex process that includes the following:

1. acquainting oneself with the phenomena to be observed for (knowledge)
2. recognizing the factors
3. describing the attributes of the factors

In the process of data collection we must use valid techniques and technologies. These are illustrated in Figure 7.4.

The writings of von Bertalanffy (1967) are helpful to nurses in conceptualizing the processes of nursing. He suggests that man is symbol-making, symbol-using, symbol-dominated. Human symbol activity has these characteristics:

1. Symbols are representative—they stand for the things symbolized
2. Symbols are transmitted by tradition, by learning processes of individuals
3. Symbols are freely created

Goal—Take an objective look at what is needed in nursing.

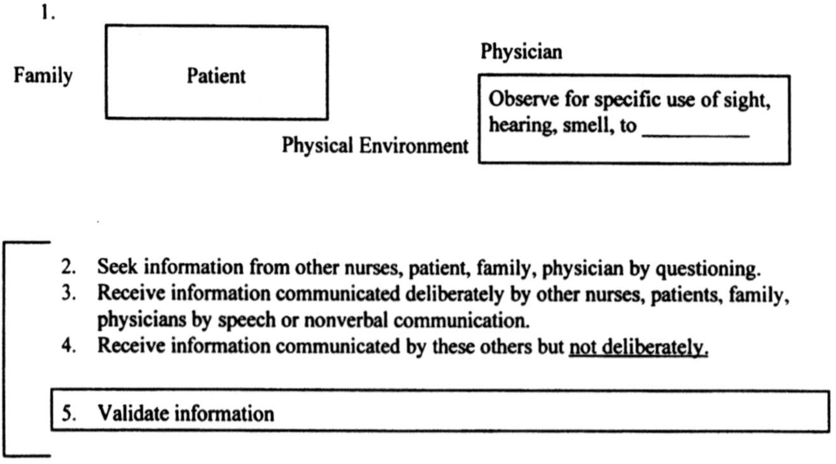

1.

Family   Patient

Physician

Observe for specific use of sight, hearing, smell, to _____

Physical Environment

2. Seek information from other nurses, patient, family, physician by questioning.
3. Receive information communicated deliberately by other nurses, patients, family, physicians by speech or nonverbal communication.
4. Receive information communicated by these others but not deliberately.

5. Validate information

FIGURE 7.4   The data collection process.

CHAPTER *8*

Design of Systems of Nursing Assistance and Plans for the Individual

A design of a system of nursing assistance is a plan for nursing in its essential outline. If we accept that a nurse may contribute to (1) accomplishing the self-care of the patient in a therapeutic manner when a patient limitation must be compensated for and (2) overcoming a patient's present *limitations*, it is possible to *narrow* action down to four types. By the arrangement of these types we can come up with four basic designs for nursing action: wholly compensatory, partly compensatory (supportive), supportive-educative, and compensatory-educative (see Figure 8.1).

A deterrent to the development of nursing system plans has been a lack of understanding of a framework for planning as well as lack of organization providing for it, time, and the conviction that it is a nursing requirement (see Figure 8.2).

Nurses utilize scientific facts and theories in describing and explaining the above. For example, this is illustrated when a totally blind elderly male patient directs a nursing student in arranging his bedside table and the food on his tray so that he can eat. This man has developed the capability for directing and guiding others. The recognition of the compensator technique that patients have worked out is important. Furthermore, we need to collect data to describe how individuals do compensate when they have a limitation.

This paper was originally presented in a series of workshops at the Catholic University of America, Washington, DC, on July 23, 1969.

61

Patient action—Type I   Therapeutic self-care action (compensatory)
Patient action—Type II Overcoming a limitation

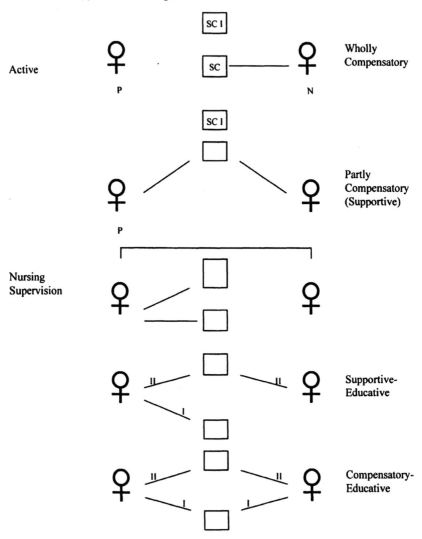

FIGURE 8.1   Variations in nurse–patient action systems.

Valid technology of assisting to compensate

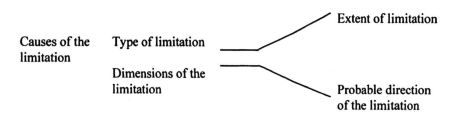

Causes of the limitation

Type of limitation

Dimensions of the limitation

Extent of limitation

Probable direction of the limitation

FIGURE 8.2 Valid technology of assisting to overcome limitations.

These models of designs are based upon types of limitation and ways of assisting. They are useful in determining the amount and kind of assistance that a patient will need, but we do not see the whole of a design until we bring the kinds of therapeutic self-care into the picture. In the process of designing a system of nursing assistance these requirements would be known prior to a selection of ways of assisting and would guide one in choosing the method of assistance to be used.

To understand basic design, we must have an understanding of ways of helping, for essentially these basic designs describe in a general way how the nurse will help the patient. Ways of helping and types of limitations are illustrated in Table 8.1.

We must know the conditions that have brought about the limitation before we can identify the most valid way of helping. Self-care requirements can be classified and named as follows

1. Universal self-care
   a. self-maintenance care
   b. protection of personal integrity
2. Health deviation in self-care
   a. derived from disease, injury, or defect
   b. related to or derived from the medical care needed and received

Let us take a look at some case material (see Figure 8.3).

In Figure 8.4 a case of a patient who had introduced a new form of self-care into her system of care is presented. In this situation the patient's body obstructed her vision.

TABLE 8.1 Ways of Helping and Types of Limitations

		Ways of Helping		Types of Limitations
(c)	1.	Acting for another	I.	Limitations of awareness and perception
(c)	2.	Guiding another	II.	Limitations of valid knowledge about self-care requisites and skills
(s)	3.	Supporting another (a) in action	III.	Limitations in initiating, maintaining, and controlling actions
(s)		(b) by providing resources		
(ed)	4.	Providing a developmental type environment	IV.	Limitations of movement necessary in the accomplishment of self-care
(ed)	5.	Teaching another	V.	Limitations of essential material resources; environmental, physical, and social conditions; and time

c—compensating, s—supporting, e—educating

I give this example to illustrate that in designing systems of nursing assistance we must meet known requirements before we can assess abilities and limitations, except in those instances where limitations are such that little or no activity is possible, as in coma or acute anxiety states.

> **A limitation is a function of the total situation viewed from the standpoint of purpose.**

DETAILED PLANNING

A plan specified (1) the person or object, (2) what is to be done, and (3) how it is to be done. This is illustrated in Figure 8.5.

1. Required observational care must be attached to each other type of requirement.

FIGURE 8.3   Patient Situation

Patient: 65 years old, mature, married woman with grown children, none of whom lived at home. Her husband was well and normally concerned and interested in his wife's health and needs.

1. { Resection of colon—4 weeks ago
      Colostomy in right lower quadrant

   { Perineal incision

2. Admitted to the hospital because of an incisional area abscess and the systemic effect of the abscess

Aging	Related to	{ New technology for bowel evacuation { New - a man-made bodily orifice to care for
Obese	Related to	Care of an incision

Patient understood colostomy care, had been supervised in giving it, and was able and did give colostomy care.

Periodic supervision of a visiting nurse in the home.

---

2. Plotting the distribution of the care required by time and place is an aid to implementation.
3. Identification of need for movement from one location to another is important for a number of reasons.
   a. Is there a need for a nurse to travel with the patient and remain with the patient?
   b. How much nurse coordination with other personnel is required?
   c. How much time is consumed?
   d. What is the effect on the patient?

Arrange therapeutic care system according to (1) the patient's requirements and preferences and (2) conservation of energy of the patient and time and energy of the nurse.

FIGURE 8.4   Patient Situation Illustrating New Self-Care System

The patient continued to give her own colostomy care using her own equipment despite weakness—the patient preferred not to give us this aspect of her care. | If not too weak

The cause of a limitation related to the patient's giving her own colostomy care was her obesity; she was unable to see what she was doing when in the bed and was too weak to be out of bed. Compensation for this limitation was made by placing a mirror on the patient's bedside table.

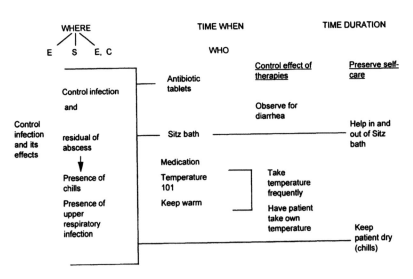

FIGURE 8.5   Planning.

E—education   S—support   C—compensatory

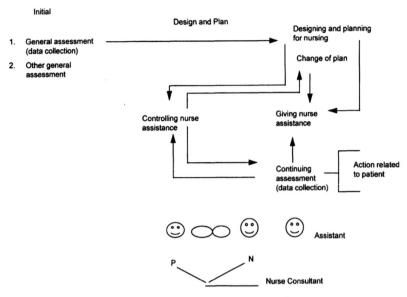

FIGURE 8.6   The nursing process as a system of action.
P—Patient   N—Nurse

GIVING AND CONTROLLING NURSING ASSISTANCE

The steps of the nursing process are related and should be seen as systems of *action*. These steps are illustrated in Figure 8.6 and include

1. Communication and discussion of the plan with patient or family (nursing is a service that is purchased).
   a. total dependence and extensive limitations
   b. moderate deficits
   c. deficits limited to measures of care
2. Giving Nursing Assistance: This step of the process *produces* nursing for the patient.

Giving

1. A set of interpersonal relations that permits nurse–patient cooperation, including a willingness on the part of the nurse and the giving of responsibility to the patient
2. Nursing knowledge and skills added to the use of the appropriate technology

3. Ability to adjust nursing assistance to the patient's state and needs
4. Continual assessment of the effectiveness of the patient's actions and the nurse's own actions

Control Activities

Control activities include evidence related to evaluation of what is being done in relation to the stated plan, and evidence related to the evaluation of the results based on the stated criteria and critical observations.

CHAPTER 9

Design, Production, and Control Operations Required for the Delivery of Nursing on an Agency-Wide Basis

Today in many nursing departments in hospitals, and in other types of health service institutions that provide nursing, attention is given to the development of statements of "philosophy" and of objectives of the nursing department, consideration being thus given to the setting of very general standards to be met by the department. All too frequently such expressions have their roots in the convictions of the individuals who write the statements but have no roots in the specific characteristics of the population in need of nursing assistance. What I am suggesting is that these are good, but not good enough. They do not suffice as guidelines for delivery of nursing to populations served by the agency.

Ensuring the delivery of nursing on an agency-wide basis to the population served is a responsibility of nurses in executive positions within the agency. This responsibility cannot be fulfilled without coordinated effort with other executives and with nursing department staff who function at the operation level.

To establish an executive or administration frame of reference I shall enumerate the three functions of executives according to Barnard (1962).

This paper was originally presented at a series of workshops at the Catholic University of America, Washington, DC, on July 24, 1969.

1. Define and limit purpose.
2. Provide and maintain essential effort.
3. Provide and maintain a system of communication.

The purpose of an agency as stated in its *statutes or articles of incorporation* is the point of departure for all subsequent definitions and limitations. The name attached to any agency, such as nursing home or hospital, is also an expression of purpose. The name carries with it certain expectations for service. A society's expectations vary from era to era. What society today expects from hospitals varies greatly from expectations of seventeenth- or eighteenth-century societies.

Executives, including nursing executives, today are faced with shortage (real or apparent) of nursing personnel, rising costs, and a more knowledgeable and sophisticated clientele. The day when patients placed their full trust and confidence in professionals seems to be waning. Many people have sufficient knowledge of health and health service to make valid observations and judgments about the quality of care received. Some patients bring to the health professional and to the health agency the time-honored admonition as relabeled in the market place *Buyer beware!* Health care is no longer provided as an expression of man's concern for his fellow man—it is presented *as a service to be purchased.*

The why, what, and how of health service, including nursing, must become of greater concern to executives. The question is how to proceed. Much of the national effort (using federal money) to bring about change in the delivery of health services is going on in or being sponsored by the large medical centers where the initiating and control of projects is in the hands of physicians and where nurses often have (for a variety of reasons) minor roles. Change in delivery of nursing can and should be going on in institutions and organizations large and small.

If we accept that *change in nursing can proceed if we have the interest and the will to make it happen,* perhaps nurses can again bring about revolutionary change in health service, at least in countries where Western medicine is the cultural norm.

WHAT ARE SOME OF THE STEPS?

1. Look at the population served in terms of similarities and differences relevant to nursing in the population over time.

2. Make tentative judgments about the kinds and number of nurses needed on the basis of these nursing-relevant similarities and differences in proper object.
3. Develop formulas and models for an effective (adequate) and efficient mixture of patients in the physical units of the facility.
4. Accept that being in residence in an institution (short-term or long; in some instances the institution is theirs) sets up a list of requirements related to daily living of practical nursing. These are not nursing requirements, but nursing must be designed in light of the requirements, and nursing functions may need to be closely coordinated with *residence functions*. These differences exist because of type of institution, type of unit, health state of patient, and so on.
5. Look at self-care performed by patients, nursing, and other forms of health care needed and then at the daily lives of patients to determine how much of a patient's day is consumed by self-care activities.
6. Develop models of nursing systems sharing relations to residence status and systems of daily living of *patients*.
7. Relate these to modes for health care systems and other systems, making adjustments as needed.
8. Begin to estimate requirements for nursing effort and time and the need for supportive clerical personnel, equipment, and supply and facility personnel. This is the day of expansion of technical evolution in health service. Let us not split up the patient and nurse more than we have already done and let us educate patients so that they are safe.
9. Begin to estimate requirements for the setting up of administration positions and in the operative levels and the module section of the organization.
10. Make decisions about the *relations of patients to nurses* established through *nurse–patient assignments*. Some questions, in light of present practices, which are not uncommon, are the following.
    a. Is a single nurse responsible from a professional nursing point of view for the overall distribution and coordination of the nursing of a patient?
    b. If the answer is yes and this person is head nurse, does she have time, knowledge, skill, and adequate channels of communication to fulfill this responsibility for the in-patient and the out-patient?

CHAPTER 10

Nursing and Nursing Education: The Problem of Relations

INTRODUCTION

The history of nursing and the history of nursing education in the United States have the relation of the one to the other as a unifying theme. The problem of relations between nursing and nursing education has been and continues to be the focus of concern for nurses and others interested in the continued development of nursing as a health service. This paper presents for the consideration of nurses some suggestions that may give direction to analyzing problems of relations.

Historically, relationships between nursing and nursing education have been described in at least two ways: (1) in terms of the status and roles of the nursing student, and (2) in terms of what the product of nursing education, the nurse, could do after completion of the educational program. During the closing years of the nineteenth and the early years of the twentieth century there were two classes of nurses: *nurses-in-training* and *trained nurses*. Student or pupil nurses were afforded the title "nurse" and were expected to provide nursing under supervision within a hospital. Upon graduation, and after a one- or a two-year period, these nurses were considered trained and, therefore, competent to nurse outside the hospital

This chapter was originally developed as a background paper at the Catholic University of America in the late 1960s, for presentation to one of the nursing groups with which Orem was meeting at the time.

in private families or to engage in district nursing. The quality of nurse training, as well as the character and prior education of the *pupil nurses*, was seen as affecting what the graduates of a particular training school could do upon graduation. The giving of the title *nurse* to students was in keeping with the expressed primary objectives of schools for nurses: to secure for the hospital a fairly reliable corps of nurses or to introduce scientifically based nursing into a hospital where the continuing care of the sick was entrusted to the unknowing, the unwilling, and the unable. The education of nurses in the latter instance was seen as the means to change a system of care, and the number of pupil nurses or nurses-in-training was a determining factor in spreading nursing to the various wards of a hospital.

As training schools were established in hospitals of all types and sizes, problems of justice as related to students and society were recognized. In 1893, with specific reference to training schools in small hospitals and sanitoria, Isabel Hampton Robb expressed to the International Congress of Charities, Correction and Philanthropy the following view.

> [T]he mere fact that they are hospitals in nowise justifies them in establishing training schools for the sake of economy, and accepting as their pupils women who, perfectly ignorant of what they need, go to them and give up a year or two years of precious time, and then find that their education has been thoroughly inadequate to enable them to fulfil what is afterwards required of them. We cannot but feel that a real injustice is often done in such cases. If the nurse had gone into such a hospital as a philanthropist it would be different, but she went there for the purpose of acquiring a certain kind of education. Again these small hospitals, not having the same number to select from as the larger schools, are apt, and in fact do take women who, not being intellectually capable of comprehending the high calling into which they have been admitted, tend to lower the standard to which we are striving to attain. (Robb, 1907)

Such consideration for the rights of persons seeking to prepare themselves as nurses was not widespread during the early years of development of nursing education when its control and the sponsorship of its programs was under the jurisdiction of hospitals and sanatoria. Of particular interest here are the relations between nursing and nursing education that were expressed or implied in Mrs. Robb's statement. Relations were expressed in economic, sociological, and educational frames of reference. That which is specifically or peculiarly nursing was expressed as what is required of them. The considerations expressed by Mrs. Robb are important in any age or in any stage of development of nursing and nursing education regardless of the types of agencies in a society that sponsor and control nursing education.

The separation of the sponsorship and control of preservice education from the hospital has moved forward in the twentieth century. Preservice nursing educational programs are under the control of various types of educational institutions as well as under hospital control. The term *nursing student* has replaced the term *student* or *pupil nurse* and the educational focus and objectives of preservice nursing educational programs are emphasized. But the movement of nursing education into educational institutions that offer occupational and professional education, in and of itself, does not solve the problems that arise from the relationships that do or should exist between nursing in a society and nursing education in that society.

THE PROBLEM OF RELATIONS

From a broad social or cultural perspective, nursing and nursing education together form a single but complex system within a society, since both are required if the society is to provide itself with nursing. This assumption or proposition is basic to any examination of relations between nursing and nursing education. The assumption is substantiated by historical evidence, past and current. Failure to make the assumption explicit and to use it as a guide in decision making can result in an *isolationism* that favors either nursing or nursing education at the expense of the provision of nursing to a society. The proposition provides a framework essential to a consideration of the relationships between nursing and nursing education.

Relations are characteristics that can be considered as belonging to two or more things when taken together, that is, when considered with reference to one another. The question of the relationships between nursing and nursing education is one that is or should be of concern to all persons in a society who are responsible in any remote or direct way for the provision of nursing in the society. The setting forth and the formal recognition of these relationships by all concerned groups and individuals is viewed as not only contributory but as essential to the continuing existence and development of nursing as a health service in the United States. The current condition of nursing and nursing education is that of complexity and change, without the availability of clear-cut and detailed guidelines to enable concerned persons to penetrate the complexities and to direct change toward defined and realistic goals. The recognition and description of the relations between nursing and nursing education would provide an instrument to aid nurses in penetrating the complexity of and in decision making relative to nursing and nursing education.

If the proposition that nursing and nursing education together form a single but complex system within a society is accepted as a frame of reference for analysis, it is possible to formulate other propositions that would set forth more specifically either the *elements* that stand at relation one to the other or the *given relations between the elements*. This is, of course, a logical exercise of attributing *qualities* and *relations* to the human endeavor called nursing and nursing education in light of available information.

Some characteristics and relations are set forth in the subsequent section of this paper. They are offered as stimuli to provoke reactions and a more formalized consideration of the problem by nurses. They are not offered with any thought that the presentation is complete or without error, or that the problem of relations between nursing and nursing education is unrecognized and untreated.

SOME QUALITIES AND RELATIONS

The following propositions, which made explicit some characteristics of and relationships between nursing and nursing education, are assumptions about the foundations of nursing in a society. The assumptions are seen as a base from which to build theoretical structures that would be useful tools in analyzing, describing, and decision making relative to constructing complex and interrelated systems of nursing and nursing education. The assumptions are presented under three headings: the provision of nursing by a society, and nursing in a society, and nursing education in a society.

The Provision of Nursing by a Society

Five assumptions are presented.

1. A society, to provide its members with nursing, requires a system of nursing practice through which nursing is provided to individuals, families, and communities, and a system of nursing education

through which schooling is provided to persons who seek initial preparation for nursing practice or to increase their preparation. The two systems are linked by the movement into nursing practice of persons who have completed programs within the system of nursing education.

2. Provision of nursing to a society requires recruitment and retention of members into nursing practice and nursing education. The conditions that prevail in nursing practice and nursing education in the society and the alternatives open to desirable recruits will affect choices.

3. Nursing considered as a health service is a *consumer service*; nursing education is a *producer service* since it prepares persons who will produce the consumer service. Both services in a society will be affected by scarcity of resources and labor, as well as by other factors related to supply and demand

4. Nursing and nursing education have different purposes and require different forms of human endeavor. However, the demands of a society for nursing, the developed and validated technologies of nursing practice, and the prevailing forms or modes of nursing practices will be influencing forces on both nursing and nursing education

5. The effectiveness and efficiency of a system for providing nursing in a society is related to (a) the degree to which the requirements for nursing in the society are or are not met, (b) the labor and resources used and conserved, and (c) the satisfactions and dissatisfactions accruing to consumers of nursing, nurses, nursing students, teachers, as well as to others in the society who finance, sponsor, and administer programs of nursing and nursing education.

These propositions are presented not because they are tenable or already recognized assumptions but because they provide a base around which nursing and nursing-relevant information can be organized in the interests of improving the condition of nursing in a society.

The assumptions are seen as foci for selecting and bringing in facts and theories from related fields and as indicators of the kinds of factual *information* needed to describe the system of providing nursing to members of a society. Much has been done by nurses and by persons from the field of social sciences in these regards. What is now important is the organization of what has been done in the interests of the formalization of available knowledge as a guide for future action. These are tasks for both scholars and researchers, tasks that must be done before a scientific approach to providing nursing can be taken by nurses and by others who bear a part of the responsibility.

Nursing in a Society

The assumptions presented are developments of selected characteristics and relationships derived from the first group of propositions.

1. The essential structural elements of an organized system of nursing practice are nurses and consumers of nursing. The elements stand in an agent–patient relationship to one another but the capacities and developed abilities of the *patient* should serve to define the role of the agent.
2. The nurse as agent is in a position of responsibility toward another; the other may be an individual, a family, a community. How a nurse views the *other* is influenced by the nurse's values and by the amount and kind of scientifically derived knowledge she can bring to bear toward gaining understanding of the other. Different bodies of knowledge must be drawn upon by the nurse when the other is an *individual, a family, or a community.*
3. The consumer of nursing is in a position of receiving service from another, *a nurse*; how the nurse is viewed will be influenced by factors operative in the individual, family, or the community being served by the nurse or in the environment in which nursing action is to take place.
4. The number of needful individuals, families, and communities receiving nursing at any one time in a society will be affected by the total number of nurses engaged in nursing practice, the manner in which their nursing efforts are distributed, and the amount of time each contributes to nursing.
5. The quality of nursing received by needful individuals, families, and communities will be affected by the nursing-relevant knowledge that nurses can bring to bear in making nursing decisions and rendering nursing care and service, by the time and resources available, and by the nurse's creativity and ability to coordinate nursing action with relevant actions of others.

The further development and utilization of these five assumptions is dependent upon making explicit the social focus of nursing by which nursing is differentiated from other health services. Ideal systems of nursing practice would align the requirements of patients for nursing with the nursing responsibilities of nurses.

Nursing Education in a Society

Five assumptions are presented. They are developments of the first group of propositions.

1. The essential structural elements of an organized system of nursing education are nursing students and teachers. The elements stand in an agent–patient relationship and the capacities and the developed abilities of the *patient* should serve to define the role of the *agent*.
2. Several types of teachers are required in a system of nursing education because nursing as a body of knowledge is developed according to areas of practice, and because nursing can only be understood and developed as knowledge from related fields as systematically applied in the development of nursing technologies.
3. Nursing education is a specific type of occupational and professional preparatory education; systems of nursing education may be composed of a number rather than a single form of the kind of education that is preparatory for the occupations and professions. The problem of the movement of persons from the system of nursing into the system of nursing practice increases in complexity with the variety of the kinds of programs offered within the system of nursing education.
4. Nursing education as a specific type or occupational and professional preparatory education requires an educational component concerned with learning occupational or professional roles in the society. This demands articulation between the system of nursing education and the system of nursing practice. This articulation forms a secondary link between the two systems, the primary link being the movement of persons who have completed programs of nursing education into nursing practice.
5. Nursing education derives its standards from the field of education as this field is grounded in scientifically derived knowledge. Since

these standards must be expressed in terms of nursing, they are developed in light of the current state of development of nursing as a body of knowledge, and in light of real and ideal conditions of nursing practice.

These five propositions serve to relate nursing education in a society to nursing considered as a body of knowledge, to related fields of knowledge, to the educational system of the society, and to the system of nursing practice. Further development of these propositions would require attention to each of these areas.

CONCLUSION

The ideas presented are the result of an accumulation of experience in nursing and nursing education. The ideas of others as verbalized or expressed in writing have been influencing factors. The recognition of the need to take a formalized approach to analysis of situations of action and to decision making is due in no small way to writers such as Chester Barnard (1962) and others who focus upon organized action in society.

CHAPTER 11

Processes in the Development of a Conceptual Framework for Teaching Nursing and for the Practice of Nursing

INTRODUCTION

In both education and practice, nurses have had considerable experience in adding things on, not unlike the television personality who, when asked about his health responded, "After fifty it is patch, patch, patch." Nursing is in a period characterized by emphasis on new approaches, new ways of organizing what should be known and done. New models, new frameworks for both teaching and practicing nursing are sought. A framework, whether it is formed from concepts, types of experiences, work operations, and so forth, is something constructed, something made. Since it is a structure, a whole theory with parts and organization, the essential process is one of forming and developing it.

If development is seen as movement from "general indeterminacy toward specific perfection" (Lonergan, 1958, p. 461) conceptual framework development involves a narrowing down of the possibilities. But the possibilities first must be identified. For example, in relation to teaching nursing, general concepts of education and teaching are narrowed down by relating them specifically to nursing toward the development of a concept of *teach-*

This paper was originally presented at the Catholic University of America Conference, Nursing Conceptual Framework, October 5, 1973.

ing nursing, which can be further developed by specifying the why and the what, leading to a setting forth of foci, limits, and constraints.

A CONCEPT OF DEVELOPMENT

Development is a process, and process implies change, movement in time and over time; it implies events and sequences and energy exchanges. Our goal, in efforts to understand development of anything, is to *master the sequence*, proceeding from the regularities of one stage to those of the next. As we know from the developmental processes of plants and animals, with development there is an increase in bulk with increasing differentiation and integration with ever more intricate arrangements and patterns until full differentiation is reached (Lonergan, 1958). As we shall see, conceptual framework development has this pattern. As an example of increasing bulk and intricate arrangement, I shall take a segment from personal experience. In 1957, 1958, and 1959, I developed and worked with a concepts of self-care and self-care limitations. This led to an exploration of types and causes of limitations. Experience has demonstrated that the higher order theories, including action theory, human organizational theory, theories about wholes composed of parts, as well as concepts of order, relations, and cause–effect series, are invaluable guides in conceptual framework development (Nursing Development Conference Group, 1973).

It is helpful to recognize that each stage of development is an integration of input that went before and each stage operates to form its own replacement (Lonergan, 1958). If we reflect on these ideas in light of what we know about development in plants or animals, we will perhaps form a general concept of development, if we do not already have one, which should serve us in thinking and action whether we are focusing on man-made constructs or natural things. The general concept is in the nature of a tool for dealing with the real world, a basis for thought and for intellectual play, if you will, as well as a guide for action for conduct. Lonergan (1958) indicates that "conception is the playground of our intelligence" (p. 8). A conceptual framework for teaching and practicing nursing is such a tool but on a much larger scale. It is made from concepts standing in ordered relationships. It is a mental construct that can be expressed in words, pictures, and so on.

Our concern is with mental constructs made from concepts and expressed in statements, definitions, diagrams. Where to begin and how to proceed in the construction of such a framework are the relevant questions.

THE SEQUENCE OF DEVELOPMENT—RELATIONS
AMONG THE STAGES

A developmental sequence can be known from the similarities and differences in events and in results that occur as the process proceeds. Not only the stages of development but the relations among stages must be identified and understood. It is proposed that in conceptual framework development, relations between the primary stages may be understood, formulated, and expressed generally in terms of (1) time of occurrence (before, after, concurrently), and (2) type of conceptual expression and integration.

Of necessity one begins where one can, that is, in accord with one's already structured knowledge, motives, and habits of thought. Ideally, one begins with a foundation for thought and scholarly action that goes beyond commonsense knowledge and desires of the moment. Some grounding in validated and structural knowledge from a range of disciplines is required, as well as motivations and a degree of self-discipline that permits for search and reflections. Insight and understanding precede conceptualization. Individuals who require the answers before they begin should not be involved in conceptual framework development except as related to specific detailed tasks or as a learner. If you have not been through the process, it is necessary to keep in mind that it is a discovery type of operation and that one works with *periods of blindness* and *periods of sight*. Once through the process you will have some vision of what you have been through and may be able to guide and support others as they engage in conceptual framework development.

As I proceed, I expect that you will become aware (if you are not aware already) that my idea of a conceptual framework extends beyond the selection of a number of general concepts and the pronouncement that these general concepts constitute the framework for a curriculum or for the practice of nursing. Ensuring that the concepts selected are valid and reliable aids in thinking about nursing, teaching nursing, and practicing nursing can be done by putting concepts to work personally or by investigating how they have been used by others. Failure to put concepts to work, to make them dynamic in thinking and action, is exemplified by selecting a specific general concept of nursing and pronouncing that it is the nursing base for curriculum development or revision. The expressed concept appears in the school or program documents but one looks in vain for evidence that it is in use by teachers or students, or that it has been analyzed to identify its substantive elements, or that the elements have been used in establishing curriculum foci or in setting boundaries and limits for educational experiences.

Conceptual framework development involves formulation or identification, selection, as well as use of concepts. It requires conceptual analysis, identification of relations among conceptual elements, and progressive development of the conceptual elements as framework development proceeds. It includes demonstration of the utility of concepts for understanding and developing the practice of nursing and for structuring and evaluating education.

MASTERING THE SEQUENCE

In addressing the question before the Institute—What are the processes through which conceptual framework for teaching and practicing nursing are developed?—I shall take a normative approach, endeavoring to express to you what should be done (an ideal path), painting, as it were, a whole picture, on the basis of my knowledge of what is being done at the present time. I predict that you will be able to identify where your own efforts fit into the model. I want you to know that preparation for this session of the Institute forced me to conceptualize the process of developing conceptual frameworks for teaching and practicing nursing. So bear with me remembering that this is the first time that I have attempted to bring all parts of the process together.

OVERVIEW OF THE PROCESS OF DEVELOPMENT: THE STAGES AND THE MODEL—TESTING

The Stages

Four interlocking stages in the development of a conceptual framework for teaching nursing or practicing nursing are suggested. In the first stage nursing is recognized as a social entity (social institution). To understand nursing we must view it in terms of how it relates to other sound institutions within whose framework it is a specific instance. We assume that the fit of teaching and practicing within the framework of these broader fields (all are human inventions) can be identified and should be identified for purposes of understanding and for purpose of making explicit the connotation and denotation of the terms teaching nursing and practicing nursing. Stages one and two contribute to the understanding of teaching nursing and practicing nursing as practice disciplines and aid in developing a framework for nursing knowledge, the conceptual and substantive structure, and together the syntactical structure (see Figure 11.1). Stages three and four address articulations with other fields, how other disciplines or

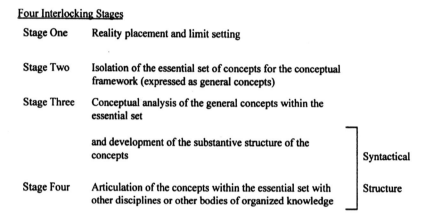

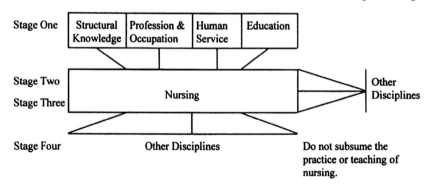

FIGURE 11.1 Overview of the process of development.

bodies of knowledge contribute to knowledge structuring in nursing, aid in problem solving, leading eventually to the identification and development of applied nursing science.

Stage One: Reality Placement and General Limit Setting

1. Locating teaching and practicing nursing in the world of man and human affairs; a minimal initial placement would include the placement of nursing in relation to (a) human services, (b) the health professions and occupations, (c) structured knowledge, and (d) education. These entities would in turn be related to community, culture, and society, and these in turn would be related to man (see Figure 11.2).

2. Exploration of the dimensions and facets of the entities proceeding from the most to the least general to form a hierarchy of aspects until the articulations with nursing are identified and in turn conceptualized. It is suggested that four concepts are necessary to begin to set forth the linkages between nursing and the types of human endeavor named in Figure 11.3: *practice disciplines, health profession and occupation, health services,* and *educational services* for the health professions and occupations. This step of stage one also includes making explicit the relations among the fields to which nursing is being related: for example, making explicit the relation between practice disciplines and other forms of structured knowledge (internal) and relating practice research to the profession and occupation.

3. Conceptualization of teaching and practicing nursing in terms of the limits and constraints revealed in steps 1 and 2 (an example of a limit would be the placement of nursing education within education for the profession and occupation; an example of a constraint would be the need for education to include attention to nursing as a practice discipline): this step should yield conceptualization and definition of the professional practice of nursing and other forms of practice (so that differences are revealed) as well as definitions of teaching as related to professional practice and to other foci of practice (to the end that differences are revealed). *Note*—This step should take us beyond imitation of sets of practices. It should lead to understanding of the character of what we do and why we do it.

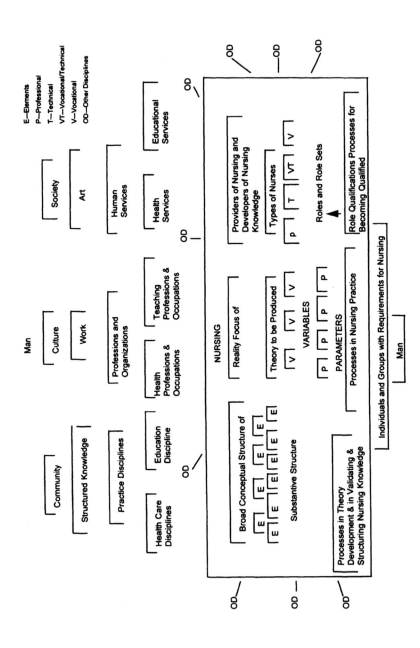

FIGURE 11.2 Guide toward the development of conceptual frameworks for nursing curricula.

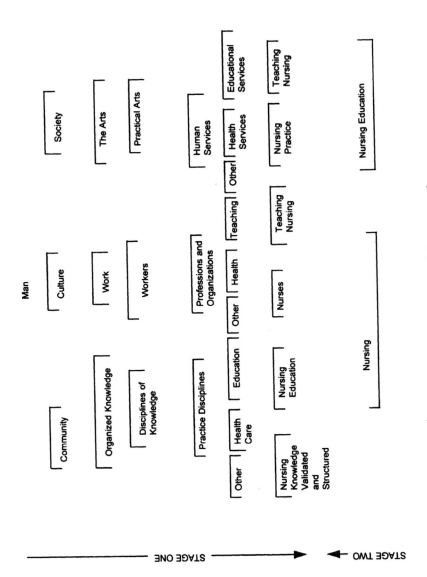

FIGURE 11.3 Links between nursing and types of human endeavor.

87

Engagement in Stage One demands knowledge of both nursing and the fields of human endeavor to which it is related. Concept framework developers may require time to explore both the literature and to arrive at insight and understandings about the fields before they can conceptualize the relations among the fields and relations between the fields and nursing (see Figure 11.4).

Stage Two: Isolation of the Essential Set of Concepts for the Conceptual Framework (Expressed as General Concepts)

1. Identification and conceptualization of persons and groups served by nursing, proceeding to the point of conceptualization of the specific object of nursing
2. Conceptualization of what nursing is: This takes in the form of conceptual elements and relations among them (see Figure 11.5).
3. Conceptualization of nursing variables and the parameters of each nursing variable within a nursing practice perspective
4. Conceptualization of the end product of nursing within a nursing practice perspective
5. Conceptualization of the producer of nursing (nurses) within a nursing practice perspective including limits and constraints
6. Conceptualization of the processes and orientations involved in learning nursing

Stage Two results in statements that incorporate the conceptualization produced; these, of course, were developed in light of, and may incorporate, concepts or conceptual elements from Stage One. Stage Three requires prior insights and understandings about nursing.

Stage Three: Conceptual Analysis of the General Concepts That Constitute the Essential Set of Nursing Concepts

1. Conceptual analysis of each concept formulated and expressed in Stage Two
2. Arrangement of concepts in accord with their relations within each hierarchy, many from the most general to the least general

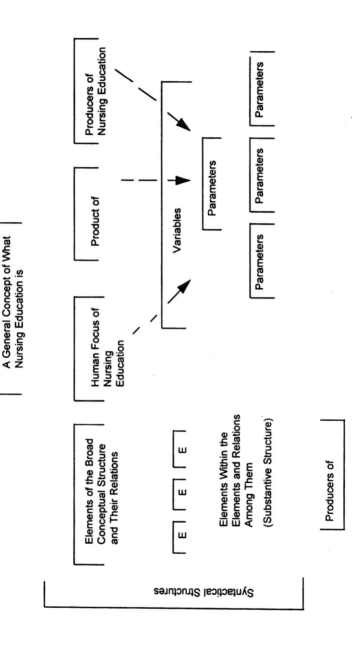

FIGURE 11.4   Conceptualizing relations between nursing and fields of human endeavor.

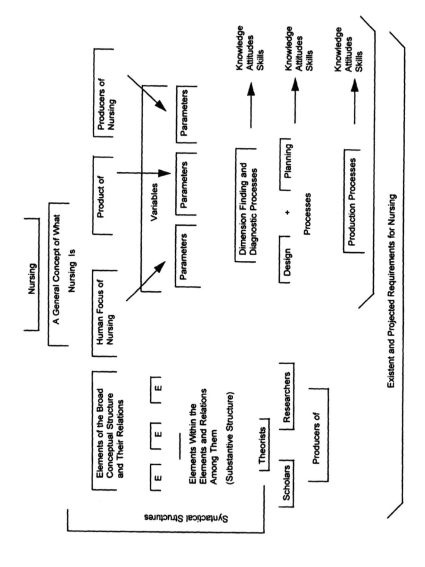

FIGURE 11.5 Conceptual elements and relations among conceptual elements.

3. Identification of relations among the hierarchal order of concepts for members of the set: for example, between producers of nursing and learning nursing

Stage Four: Articulation of the Concepts Within the Essential Set of Nursing Concepts With Other Disciplines or Other Bodies of Organized Knowledge

1. Exploration of the need for use of other bodies of knowledge in understanding the concepts with the essential set
2. Identification of the points of articulation between nursing concepts and other bodies of knowledge
3. Formulation of a statement about these points of articulation

CONCLUSION

Dependent on human effort and abilities and interests, only the thinker, the scholar, can effectively engage in conceptual framework development. Analogy: the conceptual framework is a mental map for structuring knowledge. Conceptual framework development requires time. Conceptual framework development permits for flexibility as well as constraint in the practice and teaching of nursing. Conceptual framework development identifies the view of man that it is necessary for one to take relative to teaching and practicing nursing. Conceptual framework development provides for flexibility in the ongoing search and research within identifiable limits and constraints.

RESULTS—THE PARTS OF A CONCEPTUAL FRAMEWORK

Parts of a conceptual framework for nursing are described in relation to the hypothesized stages of development. The descriptions reflect personal events and results. It is my belief that the formation, as well as the reliability and validity of the general concept of nursing Stage Two of the developmental process, is critical in conceptual framework formation. There is, of course, the possibility that the developmental process may stop while in Stage One, but whenever it proceeds and the general concept of nursing is inadequate, the developmental process is in trouble. See *Concept Formalization in Nursing* (Nursing Development Conference Group, 1973, pp. 26–30) for suggestions about standards of adequacy for general concepts in practice disciplines.

CHAPTER 12

Some Premises and Rules for Use in Curriculum Design and Development in Nursing

The current emphasis on conceptual frameworks for nursing curricula has served as a stimulus for thought about the functions of the nursing and nursing-related parts of such a framework. Some ideas formulated for, and expressed over time for a variety of purposes have been selected for presentation as sets of premises and derived rules. The premises are considered as providing valid foundations for action.

SERIES ONE

Premises

Premise 1

A general concept (theory) of nursing is the *center* from which to move in curriculum design and development for baccalaureate nursing programs (BDN) and associate degree nursing programs (ADN), which are offered in the form of high-level technical education.

This paper was originally presented on April 19, 1974, location unknown.

Premise 2

The integrity of the disciplines of knowledge is respected in education for the professions and in high-level technical education.

Rules

1. In BDN and ADN programs conducted in the form of high-level technical education nursing, students are introduced:
    a. to nursing as a discipline of knowledge
    b. to nursing-related disciplines in accord with the identified articulations of each discipline with nursing and with the distinguishing characteristics of each discipline of knowledge
    This rule cannot be followed without the formal acceptance and use of a valid general concept (theory) of nursing because of the present lack of formal structuring of accumulated nursing knowledge, hence the need for Rule 2.
2. Curriculum designers and developers in the types of nursing programs named select, accept, and use a valid general concept of nursing as the theoretical center from which to move in curriculum endeavors.
    a. The general concept of nursing accepted as the theoretical center for the curriculum is used as a guide in moving from the theoretical nursing center to known realities of nursing practice.
    b. Various aspects of the theoretical nursing center are related to facts and points of theory in other disciplines that articulate with specific aspects of the theoretical center. These aspects include conceptual elements within the general theory of nursing, relations among the elements, and relations of the conceptual elements with factors (parameters) that affect the value of the elements.
3. The accepted general concept of nursing is used by the curriculum designer to identify and make explicit the view or views of man and society that are specific to nursing.

SERIES TWO

Premises

Premise 1

A valid general concept of nursing establishes the specific nature and characteristics of nursing as (a) a field of human endeavor directed toward the achievement of specific types of results and (b) as organized, structured knowledge with a foundation in first principles arising from the nature of man and society.

Premise 2

A valid general concept of nursing by specifying the human focus and distinguishing characteristics of nursing points to broader categories of human affairs that subsume nursing: for example, disciplines of knowledge, institutionalized human services, and professions and occupations.

Rules

1. The accepted general concept of nursing is used by the curriculum designer and developer to make explicit the following:
   a. the *value* aspect of nursing
   b. the *domain* of nursing, that is, the human and social phenomena on which nursing focuses
   c. the *key concepts* of nursing
   d. the system of symbols or *language* demanded by nursing
2. The broader categories of human affairs that subsume nursing enable the curriculum designer and developer to make explicit the place and fit of nursing in the world of man and human affairs, including nursing considered as
   a. knowledge required for the achievement of nursing results
   b. a socially approved form of activity to help or assist individuals or groups in a society
   c. the endeavor of specialized workers (nurses) in a society with role responsibilities defined by their formal education in nursing and nursing related disciplines
3. The curriculum designer and developer utilizes the foregoing general characteristics of nursing (2. above) to identify models for developing the dimensions of each of the specific characteristics of nursing (1. above).

DISCUSSION

A curriculum designer and developer will become aware of the utility of the foregoing rules only by working with a valid general concept (theory) of nursing. This is a difficult undertaking for persons who have not been *thinking nursing* within the theoretical frame established by a particular general concept of nursing. However, it is a necessary undertaking if curricula are to enable nurses to *think* as well as *do* nursing. *Doers* of nursing who cannot *think* nursing are not able to practice nursing at the full professional, or even at a high technical, level of practice even though they become skilled technicians in some narrow segment of health service.

The quality of education within the various components, as well as the scope and depth of each component, determines what the professional with motivation and ability will be able to do in society. Whether he will be able to think as a scientist within his professional field or in one or more of the foundational fields will be dependent upon the educational approach taken. Today, there is an increasing demand for the established professions to take a hard look at their educational programs because of both the rapid increase of available knowledge and the demands for professional services. This is well summarized in an article that appeared in the *Journal of Medical Education* (1965).

1. To adhere to uncompromisingly high scientific standards
2. To hold to high standards for all in quality of education but making adaptations to the specific requirements of the developing country
3. To set a standard of training that would produce graduates who would function at a level between doctors and auxiliary personnel
4. To view as unrealistic in light of the present state of medical knowledge and its immediate perspective maintaining the *basic doctor* or general practitioner concept but to introduce *an educational common denominator for all doctors,* to include: (1) basic medical sciences, (2) paraclinical subjects, and (3) fundamentals of medicine. This educational denominator would be designed to produce a medical scientist who would then concentrate on some selected area of clinical subjects (Grzegorzlinski, 1965).

Today there is a trend that all forms of work-preparatory education be offered in combination with liberal or general education or be built upon it, as has been the practice in the professions. At last there seems to be consensus about the inadequacy of work-centered education to move a man toward the fullness of his stature as a man.

The form of education selected by persons constructing work-preparatory programs should bear a direct relationship to the type of worker to be obtained through education and training. When this question as to type of worker is asked and left unanswered, or when it is not asked, the selected form will not have a realistic, empirical base; the relevance of the work-preparatory program will be by chance and not by design.

Since the form of work-preparatory education is a function of the definition of work role, educational planners and curriculum designers must be aware of trends both in education and in the occupations and professions. Work-preparatory programs should be seen as dynamic and not static; what was good enough for my grandparents may not be good enough for me. We have much in our heritage to overcome. Our country did not give immediate academic attention to work-preparatory education. Not until the nineteenth century did we begin to move in the area of vocational education; technical education has come into the foreground of our thought subsequent to World War II. Sound professional education has emerged in the twentieth century. Our contribution as nurses, nurse educators, and educationists toward the development of nursing education and practice should be both realistic and creative—forward thinking and not bound by traditions. Failure to see the here and now and to project into the future can lead to the disappearance of an occupational group from society. As professionals, let us look toward the future of nursing education and practice as scientists and realists. *We construct education and practice.* What standards are to be our guides?

CHAPTER 13

Validity in Theory: A Therapeutic Self-Care Demand for Nursing Practice

I was asked to participate in the conference "Freedom for Nurses Now" because of the work that has engaged me since the 1950s, the work of acquiring insights about nursing and formulating and expressing these insights in an organized form. Nursing involves us as human beings; it involves the use of our freedom, from the point of view of our existence in time; and it involves us in the order imposed by our culture.

My general focus today (and I hope it will be your focus) is the relationship between the nurse's utilization of valid theory and the responsibility and freedom of the nurse in nursing practice. Nurses have tended to reject the notion of theory as providing a basis for practice. Knowing how to do this and that for individuals under the care of nurses has been emphasized as the central case of both nursing education and practice, by nurses and those others who always seem to know what is best for nursing and nurses. This focus on doing as an organizing center is comparable to developing a medical curriculum around drawing blood samples, giving intravenous infusions, or taking out appendixes outside a substantial frame of reference.

The orientation of the practicing nurse to individuals or groups who can benefit from nursing is in large part determined by the experiences of the nurse and by the degree to which the nurse is or is not guided by theoretical formulations about the phenomena that confront the nurse as nurse. I recall hearing Dr. Rusk (Rehabilitation Medicine) make the statement that when patients with disabilities were ready to embark on the

---

This paper was originally presented at the Georgetown Student Conference in 1976.

long, difficult, and painful process of engaging themselves again in activities of daily living, it was necessary to get the nurses out of the wards because the nurses were oriented only to taking care of by doing for. The nurses to whom Dr. Rusk referred had a narrow concept of their social role; the narrow role conceptualizations are still with us but are gradually being replaced by more comprehensive and realistic role conceptualizations based on the action capacities of and action demands for individuals who can be helped through nursing.

The title for my presentation in this session of the conference conveys the message that valid *theory* is a prerequisite condition for the kind of nursing practice that will bring a positively therapeutic return to individuals or groups. The term *Therapeutic Self-Care Demand* is used analogously to help us move toward understanding the *here-and-now* demand upon nurses to utilize reliable nursing knowledge, including *facts, theories,* and *laws* in observing and regulating the realities of self, client, and environment within situations of nursing practice.

Nursing, like any profession, has an objective field of practice. Nursing scholars, researchers, and theorists have the social roles of defining and describing this objective field and laying out the explanatory systems and laws that will serve practitioners of nursing. Practitioner roles may be combined with the role of scholar, researcher, developer, or theorist; this is needed for adequate enactment of all roles toward the survival of nursing. The roles of scholar and theorist have not been afforded the attention they require within the profession; research without scholarship and theory is on barren ground.

NURSING AS PRACTICAL ENDEAVOR

Any effort to conceptualize what nursing is or to formulate explanatory systems in nursing (and theories are explanatory systems) ideally begins with the premise that *nursing is practical endeavor.* Nursing is action, deliberate endeavor of nurses directed toward the achievement of ends or results that are sought by nurses for other individuals in the role of client or patient. Theories and laws are terms associated with *science,* with knowledge that is detailed, descriptive, explanatory, and organized. The question "Can there be a science of nursing?" is related to the question "Can there be a science of the practical?"

Dickoff and James (1968) brought the question into focus and answered it first at the Conference on Nursing Theory held at Western Reserve in the late 1960s. Their designation of nursing as a *practice discipline* and their description of kinds of theory in practice disciplines was and is an important contribution to nursing.

Jacques Maritain (1940) had this to say about science and the practical:

> The word science takes on diminished meaning when it passes over into the practical order. And yet the practical sciences are authentic sciences—involving a group of certitudes organically bound together, assigning principles and causes in a certain objective field. These sciences are essentially practical because their object is work or action to be performed . . . (they have) and they retain a speculative element up to the point at which practical knowledge becomes prudence. [p. 80]

The point at which a practitioner makes the decision to do this and not that on the basis of theoretical knowledge, knowledge of the rules and procedures of nursing practice, and reliable information about the conditions in self, client, and environment, that should affect the decision about what is to be done.

Dickoff and James (1968) are philosophers who have associated with nurses but who are not nurses. Neither they nor the philosophers of science can set forth the objective field of nursing practice, nor should we expect them to. Because philosophers look upon nursing from outside (they generally refer to it as from above), what they tell us about practical sciences and practice disciplines is not specific to any one of these disciplines but equally relevant to all the fields of practical endeavor that are dependent upon the acquisition of an inside range of substantive knowledge as well as upon skills and maturation by practitioners. It is nurses who can and should lay out the dimensions and boundaries of the objective field of nursing.

In all human services there are two actors and two roles—the practitioner and the client. Each has responsibilities and freedom within the reality situation in which their roles are enacted. It is a valid general theory of nursing that enables nurses to see with clarity about the present and with vision into the future that which can and should unify these actors and that which differentiates these roles.

The practical endeavors of the professional nurse are conducted within the frame of the objective field of nursing, and each nurse and each client of a nurse is a living, real part of the field of the real that is conceptualized by the theorist. If the domain and the boundaries of the field remain unclear, nursing cannot attain its rightful status in society, nor can it make its contribution to that society.

RESPONSIBILITY AND FREEDOM FOR NURSES

Societies give to the professions certain aspects of those human problems that individuals or families are unable to solve unassisted. Each profession formulates and structures both theoretical and practical knowledge about its objective field (for example, theoretical medicine and practical medicine). Each profession is expected to develop its own substantive body of knowledge and the members of the profession who have mastered or are mastering knowledge in the profession and in related fields are expected to be clear about their social roles and articulate those roles to others with precision. Every professional must be clear about the domain and boundaries of that professional field, for the professional's status and legitimacy in functioning in the society is confined to the institutional domain of the profession.

Nurses have been and some continue to be characterized by an inability to clearly articulate their social roles. Some nurses, while actively engaged in nursing practice or nursing education, do not hesitate to say, "I don't know what nursing is," "nursing has not been defined," or "there is no official definition of nursing." These statements amount to saying "I (or other nurses) am nursing or teaching nursing but I am unable to express the nature or character of what I am doing or teaching." The lack of clarity about nursing is evidenced in the tendency of some nurses to minimize (even in the face of evidence to the contrary) the contributions of nursing to the achievement of health results for individuals or groups. (This tendency was represented to me by a clinical psychologist who was impressed with the health care contributions of the nurses with whom he had an association.) Related to this is the low profile that some nurses afford to self as nurse. "I am only a nurse."

Responsibility and freedom will never come to nurses unless nurses understand what are and what can be the dimensions of nursing in the society and become able to articulate the social roles of nurses with clarity and precision (using symbols that are appropriate for the audience). The state of the arts and the sciences, of course, will limit what nurses can do within the field but there is no question that the professional practice of nursing is dependent upon the parallel advancement of nurses as scholars and practitioners. It should be recognized that the responsibility of the nursing profession extends to all endeavors necessary to enable nursing to serve in a society. These include the human service of *nursing practice*, nursing education, and the knowledge-producing actions of theory formulation. The knowledge-oriented endeavors are for the sake of the service endeavors or the service endeavors will be lost to society. Science or knowledge-producing and knowledge-structuring endeavors in nursing can begin with questions of such a general nature that their answers constitute general guides to all forms of nursing endeavors. These include the "why" questions.

1. Why do physicians and families seek nursing for individual family members and not for others?
2. Why do some individuals seek nursing for themselves?

The implication is that some but not all persons are perceived by themselves or by significant others as requiring or being in a state to benefit from nursing services. How do we explain that fact? We do it through a deductive argument in which the explanation is a logically necessary consequence of the explanatory premises. Premises must be based in fact. I started with the "why" questions, and this was the argument (key facts based on over 20 years of experience).

1. Nursing is not sought by or for all individuals, even for those under medical care.
2. All individuals for whom nursing is sought have continuing requirements for care that cannot at the time be met by themselves or their families.
3. This inability to meet continuing care requirements is the reason nursing is sought and needed in a society.

I had an answer, an explanation, that helped me move to answer other general questions:

What is the objective field of nursing practice?
What are the domain and boundaries of nursing considered as a discipline of knowledge?
What is nursing?

I was able to express the *focus* of nursing, and such an expression is recognized as a just requirement for systematic and scientific movement in any field of or practice.

I experienced then and I continue to experience an intellectual and personal freedom in nursing that was not a part of me until I had formally, deliberately answered the question "Why are people seeking nursing?" Prior to my formulation of a general theory of nursing, one that holds for all situations, I felt the responsibility to delineate and structure nursing knowledge but I had no freedom, for I had no way to move.

NURSING'S CONCEPTUAL FRAMEWORK

The general theory of nursing that I shall now talk about was first expressed in 1956. It was later (1958) reformulated and expressed according to the deductive argument that I presented. As I formulated the argument I had the image of the nurse as "another self" for the person under care; it was from this idea that the concept of individuals as *care agents for self* and the concept *self-care* emerged. At this time I also saw that it was necessary to differentiate self-care deficits due to age, as in infants, from self-care deficits that bring about requirements for nursing. This was done by indicating that it is the health situation and not age as such that resulted in existing limitations or deficits for engaging in self-care. The latest expression of the theory appears on page 71 of *Concept Formalization in Nursing* (Nursing Development Conference Group, 1973). The theoretical approach that resulted from my exploration of *why nursing is needed in a society* is often referred to as the Self-Care Theory of Nursing.

The theory rests upon the reality of the human condition of social dependency that casts members of a social group into the roles of the one in need of help and the helper. From the condition of social dependency (whatever its cause) is born the human services, many of which have been institutionalized in our own and in other societies. Nursing is one of the institutionalized human services.

More specifically, the theory rests upon the reality that adults do deliberately care for themselves and their dependents. The putting of food into one's mouth (or into the mouth of a child) is a voluntary action. It is an act of self-care whether it be done with or without insight about the utility of the food intake. *Self-care is action for self.* It is action through which inputs are made to self or environment—inputs that contribute to the maintenance of human functioning (to think, we must eat), to the continuance of life, health, and well-being. We may see our action in these terms or at the simpler level, the emotional level of providing pleasure or alleviating pain. Self-care may become so routine and habitual that we do things because of the time of day. But self-care is action that is a response to the functional needs of human beings, needs that are both subjectively and objectively definable.

The concept of self-care requirements was formulated and expressed in 1959. These requirements were described as being of two kinds—those that are universal to all human beings and those that arise only in relation to health deviations. A self-care requirement is an essential or a desired input to an individual or the individual's environment in order to maintain or optimize human functioning. Food intake adjusted to the functional requirements of an individual with consideration of external conditions is a *self-care requirement*. Action to meet the requirement is *self-care*. The formulation and expression of a self-care requirement is essentially the expression of a broad end or goal to be achieved. Like all comprehensive or broad ends it can only be achieved when less global ends or results are brought about in and over time through a variety of action process. It is in relation to these less broad ends or results that technologies or action processes are developed. The deliberate use of a mix of these technologies at T_1, T_2, T_3 [T = time] and so forth constitutes the means through which specific self-care requirements are met. An example is presented in Table 13.1.

Ascribing to human beings the role of self-care agent and care agent for dependents and conceptualizing their power to fulfill these roles as self-care agency and dependent-care agency are important aspects of the theory. Nurses who function in accord with the theory view and work with individuals as persons but keep an objective focus on these persons as self-care agents with operating or potential powers for self-care and with responsibility and freedom as related to self-care. This objective focus on the client involves the nurse in a three-dimensional examination of the client's abilities for self-care: as developmental, as operating, and as adequate.

Even when self-care agency is developed as in a mature adult, and when it is operable, it is only possible to determine adequacy in relation to a known demand on the individual for engagement in self-care. The concept and term self-care demand were formulated. The term has its referents in outstanding or existent universal or health-related types of self-care requirements and the action processes through which requirements can be met. Therapeutic, when utilized to modify self-care demand, is an indication that the action processes identified have a known positive utility value as related to the maintenance or regulation of human functioning.

Self-care agency and *therapeutic self-care demand* within the frame of theory are client attributes or variables. They are two of the three constant

TABLE 13.1 Meeting Specific Self-Care Requirements

Universal Self-Care Requirements	Ends or Results to Be Achieved and Actions Processes That Will Be Effective

To maintain air intake and air output at physiological levels of adequacy, qualitatively and quantitatively described	1. Maximization of alveolar ventilation within physiologically safe levels (avoidance of hyper- and hypoventilation).
	  a. Posture, positioning, turning
	  b. Deep breathing
	  c. Abdominal breathing
	
	2. Maintenance or production of clear airway and air spaces by removal of internally produced fluids and mucous
	  Deliberate coughing
	  Postural drainage
	  Cupping, clapping
	  Suctioning
	
	3. Prevention of partial to complete obstruction of the tracheobronchial tree by { action processes are developed around the type of obstruction
	  a. inspired objects as fluids
	  b. the tongue
	  c. pressure from the esophagus
	
	4. Maintenance of self in an external environment where there is air that meets physiologic standards of adequacy, or providing self with an adequate supply
	
	5. Maintaining awareness of the number and quality of respiratory excursions to the degree necessary to identify
	  a. Patterns of breathing leading to identify hypo- or hyperventilation
	  b. A pattern of dyspnea following nonstrenuous activity
	  c. A pattern of dyspnea at rest

variables in nursing systems. The other constant variable is *nursing agency*, which is an attribute of the nurse. The value of the client variables at T^0, T^1, T^2 [T = time], and so on, are affected by the human factors of age, sex, growth and developmental state, health state, sociocultural orientations, and also by externally imposed conditions, such as those imposed by the physical and other elements in the physical or social environment of the individual and family. There is a demand on the nurse engaged in nursing practice to determine the nature (values) of these factors and identify the nature of the correlation between the factor and the variable that is presently governing events or that serves as an indicator of the events that should be brought about. For example, loss of awareness in an adult correlates with non-operability of self-care agency. These correlates, as well as the cause of or reason for the loss of awareness, are indicators of events that should be brought about.

Finally we come to the central concept of the theory, *nursing agency*. This nurse variable is conceptualized as a characteristic quality of the nurse, the power that the nurse has to engage in effective nursing practice. As a concept, nursing agency includes the following conceptual elements: structural knowledge, sustaining motive, performance skills, and nursing prudence, as these relate to the practice of nursing. Nursing agency is manifested by the art of nursing, as it has been developed by the nurse. It is art that enables a nurse to compose and manage a system of nursing out of the fabric of self and the fabric of the client.

The nurse's concept of self as person and of self as nurse, the nurse's self-management abilities, and other forms of agency that nurses have developed and perfected affect the quality of nursing agency. And nursing agency, like self-care agency, is continuously affected or conditioned by the nurse's age, sex, developmental state, health state, sociocultural orientation, and externally imposed conditions.

When the nurse activates nursing agency, when she moves toward the other or client, the action system that is nursing is initiated. It is sustained to the degree that the nurse assists the client (using effective and valid ways of assistance) to enable the client to regulate, protect, or develop self-care agency and to meet outstanding self-care requirements in and over time.

SUMMARY

I have been speaking this afternoon as a nursing scholar and theorist and not as a practitioner of nursing. The point of view of the scholar and theorist differs from that of the practitioner. The practitioner as practitioner is confronted with the demand to judge, to make decisions, and to act (not later but now) for the well-being of the other, the client. The nurse who masters a comprehensive nursing theory is better able to manage the details of nurse practitioner in scientific-level observation and other details of the nursing process than is the nurse who functions without an explanatory system. A valid general theory of nursing serves as an intellectual road that keeps the nurse on a nursing course, preventing her from being lost in the maze of detail that characterizes many nursing situations. It is like a map that shows the states, the highways, and the major cities, but it will get you to the District of Columbia. It is up to nurses who are professional practitioners, researchers, developers, and theorists at the middle levels to fill in details of the map of the objective field of nursing provided by a general theory of nursing.

I shall close with some statements from Bernard Lonergan that I see as relevant to our efforts as nurses attending this conference.

> I am empirically conscious inasmuch as I am experiencing; intellectually conscious inasmuch as I am inquiring or formulating intelligently; nationally conscious inasmuch as I am seeking to grasp [the unities that exist, and the correlation that governs events] or judging on the basis of such a grasp; but I become rationally self-conscious inasmuch as I am concerned with reasons for my own acts, and this occurs when I scrutinize the object and investigate the motives for a possible course of action. [1958, p. 611]

As nurses we should know the objective field of nursing, including that which is constant and that which is changing within it and we should know our place in the field and how our talents will enable us to contribute to it. Each instance of nursing is an expression of a structuring consciousness of the nurse. There is much to do to promote effective intra- and interdisciplinary functioning. Let us as nurses move nursing; nursing cannot move itself for it is our creation.

CHAPTER 14

Nursing Theories and Their Function as Conceptual Models for Nursing Practice and Curriculum Development

I t is a privilege to speak to nurses in such numbers who are interested in nursing theories and hence in nursing science, for theories are elements of developing or developed sciences. My task is to describe for you one general theory of nursing referred to by a variety of names: Orem's Theory, the self-care theory, the self-care agency theory, the self-care deficit theory of nursing and the NDCG (Nursing Development Conference Group) theory of nursing system. The central idea of the theory (the idea of self-care demands) was formulated and expressed by me in 1958 and has undergone considerable development since that time. The Government Printing Office, HEW Publication titled *Guides for the Developing Curricula for the Education of Practical Nurses* (Orem, 1959), the McGraw Hill Book Company publication *Nursing: Concepts of Practice* (Orem, 1971), and the Little, Brown and Company publication *Concept Formalization in Nursing: Process and Product* (Nursing Development Conference Group, 1973) contain the conceptual elements and principles of the theory in the various stages of development. The first book is out of print, the second two are in print and revisions of these should be available in 1979. [*Ed. Note: Concept Formalization* is now out of print but available

This paper was originally presented at the Nurse Education Conference in New York City in December, 1978.

in some university libraries; *Nursing: Concepts of Practice* is in the sixth edition (Orem, 2001).]

The central idea of the general theory of nursing, that I shall attempt to sketch for you in a time space of forty minutes, was a response to a question that I posed for myself in order to find a way to lay out the domain and boundaries of nursing as a field of practice and as an organized body of knowledge. The question was: What condition exists in an individual or a group when judgments are made that nursing is required, that a nurse or nurses should now be related to this person or group as health care providers? The answer to the question came as a flash of insight, an understanding of why some but not all persons have health care requirements that can be met through nursing rather than through some other form of health care or service.

The insight was formulated and expressed as a concept—the concept of limitations for care of self or care of dependent family members due to health state or the nature of the health care requirements that should be met continuously in time. Such limitations render self-care or care of dependents impossible, as with a comatose person, or ineffective or incomplete, as with a mother who can give effective care to a full-term, well newborn infant but not to the newborn who is premature, or of low birth weight. The image of the nurse as *another self* for the person with requirements for nursing was a part of my process of formulation and expression of the conceptualization about why people require nursing.

The process that terminated in this concept of human limitations was a process of human knowing, moving from my past nursing experiences with their yield of information, to the question that stimulated inquiry, through imagination to insight, from insight to the formulation and expression of the concept of *self-care limitations*, to awareness and the judgment that the expressed concept indeed explains why people can be helped through nursing (after Lonergan, 1967, pp. 222–223). The foregoing exposition serves to illustrate the philosophical distinction between *knowledge* and *belief*. "Knowledge is affirming what one understands in one's own experience while belief is accepting what we are told by others on whom we reasonably rely" (Lonergan, 1958, p. 42). "Insight or understanding is activity" (p. 535).

My conceptualizing moved from an accumulation of factual information about nurses and persons who require nursing. But I also moved from a generalization, a postulate that I accepted as a premise for reasoning. The postulate was expressed in this fashion: Not all persons under active medical care or under medical supervision are under nursing care, nor does it follow that they should be under nursing care.

Accepting this generalization, I then asked the question: What is the human condition that occasions requirements for nursing? The answer came within the process just described. The answer to the question has served me and others as a naming and a specification of the *proper object of nursing*, an identification of the entity that is the proper domain of nursing, considering nursing as both science and service, an understanding of the reality that is. These views of nursing are subsumed by the concept and term *practice discipline*, that has come into use in nursing within the last three decades (see Figure 14.1).

In summary, the concept of self-care limitations expresses a deficit relationship between persistent self-care abilities of persons and the objective demand upon them to engage in self-care or dependent care under the condition that the limitation for engagement in care is health derived or health related. Two entities thus are posited: a set of abilities to act and a demand to act. When abilities at T (Time) zero are in a deficit relationship to the action demand, nursing is required, or nursing may be required when abilities are equal to or greater than the demand but a deficit relationship can be predicted for T^1 or T^2. Prenatal preparation of mothers for self-care during their labor and delivery, and preparation of mothers to incorporate preventive practices in infant and child care are examples of this.

From this point on in my discussion I shall be speaking from the perspective of *nursing science*. I suggest that you refer to the material from me which is in your folder—the naming of 5 fields of nursing knowledge,

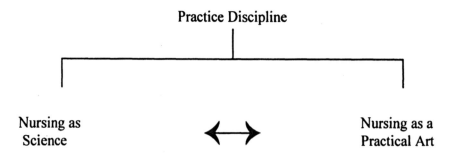

FIGURE 14.1 Elements of a practice discipline.

one of which is nursing science. [*Ed. Note*: Orem now identifies 8 fields of knowledge about nurses and nursing—nursing sociology, nursing as profession and occupation, and nursing jurisprudence, nursing history, nursing ethics, nursing science, nursing economics, and nursing administration (Orem, 2001, p. 160).] Specifically, the general theory of nursing that I shall now describe is "Theoretical Nursing Science," that is, knowledge that is theoretical, explanatory in form, and utilitarian in practice.

I hope that you will bear with me in my presentation. Some of you are advanced scholars within the theory; others may express belief in the theory; and still others are having an introduction to it. The advanced scholars can take care of themselves; you who are not advanced, please don't expect that the meaning of what I say will be simple and obvious. As one philosopher said, "The human mind moves at a snail's pace." And another, "Only the man (who) understands everything is in a position to demand that all meaning be simple and obvious to him" (Lonergan, 1958, p. 558).

THEORY: ITS CONCEPTUAL FORMULATION

The general theory of nursing, the conceptual structure of which I shall describe for you, is, as I mentioned, a unity of three theories: (1) the theory of self-care, a form of human activity essential for continued human functioning and human well-being in life, (2) the theory of self-care deficit, as predictive of requirements for nursing, and (3) the NDCG theory of the nursing system as the end product of nursing. The conceptual elements of the theory are shown in Figure 14.2. Six different concepts are symbolized by the terms that appear on the figure: These are:

1. Self-care: human action, deliberately performed by persons for the sake of self in order to regulate one's human functioning
2. Self-care agency: the human capability to give self-care
3. Self-care demands: the summation of the self-care actions that will regulate the human functioning of a person, which, if not performed, will result in death, injury, illness, or deterioration of the state of well-being
4. Nursing agency: the human capacity to design, operationalize, and manage nursing systems with and for others in need
5. Self-care deficit: the concept of a deficit relation of self-care agency to self-care demand

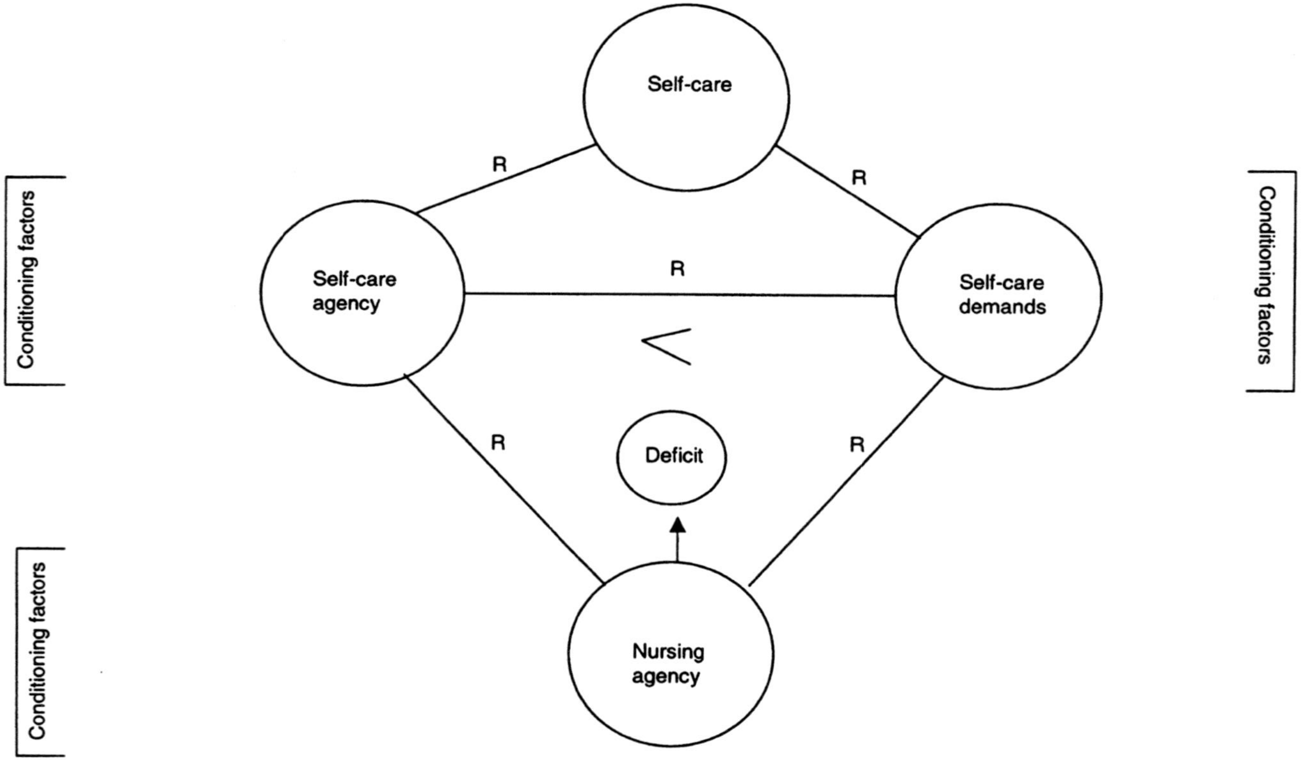

FIGURE 14.2 Conceptual model.

From "A Conceptual Framework for Nursing," by D. E. Orem, 2001, *Nursing: Concepts of Practice* (6th ed.), p. 491. St. Louis: Mosby.

6. Conditioning factors: human or environmental entities that *condition* the value of *self-care agency*, *self-care demand*, and *nursing agency* at points in time

Next, the relations (and it is important to keep in mind that nursing science is concerned with exploration of relations between entities): the most central relation within the theory is that between self-care agency and self-care demand. As indicated, there are two possible relations—*equal to* or *not equal to*, specifically, *greater than* or *less than*. To arrive at a judgment about this relationship in concrete and particular situations, it is necessary to know the constituent elements of self-care agency and the value of each element at a point in time, and to know the courses of action that constitute the self-care demand, e.g., all the courses of action to be taken to keep food intake adjusted to (1) metabolic requirements of cells, (2) operational requirements of body parts, and (3) caloric energy requirements of the person. If one uses the field theory approach as a *method* of analyzing relations and building scientific constructs in nursing, *phenomena* descriptive and explanatory of self-care agency and self-care demand separately or together will always be a part of a field, a part of the life space of an individual.

The next consideration is a triad of relations (refer to Figure 14.2).

1. Self-care agency as related to self-care demands
2. Self-care agency as related to self-care
3. Self-care as related to self-care demands

We have already considered the first. But the second, self-care agency (the capability for self-care) must be considered in terms of its *development*, *operability*, and *adequacy*. State of development and operability together determine whether the person can produce self-care actions regardless of the demand. Adequacy is specified in the first relationship. Self-care as related to self-care demand raises the questions: Are self-care actions being performed? Some are observable, others are not. Do these actions compare with the self-care demand? With respect to self-care we must always keep before us the image of man acting on self or environment for the sake of self. Self-care can be identified as existent, as equal and sufficient as related to the demand, and as effective in regulating human functioning.

Determination of the self-care demand in concrete and particular situations provides the standard against which the qualitative and quantitative adequacy of self-care actions can be evaluated.

The work of Barbara J. Horn and Mary Ann Swain (1977) and their associates at the University of Michigan fits within the triad of relations I am now describing. They utilized conceptualized systems of actions to meet the universal self-care requirement (one portion of the self-care demand) as well as conditioning factors toward the development of criterion measures of care. This exploratory research included the dimension of effectiveness of the self-care actions taken to meet the universal self-care requirements. The ability to conceptualize this triad of relations is ideally a capability of each mature person; it is within the human power, the term conceptualized as self-care agency.

The next set of relations brings nursing agency into perspective and brings us to the theory of nursing system (the third part of the general theory of nursing), as expressed and accepted by members of the Nursing Development Conference Group.

The conceptualization of nursing system is expressed on pp. 70–71 of *Concept Formalization in Nursing: Process and Product* (Nursing Development Conference Group, 1973). Some of the assumptions on which the conceptualization is based, that is, its presupposition, can be found on pp. 71–72.

A nursing system is conceptualized as a product—something made. The product comes from the deliberate actions of the person who is nurse and the person(s) who is patient. The nurse exercises nursing agency to determine the legitimacy of the person holding the status of patient and the status of nurse to this patient. This is done by determining the presence or absence of a self-care deficit in the patient, including the nurse's determining the adequacy and value of the self-care agency possessed in relation to the indications for regulation, including alteration of a patient's self-care agency and self-care demand. With respect to the patient, the activation of the components of nursing agency by the nurse to diagnose, prescribe, or regulate the value or state of self-care agency and self-care demand of the patient is nursing.

From the broadest perspective nursing is conceptualized as a hierarchy of interlocking systems, each with its own set of variables (see Figure 3.1, p. 76, in *Concept Formalization*, NDCG, 1973, 1979). The systems are named:

1. The *social* system—the variables of the system are the persons occupying the status of patient and of nurse to the patient. The relation between the persons within this context is identified as *contractual*

2. The *interpersonal* system—the variables here are the persons who occupy the status of nurse and patient in all their uniqueness as individual human beings and in the mutuality of their relations with others

3. The *technological* system—the variables here are conceptualized as two patient or client variables (I use the terms patient and client as synonymous) the human attribute self-care agency and the totality of self-care courses of action to be taken, that is, self-care demand, and the nurse variable nursing agency

The social, interpersonal, and technological systems are interactive. The interpersonal system is enabling for and interactive with both the social and technological systems. The contractual nature of social systems sets limits on the technological, and the technological provides the role content and role sets for both nurse and patient operating within that contractual and interpersonal system. My conceptualization of three types of nursing systems—wholly and partly compensatory systems and supportive-developmental systems—is an expression of three modes of interactiveness of the variables.

1. In a wholly compensatory nursing system, self-care agency is not interactive or is negatively interactive with self-care demand. It may be interactive with nursing agency. Nursing agency is interactive with the self-care demand in generating a system of action that meets the demand and at the same time is operative to protect and preserve the person's self-care agency.

2. In partially compensatory systems, both self-care agency and nursing agency variables are interactive with self-care demand, and nursing agency will be directed to assist the person to withhold use of, or further develop, self-care agency.

3. In supportive educative systems, nursing agency is interactive with self-care agency and self-care agency is interactive with self-care demand.

I shall move now to the sixth conceptual element, namely, *conditioning factors*. The term appears in Figure 14.2, adjacent to the two patient or client variables and the one nurse variable. Conditioning factors are not seen as explanatory of the structure of the entities named but are interactive with them and affect their values at points in time. The Nursing Development Conference Group has worked with a set of eight factors:

1. Age
2. Sex
3. Developmental state
4. Health state
5. Sociocultural orientation
6. Health care system elements, for example, being hospitalized or being under medical care
7. Patterns of living, life style
8. Resources

In a concrete and particular nursing situation, one or some combination of these factors can be operating dynamically to change the values of the time patient variables. Other factors may be relatively static. The term *basic system* was introduced by the Nursing Development Conference Group to refer to the process by which a basic conditioning factor affects the value of the patient variables. This raises questions such as: How does developmental state affect self-care agency? Does or how does this or that pathological process affect self-care agency or give rise to new requirements for self-care?

The number of basic conditioning factors that are dynamic in affecting the values of the patient variables and the rapidity of changes in them is an index of the complexity of a nursing situation. The conditioning effects of the named factors on the patient variables will determine the value of nursing agency that is sufficient to diagnose, design, and produce an effective nursing system with and for the person in need of nursing. But at the same time, with respect to the individual nurse, for example, age, health state, or resources may be directly conditioning the nurse's ability to produce nursing.

This concludes my presentation of the broad conceptual structure of the theory.

CHAPTER 15

Scholarly Endeavors: Eight Sets of Work Operations for Advancing One's Scholarship

SET ONE: DEFINING THE DOMAIN OF CONCERN

1. Identifying the area or the related areas of a field of knowledge to be investigated
2. Identifying known or posited points of articulation with other fields of knowledge
3. Identifying the aspects of the real world that the areas of knowledge describe and explain

SET TWO: INVESTIGATING SOURCES OF INFORMATION

1. Identifying sources of knowledge by fields
   a. primary
   b. secondary
   c. sources not identified as primary or secondary
2. Preparing a working bibliography
3. Preparing a list of advanced scholars

This outline was written in 1970 and revised May 22, 1979. It was initially developed and received as part of a Georgetown University School of Nursing Project on Work Operations of a Nursing Faculty.

SET THREE: BUILDING KNOWLEDGE

1. Reading and analyzing written source materials
   a. formulate and express questions for reflection
   b. formulate and express questions for further investigation
2. Attending scholarly lectures and discussions
3. Seeking information from advanced scholars
4. Identifying terms and clarifying the meaning attached to them by particular persons in the field(s)

SET FOUR: ACHIEVING UNDERSTANDING

1. Expending effort and energy in clarifying and synthesizing knowledge
   a. discussions with colleagues
   b. identifying key ideas
   c. identifying the real world entities being dealt with
2. Formulating and expressing in speech or writing the insights one has at particular times
3. Formulating and expressing perceived issues and unanswered questions
4. Evaluating oneself for consistently correct use of terms

SET FIVE: ESTABLISHING AN AUTHORITATIVE SET OF SOURCES OF INFORMATION

1. Preparing a definitive bibliography for oneself (or identification of preferred works in existent bibliographies)
2. Preparing a listing of authorities by areas of particular fields of knowledge and by their adherence to a particular theoretical position(s)
3. Expressing one's own position(s) about the area of knowledge under investigation
   a. in discussions with colleagues
   b. in discussion with advanced scholars
   c. in essays

SET SIX: CONSTRUCTING A FRAMEWORK FOR INVESTIGATION OF A DOMAIN

1. Formulating and expressing the conceptual framework for an area or a segment of an area of knowledge
2. Developing a glossary of essential explanatory terms
3. Establishing the validity and reliability of the expressed conceptual framework in investigating aspects of the real world
4. Developing a glossary of descriptive terms

SET SEVEN: ELABORATING AND COMMUNICATING THE FRAMEWORK

1. Keeping abreast of developments in the areas of the fields of knowledge in which one has achieved scholarship and in significantly related areas by
   a. reading periodical literature
   b. new works
   c. continuing dialogue with advanced scholars
2. Formulating and expressing one's mental position of certitude about an area of knowledge or a segment of an area
3. Formulating and expressing the assumptions basic to the position one takes about an area of knowledge or a segment of an area
4. Engaging in the writing of scholarly papers, monographs, or other texts that bring together major developments in an area of knowledge or a segment of an area

SET EIGHT: FORMALIZING THE DOMAIN OF CONCERN

1. Utilizing one's scholarship in an area(s) of knowledge in the formulation and expression of
   a. unanswered questions
   b. meanings for practical endeavors
      (1) rules to guide practice
      (2) technologies of practice

2. Utilizing one's scholarship in an area(s) of knowledge to guide research
3. Utilizing one's scholarship in an area(s) of knowledge in theory building

CHAPTER 16

The Structure of Antecedent Nursing Knowledge

ecause of the diversity and complexity of nursing cases, Nursing
Development Conference Group (NDCG) members have been atten-
tive to the need to structure existent knowledge in forms useful to
nurses engaged in nursing practice. Nursing cases can be grouped on the
basis of resemblances among them. As a genus within the occurrence of
requirements for human services, nursing cases should be understood and
can be classified in terms of differences in ends sought and in the actions
required to achieve the ends. Knowledge that is antecedent to nurses'
engagement in nursing practice should be structured to make these differences explicit.

One position to be taken is that antecedent knowledge should be organized and expressed according to degrees of invariance with respect to
instances of individual and group health care requirements that can be
met through nursing. As previously stated, some antecedent knowledge is
invariant for all nursing cases but other antecedent knowledge is invariant
for some types of nursing cases when specific factors are exercising a
conditioning influence on the nursing system variables.

Three examples of NDCG members' endeavors to structure antecedent
knowledge required by nurses are presented. All the examples assume the
acceptance and use by NDCG members of (1) self-care deficit to explain
why individuals require nursing, (2) nursing systems as products designed
and produced by nurses to achieve nursing goals, and (3) the conceptual

This paper was previously published in 1979 in the Nursing Development Conference Group's
Concept Formalization in Nursing: Process and Product, ed. D. E. Orem, pp. 248–272. Boston:
Little Brown.

constructs of therapeutic self-care demand, self-care agency, and nursing agency, viewed as qualities of persons that operate as variables within the technologic subsystems of nursing systems. The examples differ in focus and in scope. All are illustrative of the effort and the nature of the work involved in the structuring of knowledge that is antecedent to nursing practice.

NURSING SYSTEM VARIABLES AND CEREBROVASCULAR ACCIDENTS

An effort was made by Hartnett-Rauckhorst (NDCG, 1979) from 1977 to 1978 to organize (i.e., structure) knowledge about cerebrovascular accidents derived from the fields of neurophysiology, pathology, medicine, psychology, sociology, nursing, and physical and occupational therapy around the nursing system variables of therapeutic self-care demand, self-care agency, and nursing agency. The occurrence of a stroke was viewed as a basic conditioning factor that sets up the requirement for development of a nursing system. This is an example of bringing together existing knowledge derived from the literature of nursing and nursing-related fields into a nursing framework and applying the NDCG's theory of nursing system to a particular patient population.

From the perspectives of pathology and medicine, a cerebrovascular accident or a stroke is the cardinal feature of cerebrovascular diseases. A stroke is the sudden development of a focal neurologic deficit resultant from the effects of pathologic processes in one or more blood vessels of the brain on brain tissue. Cerebrovascular accidents range in degree from very severe to very mild. The occurrence of a cerebrovascular accident and the time sequential occurrence of subsequent events are referred to as the time profile or the stages of cerebrovascular accidents.

Five stages were utilized in the work of organizing existent knowledge about stroke around the nursing system variables. These stages are referred to as

Stage I   Being at risk for cerebrovascular accidents or having premonitory signs

Stage II   Acute stage of a cerebrovascular accident (severe stroke)
             A. unconscious phase
             B. returning consciousness phase

Stage III   Convalescent stage of cerebrovascular accidents
Stage IV   Rehabilitation stage following cerebrovascular accidents
Stage V   Health maintenance or continuing care stage following cerebrovascular accidents

In using the foregoing time dimensions that mark the patterns of occurrence of types of events and results associated with stroke, it is important to understand that for particular individuals the time profile need not extend over the five stages. For example, some persons at risk (Stage I) do not have cerebrovascular accidents; individuals may die in the acute stage (Stage II), or the stroke may be mild rather than severe; or individuals may be arrested in Stage III, not able to progress to Stage IV or to Stage V.

The results of knowledge structuring using the selected basic conditioning factor, cerebrovascular accident, were formulated and are presented as (1) a changing of the degrees of operability of self-care agency by stages of cerebrovascular accidents; (2) an example of the demand for the operation of self-care agency associated with one stage of stroke, Stage I; (3) descriptive models of the characteristics of the nursing system variables by stages of cerebrovascular accidents; and (4) a charting of variations in nursing goals, nursing systems, and nursing roles in the five stages of cerebrovascular accidents.

These models are an initial attempt to organize knowledge about cerebrovascular accidents around the NDCG's conceptualizations of nursing system variables. They provide a basis for further study and refinement of the characteristics and components of the nursing system variables at each stage of stroke. Valid and reliable assessment tools for gathering evidence about nursing system variables can then be developed. This evidence would contribute to the development of a body of theoretical knowledge descriptive and explanatory of the nursing system variables at each stage of stroke. It would also provide a basis for the development of a body of practical knowledge that can provide guidance and direction to nurses who are confronted with questions of practice regarding the design and delivery of nursing care to persons at each stage of stroke.

OPERABILITY OF SELF-CARE AGENCY

Following strokes, there can be a great variation of effects on the power components of self-care agency, since the effects of strokes on human functioning vary over a wide range.

The medical literature reports effects of stroke in terms of signs and symptoms and the anatomic structures involved. On the basis of signs and symptoms identified in the literature, judgments were made about their association with human capabilities and dispositions in self-care (NDCG, 1979). On the basis of these judgments, inferences were made about how the degree of operability of self-care agency could be affected in each stage of stroke. In the box, the progression of knowing and the conceptual constructs used are described. The progression of knowing illustrated below and the use of the literature as the resource for obtaining knowledge of signs and symptoms of stroke parallel the progression of knowing of nurses in practice who must identify and then attach nursing meaning to the concrete and particular signs and symptoms of individual patients.

Having knowledge of signs and symptoms of cerebrovascular accidents	Having insights and making judgments about associations of signs and symptoms with human capabilities and dispositions basic to human action	Making inferences about degree of operability of the power components of self-care agency by stages of cerebrovascular accidents

The common and gross patterns of operability of self-care agency associated with the stages of cerebrovascular accident are shown in Table 16.1. The degrees of operability of self-care agency are indicated by the terms *fully operative, partially operative,* and *not operative.* Table 16.1 should be read with the understanding that the represented patterns of operability of self-care agency are inferences about the effects and results of cerebrovascular accidents on the operability of each power component of self-care agency. In concrete situations of nursing practice, other factors may be conditioning one or more of the power components.

Table 16.1 does not express patterns of adequacy of self-care agency as related to a therapeutic self-care demand. For example, power components of self-care agency may be fully operative in Stage I but not adequately developed in relation to specific self-care operations. This is demonstrated in the following section.

NEW DEMANDS FOR SELF-CARE OPERATIONS: STAGE I

Being at risk for a cerebrovascular accident operates as a factor that changes the objective value of an individual's *therapeutic self-care demand.* New

TABLE 16.1 Common Patterns of Operability of Self-Care Agency Associated with the Five Stages of Cerebrovascular Accidents

Power Components of Self-Care Agency	Patterns of Operability Cerebrovascular Accident Stages				
	I	II	III	IV	V
1. Maintenance of attention and vigilance	PO	NO/PO	PO	PO	PO/FO
2. Controlled use of available physical energy	FO	NO	NO/PO	PO	PO/FO
3. Control of position of body and its parts in execution of movements	FO	NO/PO	NO/PO	PO	PO/FO
4. Reasoning within a self-care frame of reference	FO	NO/PO	NO/PO	PO	PO/FO
5. Motivations or goal orientations to self-care	FO	NO	NO/PO	PO/FO	PO/FO
6. Decision making about care of self	FO	NO	ON/PO	PO/FO	PO/FO
7. Acquiring, retaining, operationalizing technical knowledge about self-care	FO	NO	NO/PO	PO	PO/FO
8. Having repertoire of self-care skills	FO	NO	NO/PO	PO	PO/FO
9. Ordering discrete self-care actions	FO	NO	NO/PO	PO	PO/FO
10. Integrating self-care operations with other aspects of daily living	FO	NO	NO/PO	PO	PO/FO

Fully operative means operation is *unaffected* by the cerebrovascular accident.
Key: FO = Fully operative; PO = Partially operative; NO = Not operative; / = or

125

self-care requirements arise or there is need for adjustments in existent requirements. The self-care requirements occasioned by being at risk for stroke increase the demand on an individual both for the exercise of self-care agency and for its further development. This is a different situation than those that exist during and following the occurrence of a stroke. In these later situations the *demand* for the *exercise of self-care agency is increased* at the same time that the power components of self-care agency are rendered *not operative* or *partly operative* by the effects of the stroke.

The following is an example of new courses of self-care actions that are required if the condition of being at risk for cerebrovascular accidents is to be regulated. New estimative, transitional, and productive self-care operations contribute to meeting the self-care requirements for *prevention of hazards* and *being normal.*

New Estimative Self-Care Operations and Results

1. Investigation of the aging process and associated risk factors, especially factors that increase risk of stroke (e.g., age, weight, life style, and habits; stress, hypertension, diabetes, arteriosclerosis)
    Result: Acquired technical knowledge that points to the need for periodic health checkups and use of valid means of control of risk factors
2. Investigation (including health evaluation) to become aware of those internal and external factors that increase risk for stroke that are probably operational in self
    Result: Knowledge of factors that are or could be putting self at risk for stroke

Associated Transitional Operations and Results

1. Reflecting on the technical knowledge acquired to determine the course of action to be followed
    Result: Judgments about the need for periodic health checkups, the best place to secure them, and the best time for them
2. Deciding about what will be done with respect to periodic health checkups
    Result: Decision to have or not to have periodic health checkups

3. Reflecting on empirical knowledge of self and those internal and external factors that are probably making one at risk for stroke
   Result: Judgment that self is at high or low risk for stroke
4. Deciding what courses of action to follow with respect to regulation of risk factors
   Result: Decisions about following or not following courses of action that will not keep risk factors under a degree of control

Associated Productive Operations and Results

1a. Make and keep appointments for periodic health checkups
1b. Actively participate in the procedures associated with each health checkup
1c. Receive information from each health checkup
    Result: Having information about health state
2a. Engage in regulatory action to reduce risk of stroke
2b. Monitor self for own performance of regulatory actions and for evidence of effects and results of the action
    Result: Knowledge that self-care requirements are being met with some degree of effectiveness or are not being met; knowledge of the presence or absence of evidence of the effects and results of the courses of action taken to meet self-care requirements

An application of the foregoing is expressed in relation to a 34-year-old woman. As a result of the *estimative* self-care operations, a 34-year-old woman, with a family history of hypertension and stroke who is 15 pounds overweight, will gain empirical and experiential knowledge of known risk factors and how they constitute a threat to her life and health and a realization that some of these factors (e.g., weight and blood pressure) can be modified to reduce the risk. She recognizes that diet modification (in terms of calories and sodium intake) is an effective means available to regulate existing risk factors. As a result of *transitional* self-care operations, this woman judges that she should modify her diet and decides that she will perform the regulatory self-care operations this entails. As a result of *productive* self-care operations, this woman will learn what foods are high and low in calories and sodium, develop a diet plan and menus, and plan for food buying and preparation. With a daily and weekly time frame she will buy, prepare, and eat a diet lower in calories and sodium. She will monitor food labels, size of portions, cooking procedures (especially if prepared by others), and check her weight regularly to obtain data about whether she is losing weight at a safe rate or whether weight loss is not being achieved. She will ascertain her blood pressure reading at each contact with health professionals. She will reflect on the evidence of the results and decide whether to continue with the present diet modification, to adapt it further, or to discontinue it.

This example of how being at risk for stroke generates new self-care requirements to be met through new self-care operations is further elaborated in the following analysis.

CHANGING VALUES OF NURSING SYSTEM VARIABLES

Six models were developed to express in a modified way the range over which the values of the two patient variables (therapeutic self-care demand and self-care agency) are known to vary and the range over which the nurse variable (nursing agency) should vary during the stages of stroke. Components of the *therapeutic self-care demand* associated with stroke are expressed as *courses of action* that should ideally be performed. Limitations of *self-care agency* are expressed in terms of inappropriate courses of self-care action commonly taken, as inadequate power components of self-care agency, or as interferences with the basic capabilities or dispositions for self-care. Components of *nursing agency* are expressed as kinds of knowledge and skills. The knowledge expressed in the models in relation to three nursing system variables was extracted from the literature and *should not be considered as necessarily complete, definitive, or precisely organized*.

The models included expressions about the populations to be served and general goals for health care for these populations (goals common to all persons involved). Levels of prevention of disease and injury were used to express general goals for health care. The levels of prevention paradigm proved useful in organizing the material within the sequential stages of cerebrovascular accident, a pathophysiologic event.

Prior to the onset of a stroke, the focus is on primary prevention for the entire community and secondary prevention for individuals with high-risk profiles or with evidence of premonitory signs. During the acute, convalescent, and rehabilitative stages, the main focus is on tertiary prevention with concern for primary and secondary prevention in terms of preventing the onset or minimizing the effects of new pathologic change. In the health maintenance or the continuing care stage, the main focus is on secondary prevention with continued concern for both primary prevention of new pathologic changes and tertiary prevention in terms of continuing restorative and rehabilitative goals.

During the development of the models, it became clear that the demand on nurses to think using particular combinations of views of man varies with the stages of stroke. In Stages I and V there is a demand on the nurse to think primarily with the combination of person-agent-symbolizer-organism views and, in a more limited way, to think within the view of *object* (i.e., man) subject to physical forces. In Stage II, thought processes move within the organism-object combination and within the person-agent-symbolizer combination in relation to achieving goals of primary and secondary prevention.

Development of these models involved thinking in the person, agency, and action frames of reference (Nursing Development Conference Group, 1979). In the *person* frame of reference, a range of life styles and habits were seen as indicative of states not enabling deliberate action in the prestroke phase. The acute phase of stroke (in severe strokes) was seen as putting the person in a state that is completely nonenabling for deliberate action. In the convalescent and rehabilitation phases, the person was seen as being in a series of states that were partially and progressively more enabling for action. In the *agency* frame of reference, self-care agency is considered from the viewpoint of self-care agency limitations, which are expressed at (1) the level of self-care actions, (2) the more basic level of power components of self-care agency, or (3) the foundational level of human capabilities and dispositions basic to engagement in self-care.

It is grossly evident from the models that the operability and redevelopment of self-care agency can vary greatly in the stages of cerebrovascular accident. The type or degree of self-care deficit that can exist at each stage of stroke and because of the stroke is indicated. A self-care deficit as a nursing diagnosis means that self-care agency is inadequate to meet the therapeutic self-care demand in the *action* frame of reference; the therapeutic self-care demand expresses the self-care actions required to maintain and promote life and health at each stage. These discrete self-care actions would have to be organized within the more comprehensive self-care system.

As indicated, the organization of knowledge extracted from the literature around the nursing system variables is the result of an initial effort. If the paradigms are useful they can serve as guides for the further structuring and refinement of this area of knowledge. (These descriptive models are reproduced in the appendix at the end of this chapter.)

Nursing Systems and Nursing Roles

The structuring of knowledge around the nursing system variables according to the time profile for cerebrovascular accidents contributes to the identification of the ranges over which the patient variables can vary and over which the nurse variable should vary. The *relation* between the *two patient variables* during each of the stages of stroke was expressed in terms of *presence* and extent of *deficits* for engagement in self-care. A deficit relationship between self-care agency and therapeutic self-care demand is the condition that legitimates the exercise of nursing agency toward the formation of a nursing system. *Nursing agency*, when considered as a variable in a nursing system, is interactive with both patient variables of the technologic nursing system and the existent relation between them.

Two questions still needed answers. The first was: What would be the form and goals of nursing systems to be produced by nurses for individual members of populations designated by the stages of cerebrovascular accidents in models for Stages I through V? The second question was: Accepting the division of labor in nursing practice resultant from the availability of nurses with different kinds of preparation, what would constitute a rational distribution of nurse roles in nursing situations where persons in the five stages of stroke are under nursing care? The formulation and expression of answers to these questions were guided by Orem's categories of nursing systems (Orem, 1971) and Cleland's (1972) proposal for the categorization of nursing roles and levels of specialization.

> *General Nurse:* A nurse with less than baccalaureate level of preparation who is accountable for daily assignments that are often functional in nature, and whose range of tasks has a high level of predictability and may be done with accuracy and speed; works in structured settings for an eight-hour day.
>
> *Nurse Practitioner:* A nurse with baccalaureate level of preparation who is accountable for a caseload of clients during their hospital stay, or on a continuing basis in an ambulatory setting; who has a wide scope of practice and range of cues used in decision making; utilizes the nursing process in working with the client and family during the entire course of illness.

Nurse Specialist: A nurse who may have less than baccalaureate-level preparation and who has mastered particular diagnostic or therapeutic procedures in a specific area of practice; who has a restricted area of practice and range of cues utilized in decision making, although the nurse's knowledge base in this specialized area is more extensive than that of the general nurse.

Nurse Clinician: A nurse with master's degree level preparation who is a generalist but who may have an area of concentration. This nurse assumes an expanded role and utilizes a very broad range of cues in decision making. Although a nurse may concentrate on caring for a specific type of client, the involvement is very broad in scope. Independent prescription of nursing care, sophisticated use of the nursing process, and colleagueship with other health professionals are characteristic of this nurse's practice.

Based on the values of the patient variables and the relations between them for each stage of stroke, goals of nursing were formulated for each stage. These goals are expressed in terms of (1) a self-care system that is related to some preventive health care goal, (2) compensation for self-care deficits, (3) patient involvement in self-care, (4) overcoming self-care limitations and promotion of adequacy of self-care agency, and (5) maintaining or promoting the adequacy of self-care agency as related to the demand for self-care (therapeutic self-care demand). The nursing goals are expressed in relation to the type(s) of nursing system that would effect the desired interactiveness of the variables to achieve each expressed nursing goal. [*Ed. Note:* See NDCG 1973, pp. 268–271 for a complete description of the categorization of nursing roles.]

Given the values of nursing agency expressed in the six models derived from the analysis of therapeutic self-care demand and self-care limitations, and given the projections of nursing goals and nursing systems for each stage of stroke, projections about the types of nurses could be made. The projections suggest types of nurses who would have requisite powers of nursing agency for persons under nursing care during the five stages of stroke.

The patterns of knowledge and skill required for the roles associated with types of nurses need to be made more explicit in order to guide (1) the delivery of nursing to persons in various stages of stroke, and (2) educational program planning at all levels of nursing education.

Further analysis and research are needed to differentiate the elements of knowledge and skills (and also orientations of nurses) that would be indices of the adequacy of nursing agency in each of the five stages of stroke. For example, the nurse specialist would need to have depth of knowledge and skill in neurologic assessment and physical care requirements in the acute stage of stroke. The nurse clinician would need to have broad knowledge of these areas, and to have more depth in the knowledge and skills associated with crisis theory and intervention and the integration of a comprehensive, long-term focus in the nursing plan for the acute stage. In the convalescent stage, the general nurse would need a minimum level of knowledge to carry out a prescribed nursing care plan for this population and well-developed skills commonly required in the day-to-day care of this population. The nurse practitioner would have a broad preparation similar to that of the nurse clinician and be able to be more comprehensive in approach, but would have less depth of preparation.

SUMMARY

This construction and analysis of nursing system variables as related to the stages of cerebrovascular accident is offered as a beginning attempt to organize existing knowledge about a specific patient population within a nursing framework. It suggests goals of nursing and the design of nursing systems for individual patients and the design of delivery systems for providing nursing to groups of individuals who are at risk for or who have sustained a cerebrovascular accident. Further development and refinement of the models can lead to the identification of fruitful areas for research and hypothesis testing.

The review of the literature from a number of disciplines with respect to the entity cerebrovascular accidents and the organization of extracted items of knowledge around the nursing concepts from the NDCG theory of nursing system suggest that (1) these nursing concepts are good subsumers, and (2) specific pathology, in this instance a neurologic deficit with its sequence of events and results, does condition, at points in time, the values of the patient variables of therapeutic self-care demand and self-care agency.

The basic conditioning factor, cerebrovascular accident or stroke, is known to be associated with chronologic age and changes that occur with the aging process. The common expectation is that a health care or nursing population defined by the stages of stroke will be an adult population. The influence of the adult status of the individuals or groups under nursing care during the stages of stroke on technological and interpersonal nursing systems should be subjected to study.

APPENDIX: DESCRIPTIVE MODELS OF NURSING SYSTEM VARIABLES IN THE STAGES OF CEREBROVASCULAR ACCIDENT

Stage I: Being at Risk for Cerebrovascular Accidents or Having Premonitory Signs

Population
Individuals with high risk for cerebrovascular accidents or with premonitory signs; the community as a whole

Health Care Goals
Secondary Prevention
$\updownarrow$
Primary Prevention

Components of the Therapeutic Self-Care Demand
Seeking of regular health checkups

Acknowledgment of risk profile

Adaptations of life-style to reduce risk

Types of Self-Care Agency Limitations
Seeking of only episodic health care
Ignorance of risk factors and effective preventive measures
Denial of threat presented by the risk profile
Lack of motivation to change lifestyle

When the above named self-care agency limitations are existent, there will be a partial self-care deficit.

Components of Nursing Agency

Theoretical knowledge of
  Stroke risk factors and premonitory signs
  Normal parameters of variable reflecting risk of stroke (e.g., blood pressure, weight)

Patterns of behavior of individuals, small groups, communities
Teaching–learning theory
Theory and strategies of change

Skills for
Health assessment screening, case-finding, referral, and follow-up of high risk individuals
Assessment of population groups re: risk profile characteristics and community resources
Public relations
Community planning
Preparation and use of media or mass communication
Teaching and support of individuals and groups

Stage II: Acute Stage of Cerebrovascular Accident

A.   Unconscious phase (severe stroke)

Population
Individuals who have had a severe stroke recently

Health Care Goals
Tertiary Prevention
$\updownarrow$
Primary ↔ Secondary
Prevention   Prevention

Components of the Therapeutic Self-Care Demand
Modification of entire range of universal self-care requirements
Frequent monitoring of multiple physiologic variables
Administration and monitoring of effects of specific drugs (e.g., antihypertensives, anticoagulants)

Detection and management of life-threatening complications (e.g., shock, hyperthermal convulsions)

Types of Self-Care Agency Limitations
Lack of awareness of environment and inoperative mental processes
Inoperative protective reflexes

Immobility (with its range of hazards to the structural and functional integrity of the organism)

Self-care agency will not be operative in persons who have had severe strokes, and the deficit for engagement in self-care will be complete qualitatively and quantitatively.

Components of Nursing Agency

Theoretical knowledge of
  Pathophysiology of stroke
  Normal parameters and interrelationships of variables reflecting health
    state; deviations from the norm that require immediate referral and
    action
  Effects and consequences of immobility
  Causes and effects of unconscious state
  Rationale for and therapeutic and untoward effects of medical treatment
    modalities
  Crisis and crisis intervention theory

Skills for or in the nature of
  Techniques for meeting universal self-care requirements (to maintain
    circulation and oxygenation of tissues, nutrition and fluid balance,
    musculoskeletal integrity, skin and mucous membrane integrity, elimi-
    nation, a balance of rest and sensory social stimulation, and safety of
    environment) in unconscious individual
  Assessment of family's level of coping
  Crisis intervention techniques
  Assessment of neurologic status and other body systems reflecting
    health state
  Administration of special treatment modalities (e.g., hypothermia)
  Recognition of condition changes that indicate life-threatening emergen-
    cies and require immediate intervention or referral
  Designing, operationalizing, and managing complex wholly compensa-
    tory nursing systems through which the universal and health deviation
    self-care requirements within the therapeutic self-care demand are
    integrated and met through nurse action

B. Phase of Returning Consciousness (severe stroke)

Population   *Health Care Goals*
Individuals who recently sustained   As in Phase A
a stroke and who are not yet
medically stable but are regaining
consciousness

Components of the Therapeutic Self-Care Demand	Types of Self-Care Agency Limitations
Self-monitoring and universal self-care modifications still required as in Stage II A with reemergence of need to be normal	Mental confusion, memory gaps, and/or emotional lability (that will impair judgment and decision making)
Reorientation of self to persons, places, things in environment	Denial of paralysis; neglect of affected side
Cooperation with performance of measures of care associated with the therapeutic modalities	
Avoiding activities that may increase intracranial pressure	
Acknowledgment of changes in self	Some combination of sensory, perceptual, motor, and communication (language) impairments
Reestablishment of communication systems	
Beginning resumption of aspects of integrated human functioning requisite to self-care agency (e.g., decision-making)	

Extensive deficit for engagement in self-care due to the stroke; extent of self-care deficit varies with severity of the stroke

Components of Nursing Agency

Theoretical Knowledge
  All types required for Stage IIA plus
  Usual patterns of recovery from stroke and of return to conscious state
  Theory concerning human sensation, perception, cognition, memory, emotion, motivation, body- and self-image, experience of loss, and stages of the grieving process
  Major types of sensory, perceptual, cognitive, emotional, motor, and communication deficits that occur following stroke

Skills
  All types required for Stage IIA plus
  Assessment of signs of returning consciousness and types and severity of deficits for action

Reorientation and remotivation techniques

Assessment of signs of readiness to participate in self-care and/or contra-indications to increasing participation

Establishment of communication systems and supportive interpersonal environments

Stage III: Convalescent Stage of Cerebrovascular Accident

Population

Individuals who have survived acute stage and whose medically defined condition has stabilized

Health Care Goals

Tertiary Prevention

$\updownarrow$

Primary $\leftrightarrow$ Secondary
Prevention   Prevention

Components of the Therapeutic Self-Care Demand

Need to be normal requires increasing participation in activities of daily living to meet universal self-care requirements

Expending effort to pay attention to and to perform initial rehabilitative tasks

Coping with changes in self (body and self-image, dependency, role loss) with hope for functional improvement and acknowledgment of own role in this

Reestablishment of relationships with family or loved ones

Working for limited, short-term goals with tolerance for slow progress or set-backs

Learning to relate to affected side and use it in accomplishing self-care (if possible)

Development of realistic goals that have meaning for self

Types of Self-Care Agency Limitations

Residual neurological deficits become more clearly defined re: how they affect self-care agency. For example, hemianopsia (unaware of things in one-half of visual field); distortion of depth perception and of vertical-horizontal planes (balance problems, bumps into things, drops things); short attention span, persisting disorientation or memory gaps; continued denial of or development of depressive reaction to changes in self; paralysis, weakness, and/or spasticity of muscles on affected side; aphasia (receptive and/or expressive) or sysarthria

Extensive deficit for engagement in self-care due to the stroke; extent of the deficit varies with the severity of the stroke

Components of Nursing Agency

Theoretical Knowledge
  All types required for Stage IIB plus
  Phases of recovery and potential ranges of functional return from common neurologic deficits after stroke
  Functions and goals of the rehabilitative therapies (occupational, physical, and speech)
  Ways to compensate for or minimize effects of various neurologic deficits
  Teaching-learning of neurologically impaired
  Normal adult growth and development

Skills
  All types required for Stage IIB plus
  Ability to shift from predominantly "doer" to "observer-teacher" role
  Coordination of supportive-developmental or partly compensatory nursing system with rehabilitative therapies
  Assessment of developmental status and response to losses of function and roles
  Techniques to compensate for neurologic deficits and promote return of function
  Techniques for teaching neurologically impaired

Stage IV: Rehabilitation Stage of Cerebrovascular Accident

Population
Individuals whose action deficits are established and potential for restoration of function largely predictable

Health goals
As in Stage III

Components of the Therapeutic Self-Care Demand
Same as for Stage III but with increased focus on need to be

Types of Self-Care Agency Limitations
Number and severity of the limitations vary with each

normal and to resume usual activities of daily living and life roles (to extent possible) Learning how to monitor own health state and to incorporate rehabilitative and medical regimen requirements into self-care system

individual and with right- and left-sided cerebrovascular accidents Rate of recovery and decrease in number of limitations vary with each individual

Extent of the deficit for engagement in self-care due to the stroke varies for individuals

Components of Nursing Agency

Theoretical Knowledge
    All types required for Stage III plus
    More in-depth knowledge of rehabilitation modalities for various types of neurologic deficits
    Patterns of adaptation to long-term illness and disability

Skills
    Same as for Stage III plus
    More specific technical skill in implementing nursing rehabilitation modalities
    Adaptation of helping techniques to enhance self-care agency and other forms of agency
    Interpersonal style, which promotes healthful adaptation to long-term illness and disability
    Ability to set realistic shorter goals and work for limited results
    Ability to work with patient and family re: planning for future life style and adapting self-care system to residual neurologic deficits
    Ability to assume team member or colleague role on rehabilitation

Stage V: Health Maintenance, Continuing Care Stage of Cerebrovascular Accident

Population
Individuals whose functional abilities have been brought to an optimal level following a stroke

Health Care Goals
Tertiary Prevention
$\updownarrow$
Primary $\leftrightarrow$ Secondary
Prevention   Prevention

Components of the Therapeutic Self-Care Demand	Types of Self-Care Agency Limitations
Monitoring self for changes in health state, functional ability	Persistence of any combination of limitations identified in Stage III; each individual will have a unique quantitative and qualitative pattern of residual limitations
Continuing prescribed therapeutic regimen (e.g., exercise, medications)	Persistence of excessive dependency
Seeking regular, periodic professional health assessment and care	Resumption of life style associated with high risk for another stroke
Resuming system of daily living and of self-care with necessary adaptation	Pattern of seeking only episodic health assessment and care

Extent of deficit for engagement in self-care due to stroke varies for individuals

Components of Nursing Agency

Theoretical Knowledge
    Same as for Stage I plus
    Common post-cerebrovascular deficits and rehabilitative modalities
    Rationale and expected effects of continuing treatment regimen
    Family interaction

Skills
    Ability to monitor health status with use of history taking and physical examination and to detect signs of functional deterioration or impending recurrence of stroke
    Home, family, community assessment
    Use of community resources; making of referrals
    Health counseling techniques for individuals and small groups
    Basic family therapy techniques
    Ability to develop trusting, long-term, supportive relationship and to be client advocate

Ability to assume colleague role with other professionals involved in continuing care

Ability to monitor adaptations of self-care system for effectiveness and to help client readapt as necessary

CHAPTER 17

Nursing: A Dilemma for Higher Education

I t is an honor to be a participant in the Centennial Academic Convocation of Incarnate Word College. I have come to know the work and reputation of the college since the year 1959 when I had my first contacts with Sr. Charles Marie Frank, who was at the time the Dean of the School of Nursing, The Catholic University of America. As a faculty member and program director for educational administration in nursing, I was associated with graduates of Incarnate Word College: Sister Teresa Stanley, Hector Gonzalez, Marine Cadena, Carolyne Patino, and others. Later I served as consultant during various phases of the curriculum revision project. I also participated in the development of a self-test for public health nurses, a federally sponsored project of the college. During the period of my consultations, I became aware that the college was confronted with the same issues and questions as were other four-year colleges and the universities. In the District of Columbia and the Maryland areas, I saw colleges close and colleges survive and renew themselves. Factors, internal as well as external to these institutions, affected the making of the decision to close college doors or keep them open. Since the 1960s much has been written about the situation of higher education in our country, with special references to the colleges and universities. The internal situation of these institutions, as well as the import of the changed and changing social and political scenes, has been explored, described, and explained in the literature. Prescriptions for action have been offered, sometimes with hope and sometimes with considerable despair. For example, Stephen Mueller,

This paper was originally presented as part of the centennial celebrations of Incarnate Word College, San Antonio, Texas, 1982.

"Education or Higher Skilling" (1974), suggested ...tion for higher education: (1) reserve higher ...inority, (2) abandon education and concentrate ...ling, or (3) "attempt to restore the possibility of ...would allow large numbers to benefit from what ...ew" (p. 151). Mueller indicated that the first possibil- ...active and least likely, the second was the most likely, ...most attractive and the most difficult. Mueller's summa- ...backdrop for consideration of the question: What place do ...liberal arts colleges within universities have in education for ...ons and occupations? Is it within the domain and the general ...of these institutions to provide education for practice fields such ...ng? I use the term *education for practice fields* to differentiate it ...offerings with a pure training focus, where the concern is on-the-job training and task performance under relatively unchanging conditions and circumstances. I thus exclude from the societal purposes of senior colleges, in or outside of universities, the function of training for specific jobs. Liberal arts colleges traditionally have viewed education for certain professions as outside of their domain. However, some colleges have long-standing and highly respected programs of education in practice fields such as teacher education, nursing, medical technology, dietetics, home economics, and business administration. Furthermore, the liberal arts colleges have provided the liberalizing general education base for professional programs, whether conducted by the college or by a professional school. And some colleges have provided specific pre-professional programs, for example, pre-medicine. It should be noted that the professional education offerings of liberal arts colleges have been in those fields where entry to practice demands or is facilitated by the holding of the baccalaureate degree with a concentration in the disciplined knowledge that must be mastered prior to practice.

Before exploring the matter of nursing and the liberal arts colleges and as introductory to the exploration, I make the following assumptions about liberal arts colleges.

1. Curricula for programs within the college are education and not training oriented. When I say this, I am not minimizing the importance of training. Those in a practice field, including those who engage in research in the various sciences, must train themselves, and they must have experiences that permit them to train themselves

to develop and use the skills that are essential in the work of the discipline. This assumption is not anti-training, but it is an assumption that emphasizes the educational purpose of liberal arts colleges.

2. College faculties recognize the uniqueness of disciplines as well as the articulations among them.
3. Communication of faculty members across disciplines is recognized as a special and a growing problem in the colleges and universities.
4. Results achievable by persons enrolled in college programs vary with their cognitional structure and preferred modes of thinking and with their social readiness to participate in liberalizing education.
5. Colleges ideally provide developmental-type environments in which both faculty and enrolled students can mature as persons and as scholars.
6. College faculties act to preserve the integrity of their colleges as institutions of higher education.
7. Educational offerings of colleges are grounded in the needs of individuals of diverse backgrounds to prepare themselves and others intellectually for a mature life, including the process of imparting general knowledge and developing powers of reasoning and judgment. Skill acquisition is one part of such preparation.

In conclusion to this introduction, I submit that liberal arts colleges can participate in the provision of education for the practice fields without violating their nature. I recognize, at the same time, that the development and offering of programs such as nursing places colleges in situations where having or not having a program can be or can become equally unpleasant and unsatisfactory. The offering of nursing, as well as programs in other practice fields, at times does place the college in a dilemma.

I shall talk now about the practice disciplines and the special case of nursing. I begin with the case of nursing in the liberal arts college with a set of assumptions not infrequently held by and operational in some members of college and university faculty. I have personally experienced the verbalization of these assumptions so I am speaking from experience. An assumption that is sometimes made is that education for the professions is inferior to education in the humanities, sciences, and fine arts. Another assumption is that nursing is servile in nature and can never be a learned profession. Another is that there are no, nor can there be, practice disciplines or sciences of the practical. The holding of such assumptions may not preclude decisions to offer nursing, but it does preclude wholehearted acceptance of a nursing program and a nursing faculty within a college or a university.

Furthermore, while a nursing program may recruit students to a college, the academic, the legal, and the financial requirements may be initially an unpleasant shock and, eventually, an unwelcome burden when compared with traditional concentrations or with practice fields that are less complex than nursing. Lack of understanding both of the essential components of professional education and of nursing as a disciplined field of knowledge and practice, on the part of both faculties and administration in colleges and universities, has contributed to off-again, on-again attitudes and to the sometimes less than whole-hearted acceptance of nursing programs.

The movement to offer nursing education in universities and colleges, particularly colleges for women, took on momentum in the 1930s and '40s. This was the period when nursing, as well as other health services, moved from conditions of relative stability to almost constant change and increasing demands for services. Preparation for nursing in hospital schools continued during this period as it continues today. I was in nursing at this time and knew the three-plus-two programs (three years in a hospital school, two years in a liberal arts college), and the two-plus-three programs (two years in a liberal arts college, three years in a hospital school of nursing). Later, generic five- and four-year programs in nursing replaced the two-plus-three programs both in the colleges and in the universities.

As you well know, variations of the three-plus-two pattern continue today and sometimes I think I am back in the '30s.

Some nurse educators have taken and continue to take the position that only university schools of nursing should offer education for nursing preparatory for movement to professional-level practice. Sometimes, the specification is made that nursing be offered only in universities where there are large health or medical centers with schools of medicine, dentistry, and nursing, as well as hospitals and clinics, both general and special. The taking of these positions would limit the roles of liberal arts colleges to the offering of general education components for professional programs and to pre-professional education in science sequences that are basic to certain professional fields. It should be clear at this point that liberal arts colleges cannot be excluded from education for practice fields. It should also be clear that downgrading the quality of education in the humanities, arts, and sciences in these colleges will at the same time diminish the base for professional education.

However, there is one point to be noted, and that is that some professional schools require only a higher education base in the sciences that are basic to the field. For example, engineering schools may require only sciences and mathematics. A few years ago, I encountered this position in a nursing school in a Canadian university where part of the curriculum revision project was to move to get the liberal arts and humanities into the general education base for the nursing program.

The growing recognition among nurses of the need for a general liberalizing education base for nursing education and practice gave impetus to the movement of nursing education into the colleges and universities. This started, as I mentioned, in the '30s and '40s and is still continuing. The practicing nurse recognized and continues to recognize the contributions made by the humanities, sciences, and arts to development of the ability to nurse in constantly changing and complex situations. The increases in knowledge about human development, human relationships, and new and deepening understanding of rehabilitation of the disabled and the handicapped brought about an increased emphasis on the many human and interpersonal facets of nursing practice.

I think nurses should take heart from the fact that in nursing, among the various human services, there was early and effective work in introducing these aspects of practice into nursing curricula.

My own reflections in the 1950s on how I understood nursing were occasioned by the rehabilitation movement and the perceived inadequacies of nurses to participate effectively. It is to be recognized that nursing is an extremely complex field of practice, but at the same time we have lay people and persons advanced in other fields who consider themselves to be experts in nursing. Why is this so? I believe it is so because nursing touches on so many facets of human living. This makes it complex, but it also helps people from many diverse fields feel that they have something to contribute to nursing. I believe that we should take account of this in terms of gaining ideas and working with them, but not taking the position that nurses took a few years ago of deferring nursing decisions to persons in other fields.

Nursing is complex because of its focus on human beings as regulators of their own human functioning. This is something that we don't often think about. Through the care we give to ourselves each day, which I name *self-care*, we are regulating our own human functioning. We are also subject to deficits, to limitations for engaging in this care. These deficits may be associated with our own health state or with the nature of the health care requirements that we meet through our own actions.

Nursing is complex because understanding man as capable of voluntary or deliberate action demands knowledge of man as a mature, developing individual, as rational, as symbolizer, as organism, and as subject to social, biological, physical, and environmental forces. Because of the complexity of nursing and because of the inadequacies of the education of nurses over the years, disciplined verified nursing knowledge has been slow in development as well as in expression. Expression has been hindered by lack of a vocabulary. I had a telephone call from a graduate student at an eastern university last week. The student was taking a course in nursing theories and she asked whether I had time to answer some questions. One of her questions related to some of the circumstances or conditions that caused me to become involved in the expression of my concept of nursing and in its continued development. I said that during my years with the Indiana State Board of Health in the Hospital Division, in my contacts with and work with nurses, physicians, hospital administrators, and members of boards of trustees, I had come to the conclusion that nurses could not talk about nursing to hospital administrators, to physicians, to members of boards. They were able to nurse, but they were not able to communicate about nursing. And this young woman said to me, "I have had the same experience. I am in psychiatric nursing. I have learned to help patients by doing certain things, by taking certain approaches. Recently a physician said to me, 'This is good; tell me what you're doing.' I was unable to express my approach to care."

If we cannot convey to others what nursing is, I raise the question, how ready are we for nursing education? I think we are ready. Structured, verified nursing knowledge has not been readily available for educational purposes. Most of it was in nurses who could nurse effectively; however, they had not developed the capability to think and communicate about nursing in an explicit manner. The old rule that the arts are not very teachable still holds. It is only when knowledge antecedent to practice has been formulated, expressed, verified, and organized that there is a sound basis for education in the practice field. Nursing, as well as other practice fields, has suffered this lack.

As you know, for many years inside and outside of colleges and universities, nursing was, and to some extent still is, conceptualized and taught in terms of tasks that nurses perform, not in terms of the technologies that would bind series of tasks into operational systems. A movement to organize nursing courses around the constant human elements of nursing situations and the particular values of these elements is slowly developing.

Some nurses have accepted that nursing does have a proper object or focus. This proper object is implicit in what nurses do today and what they have done over the years. It's also implicit but not explicit in some of the currently used definitions of nursing. Virginia Henderson, still active in nursing, was the first to begin to make nursing's proper object explicit within her 1955 definition of nursing. Working independently in 1956, 1958, and 1959, I expressed the proper object of nursing as *human beings subject to self-care deficits due to their health states or health care requirements.* It has become very clear to me that the acceptance of this object or focus of nursing is necessary for the beginning development of organized and verified bodies of nursing knowledge.

Since the 1960s a concerted effort has been made by some nurses to structure nursing knowledge. The efforts of nurses at the Yale University School of Nursing and at the School of Nursing at The Catholic University of America are two instances of such efforts. It is to be noted that at Yale, the nursing faculty worked with the philosophers Dickoff and James. At The Catholic University of America, the nursing faculty were assisted by William O. Wallace, philosopher of science, and by Eamon P. O'Doherty, psychologist and philosopher.

The work I started in 1958, to lay out the domain and boundaries of nursing on the basis of why people needed and could be helped through nursing, was continued with colleagues at The Catholic University of America and still later with members of the Nursing Development Conference Group.

Today there are beginnings of disciplined bodies of nursing knowledge organized around elements of the self-care deficit theory of nursing. These are used and in some situations are under continuing development by nurses located in various parts of our own country, in Canada, in some European countries, and in Japan. The nursing courses at Incarnate Word College are organized around elements of these beginning bodies of nursing knowledge. The self-care deficit theory of nursing and the associated theories of self-care and nursing systems are expressive and explanatory of what nursing is and should be in a society. It has a tremendous value in giving focus and direction to nursing practice and nursing education.

All of us should recognize that the contribution that nurses can make in our society is necessarily limited. Nursing is one of many human services and is supported by society to meet only some needs of the people for human assistance. Nurses must know under what human and environmental conditions individuals can be helped through nursing rather than through some other human service. Nurses act to create, that is, to make, nursing. Nursing will never exist unless nurses make it. Unless nurses know the nature of what is to be made for others and from what it is to be made, there may be some task performance for individuals under health care, but there will not be nursing.

Nursing is not readily concretized. Nursing is made from this action and that action, deliberately selected and performed to achieve specific results for and with others. Sometimes both the nurse and the person under nursing care are active as agents in the process. The behavior both of nurses and those under care can be affected by external environmental factors, and the environment may play a major role in determining what is forthcoming if control of environmental factors is not something that nurses or those under care can accomplish. The degree to which nurses can think, speak, and make nursing for individuals and groups will determine the future of this human service. But nurses must be educated; nurses must have the freedom to practice nursing in health care settings; and nurses must have career pathways to advance themselves as nurses. There is much to be done. Collaboration among educational and service institutions is essential. We shall not speak to that issue today, but shall turn attention to the role of the liberal arts college in education for nursing and other practice disciplines with a view toward shaping the future.

The future of nursing depends in large part upon nurses deepening their understanding of nursing as a body of knowledge and a field of practice. The liberal arts college can contribute to this in a number of ways.

1. By continuing to offer and by enhancing the quality and relevance of courses in the humanities, arts, and sciences.
2. By offering courses and sequences of courses that treat the human and social foundations for the human functions of self-care and the interpersonal function of dependent care. Such courses would develop or build upon the themes of deliberate or voluntary human action, conceptualizations of self as self-care agent and dependent care agent, self-care as a regulatory function, and the classes of self-care requisites.
3. By developing sequences of courses that focus on the social and interpersonal aspects of helping and the ways of helping—doing for another, guiding and directing another, providing physical and psychological support, teaching, and providing a developmental-type environment. These ways of assisting are common to all the

service professions and occupations. In such courses, a focus would be maintained on the effects of the developmental states of individuals, on the selection of appropriate ways of helping, and on the roles and relations of persons in helping situations.

4. By offering courses in ethics with a concern for the final decision in all practical endeavors, the decision that answers the question "What should be done?" It is clear, as Bernard Lonergan (1958) specifies, that practical insight, reflection, and decision are truly legislative functions within individuals.

5. By developing and offering courses in the history and economics of human services with special concern for nursing as a human service.

6. By having course sequences in human physiology, psychology, and human development jointly culminate in an interdisciplinary course on adulthood. For an exposition of the need for such courses refer to "Preface to the Issue 'Adulthood,'" *Daedalus*, Spring, 1976, pp. v–viii.

7. By ensuring that existing programs in nursing and other practice fields leading to the baccalaureate degree provide experiences that are enabling students to acquire (1) a base in the humanities, the arts, and the requisite basic sciences; (2) knowledge in the sciences foundational to understanding nursing courses (some of the suggestions I made about courses that would focus on self-care, dependent care, and helping would be foundational courses); and (3) theoretical and practical knowledge of nursing through nursing courses in which the student would be helped to develop a dynamic concept of self as nurse engaged in the process of becoming professional.

The first six suggestions, if pursued, would contribute to the achievement of the usually accepted purposes of the liberal arts college and at the same time make available courses that are foundational to both nursing and other human services. The last suggestion relates to ensuring that offerings in the practice disciplines conform to the standards for professional education. The first six suggestions do not appear, at least to me, to be outside the range of economic feasibility. They should attract not only students from the health fields but from other concentrations. They may also attract adults into the college. Some of the courses suggested would provide opportunities for nursing faculties to contribute to courses that are open to all college students.

I have other thoughts about offerings that would help people today, especially people in the helping services. For example, over a period of time I have perceived a need for in-depth treatment of the virtues, with concern for prudence and justice in their significance for practice fields; treatment of the virtue of charity in human relationships; and faith and hope in illness and under conditions of stress. Last week, in reviewing some material that had been compiled some years ago by Joan Backscheider, I came across a quotation from a woman with whom Joan was talking. The woman, who had undergone a major surgical procedure, said, "I knew the Lord would be with me when I walked in the valley of sickness and death, but I certainly didn't know what the valley would look like." Here we have an example of the use of metaphor. We have belief; we have an expression of absence of empirical knowledge. What do such statements mean to nurses? Do they give clues or lead to insight into what an individual is going through? Within certain cultural groups and groups with particular religious orientations, the religious beliefs of a patient may play a major role in interpersonal situations with nurses. Nurses need to be helped to know when it is imprudent to introduce their own beliefs and when it may be helpful to do so.

Another area that is important, and an area to which the liberal arts college has a contribution to make, is the whole matter of spiritual development. It is important that college students, including nursing students, be helped to develop insights about spiritual development in a way that is compatible with what they are learning about human development and personal maturity. I think that sometimes what we do in courses in religion does not necessarily touch the matter of spiritual development.

I shall close my remarks with my expression of gratitude to the board of trustees, the faculty, and the administration of Incarnate Word College for this opportunity to participate in the celebration of the centennial of the college.

CHAPTER 18

A System of Concepts About Nursing: A Personal History

The objective of history is to establish how things come to be as they are. The thing of interest to us is the system of concepts that forms the structure of the self-care deficit theory of nursing. My purpose this morning is to talk about some of the events that occurred during the periods preceding and following the formulation and expression of the idea that led to the eventual formulation of the conceptual system. My perspective is personal. What I say is dependent upon recall and my interpretation of events and my attachment of meaning to them.

I have charted some of my experiences to serve as landmarks to which to attach events and the conditions and circumstances associated with them. During the years that I have been in nursing I have worked in three areas of endeavor. In Figure 18.1 these areas are designated by the numerals 1, 2, and 3.

Area 1: Nursing
Includes staff nursing, private duty nursing, nursing service administration and consultation research in nursing service administration
Area 2: Education
Teaching biological sciences, teaching nursing, nursing education administration, curriculum development, teaching the administration of programs of nursing education, teaching a

This paper was originally presented at the Summer Self-Care Institute, University of Missouri-Columbia, June 11, 1984.

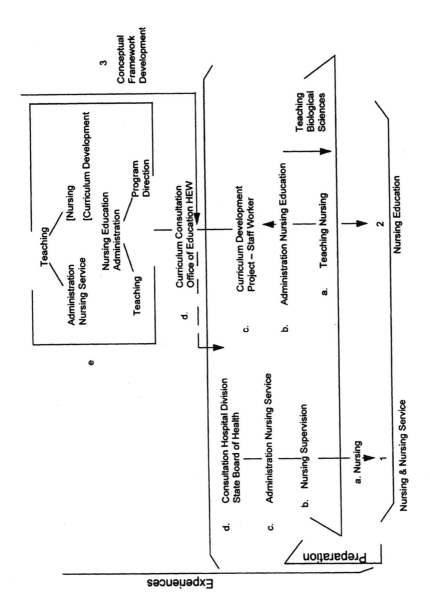

FIGURE 18.1   Three areas of endeavor in nursing.

153

seminar in nursing service administration, teaching curriculum development in associate degree nursing programs

Area 3: Conceptual framework development
         A base toward the development of nursing as structured nursing knowledge

The cited experiences within the three areas of endeavor are designated by letters. My approach is that of expressing events that I see as contributing to the formulation and expression of the self-care deficit theory of nursing. My remarks are organized in two areas: preparation for nursing and career experiences.

PREPARATION FOR NURSING

My initial preparation for nursing was in a three-year hospital associate program and continued in one of the early university programs with the achievement of the baccalaureate and master's degrees. I started university education soon after graduation and pursued it on both a full-time and part-time basis. My career endeavors in nursing, excepting staff nursing and private duty nursing, did not begin until after the completion of the baccalaureate degree and the beginning of work on the master's degree.

Certain experiences during the three-year hospital program were enabling for my developing a number of governing ideas, governing in the sense that they led me to think about things in particular ways and provided me with an empirical base for later theoretical understanding. These included the idea that nursing is distinct from but must be coordinated with medicine; the recognition that nursing was more than a series of tasks performed for patients, that nursing is for individuals who at particular times are in specific states and experiencing specific events; and a beginning base for understanding human organizations, including role specification, clarification of role relationships, cooperation, and coordination of actions.

In the period of university preparation I was involved in sorting out and distinguishing a number of areas. But it was not necessary for me to distinguish nursing from medicine, since in the three-year program I and other nurses in the program were able to distinguish nursing from medicine and to make right nursing judgments and decisions on a task basis. I knew that a nurse was responsible for his or her acts and that in the hospital setting nurses act to protect not only their patients and themselves as nurses but also the hospital that bears responsibility for the presence and the qualification of nurses as well as physicians. The chain of command for the nurse and nursing student was different from the chain of command of the physician but both chains ended in the hospital board of trustees. It is important, I believe, to note that I also developed understanding of the structure and functioning of a well-organized and effectively operated medical staff that regulated the privileges of the members and audited and judged their performance.

During my beginning period as a nursing student in the baccalaureate program, I was involved in distinguishing nursing from nursing education. The object and focus of the education of nurses were not adequately distinguished from the object and focus of nursing care for patients. Since nursing was introduced into hospitals and homes in our country in the nineteenth century through the presence and work of nursing students, these two lines of endeavor were not adequately distinguished.

Another relevant university experience was the writing of sets of beliefs about nursing. This effort was associated with Eugenia K. Spalding's courses in curriculum development in schools of nursing. These courses were heavy with subject matter on curriculum and light with nursing. Nursing was expected to come from enrolled students. The statements of beliefs focused on man, man's needs, and on the preventive focus of nursing as a form of health. One project carried out by a group of students resulted in a series of statements about nursing, a version of which later became known as Sister Olivia Gowan's definition of nursing.

In both the baccalaureate and the master's program, I carried a major in biology as well as in nursing. As a result I became aware of the structuring of knowledge into specific sciences within this broad science of biology. Also a kind of learning that had been started in high school was reinforced, namely that one learns a science through observation and experiment, not just by reading a textbook.

CAREER EXPERIENCES

An overview of career experiences is presented in Figure 18.2. I shall recount some experiences in Areas 1 and 2 before I move to Area 3 or the d and e of Area 2. In staff nursing and private duty nursing I became aware of what I knew and did not know and what I could do. Later, this knowledge was expressed in a statement that went something like this: Nurses know

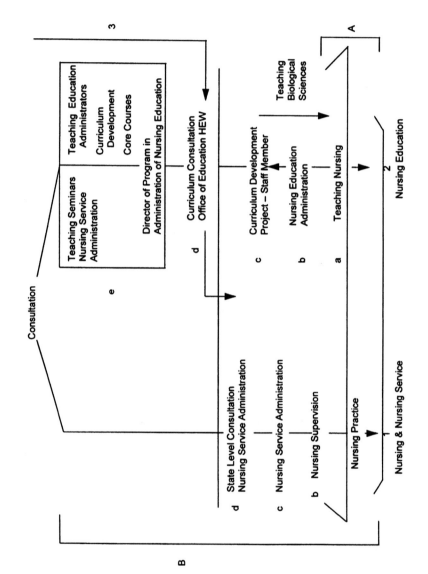

FIGURE 18.2 Experiences in education and administration.

a little about many things but do not have sufficient knowledge for action in a number of areas.

In nursing supervision I continued the development of my awareness of the functions of hospitals and the place of nursing in the hospital. I became aware of some of the financial operations of the hospitals and the relationships of physicians and hospital officers to external agencies including the health department, the coroner's office, and so on.

I want to concentrate a bit on the c and d of Area 1 and b of Area 2. I was both an assistant to a director of nursing service and a director of nursing service, the first in a 350-bed hospital, the second in a hospital of 600 beds. Both were dual positions with responsibilities for nursing education. In the second situation I was the director of both the school and the nursing service. These were some relevant learnings.

1. How to conduct a complex project and carry it through to completion
    a. beginning awareness of factors that contributed to the complexity of a field of endeavor
    b. the function of policies in the operation of complex organizations
2. The need to incorporate practices to meet the developmental needs of infants and children into both nursing service programs and into nursing education
3. The special requirements of some types of patients for nursing and the essential of meeting these requirements as individuals move from place to place
4. Beginning understanding of the satisfaction and productivity associated with working with colleagues
5. Respect for the boundaries of my own responsibility and the boundaries of areas of responsibility of others
6. Awareness that knowledge of the subject matter of curriculum development and curriculum revision did not provide the basis for answering questions that arose in the curriculum development process
7. Understanding of the necessity of individuals to have freedom to suggest, discuss, and plan and execute projects after deliberation and decision, but at all times with support and the provision of the resource required
8. The importance of forward movement rather than protection of the status quo

9.   The importance of and sometimes the essentiality of having knowledge about individuals before decisions are made about their placement for student learning experience or for work assignment
10. That the mode of thinking required for the administration of nursing service was different from the mode of thinking required for administration of nursing education. Each dealt with different realities and I, at least, could not mix them
11. The importance of working with a university school of nursing within the community toward the enhancement of nursing care and nursing education (Wayne State University). In both positions there was association with a university school of nursing—Wayne State University truly worked to advance nursing
12. Awareness of the injustice done to nursing students by not having nursing education in four-year colleges or universities

CURRICULUM DEVELOPMENT PROJECT (2. C.)

1.   Continued work with expressions of beliefs about nursing and expression of point of view about man of importance in the provision.
2.   Increase in knowledge about the professional form of education and the importance of the liberal arts, humanities, and science components.
3.   Seeing the development of a curriculum design to meet educative needs of RN students in a baccalaureate program.
4.   A first awareness of the level of intensity that professional jealousy and rivalry could reach. (I was a staff worker on the project) so it was not so much directed to me but to the project as a whole and the chairman of the project.
5.   Seeing decisions made to maintain the status quo with respect to curriculum design for RN students in baccalaureate programs.

Consultation, Hospital Division, State Board of Health

One general result of this six-year experience was a keen awareness of the state of nursing as a health service and some problem areas in this occupation and nursing profession that required resolution and solution, another result was my assessment as a scholar in the field of organization and administration. In these fields in the 1950s sources were limited but I had ready access to what was available. Someone remarked recently about the vast literature in the field of administration. This is a development. During this period, I searched for some means to put things together, an organizer, a set of good subsequent concepts. I found it in an expressed philosophical position about *types of wholes* and the four points of order posited for wholes composed of parts.

The ordering of the whole in its extrinsic end
The ordering of each part to do similar operations
The ordering of part of other parts
The order of this part to the functions of the whole

This led me to understand the human organization needed for large-scale and some small-scale endeavor, and aided me in understanding the "patient case function of hospitals" to which individuals in many professions and occupations contributed. It brought me to the use of a broad conceptual structure (four points of order in the whole composed of parts), handling detailed knowledge of the realities with which one dealt in nursing and in hospital functioning. I had an initial tool to aid in dealing with the realities of complex entities. I later was able to express the understanding that one had to have knowledge of the reality that one was dealing with in order to use intellectual tools of such broad dimensions.

To return to nursing, these are some of the conclusions I made about the state of nursing.

Background—Nurses Accepted Responsibility for All Ills in the Health Care Field

1. Nurses are able to provide nursing but they are not able to talk about nursing to patients, physicians, or hospital administrators. Nurses are not able to express in a precise manner results they expect patients to attain.
2. Physicians in rehabilitation reject nurses as essential for work in phases of rehab when patients must engage in their own care.
3. One must have some point of departure, some starting point, to engage in planning for nursing care.

4. Hospitals are large-scale enterprises but there is no large-scale design or planning for the productive operations of the hospital as a whole or for nursing.
5. Studies
   a. variation in the organizational structure of hospital nursing service by size of hospital
   b. variation in hospital population by size of institution
      1) number of admissions by admitting diagnosis
      2) number of admissions by physicians
      3) variation in length of stay by admitting diagnosis and admitting physicians; actions engaged in by nurses in administrative positions in a general hospital
6. There was evidence that some hospital administrators did not want their population to be studied.

And finally, a writing of a chapter on the characterizing features of hospital nursing service. This chapter, written in 1956, includes the following statement:

> Nursing is an art through which the nurse, the practitioner of nursing, gives specialized assistance to persons with disabilities of such a character that more than ordinary assistance is necessary to meet daily needs for self-care and to intelligently participate in the medical care they are receiving from the physician. The art of nursing is practiced by doing for the person with the disability, by "helping him to do for himself" and/or by "helping him to learn how to do for himself." (Orem, 1956)

Later, this was refined in the *Guides for Developing Curricula* (1959). Associated with the production of the Guides was a search of the literature that treated of the *practical arts* (or in Aristotle's terms, the servile arts). This involved me in the whole concept of *deliberate action* to which I had been introduced in philosophy.

Subsequent to this publication of the *Guides*, I was asked by McGraw-Hill to write a nursing textbook. As a result, I continued to work with the fundamental conceptual elements that had been expressed. This would continue from 1959 to the publication of the first edition of *Nursing: Concepts of Practice* in 1971.

LINES OF SCHOLARLY EDUCATION

I went to The Catholic University of America (CUA), 1959–1970. The focus of scholarly endeavor and the resources influencing my studies at this time are listed below.

a. The field of organization	C. Barnard, theory of strategic action (Barnard, 1962); T. Parsons, theory of the unit act (Parsons, 1951, 1964); Sorokin (1957)
b. Deliberate action	Barnard, Parsons
Prudence	Kotarbinski, *Praxiology* (1965)
c. Decision-making	Macmurray, *Persons in Relation* (1961), *The Self as Agent* (1957)
d. Practical arts	W. Wallace (CUA)
Practical sciences	J. Maritain (1959)
Philosophy of science	Eamon O'Doherty
	V. Ed Smith (Fordham)
e. Systems theory	Ashby writing on cybernetics (1964)

CURRICULUM

Nursing as a discipline is the organizer for the nursing content of professional and high-level technical programs.

1. Content in preservice nursing curriculum
2. Conclusions I arrived at
   a. One could not teach curriculum development in nursing to graduate students in clinical specialty areas in the absence of a conceptual framework for nursing.
   b. Curriculum organization is a product that results from the actions of the people involved.

SUMMARY AS RELATED TO THE SELF-CARE DEFICIT THEORY OF NURSING

1. As the result of an *insight*, I was able to conceptualize and express the reason people could be helped through nursing. We could label this, if properly expressed, as an empirical law. Expression of a statement about what nursing is—an empirical generalization.
2. The development of a theoretical conceptual structure
3. Conceptualizing the product of nursing as a nursing system
4. Development of *classification* as the conceptual elements were developed to the point of detail that conform to reality

CHAPTER 19

Self-Care Model of Standards for College Health Nursing

INTRODUCTION

College health nurses practically should address two questions: What are the objectively discernible requirements for nursing presented to college health nurses by changing populations of enrolled students? and How can such nursing requirements be accurately described? Given the introduction and use of a process that includes continuous data collection and analysis to yield accurate descriptions of why college students need and can benefit from nursing, there is another question to be addressed: Are these needs being met, and if so with what degree of effectiveness and efficiency?

In college health units, there should be standards to guide nurses in the description of students from a nursing perspective, and in the provision of nursing to individual students or to groups of students. Since college health nurses' duties may extend beyond nursing to include the operation and management of college health units, as well as other tasks, it is important to keep in mind that the subsequent section on standards addresses only standards for nursing.

STANDARDS FOR COLLEGE HEALTH NURSING

The word *standard,* in a somewhat loose sense, means a pattern or an exemplar, a design or a model that is worthy of imitation. For example,

This paper, here abridged, was originally presented at the annual meeting of the American College Health Association, joint luncheon of the Junior Community Colleges and Nursing Sections in New Orleans, May 30, 1986.

[*Ed. Note*: Portions of the original presentation that duplicated other papers appearing elsewhere in this book or in other publications have been deleted.]

if an institution of higher education has an effective system of operation of its academic departments or its service units, it may be held up as a model worthy of imitation. However, in the context of this paper, the term *standard* is used in its technical sense to mean rules, principles, or established levels of excellence, based on some authority, that are set up as a means for determining what a thing should be or whether something is correct.

When working toward the formulation and expression of standards, standards should be distinguished from criteria. The word *criterion* stresses employment as a test. When a rule or a principle is used for making a correct judgment about how something approaches a standard of perfection or in making a judgment about the exact characteristic of the thing, the rule or principle is identified as a *criterion*. Criteria are the measures used by a critic of something that is accomplished. Standards are for the guidance of those who are to make or do something.

In college health units nurses should recognize the need for standard setting to guide them in providing nursing that is needed by students as well as for development and use of criterion measures to determine if this kind of nursing is provided. The Horn and Swain (1977) report, *Development of Criterion Measures of Nursing Care*, is an excellent example of the development and use of criterion measures in a study designed to determine the quality of nursing care provided to segments of hospitalized populations. The self-care deficit theory of nursing and models derived from it served as the source of standards of what nurses should have accomplished with and for patients who were study subjects.

The general rules of nursing practice presented in the third edition of *Nursing: Concepts of Practice* (Orem, 1985, pp. 240–244) are examples of standards about what nurses should make or do in nursing practice situations. These general standards or rules of practice can be made specific to specialty areas of nursing practice, such as college health nursing. Rules are developed in five sets that relate to (1) nurses' initial contacts with patients, (2) continuing contacts, (3) the quality of interpersonal situations, (4) the production of nursing, and (5) relationships with nurses and other care providers.

Rule is used in the sense of a principle that governs the conduct of nurses in practice situations by specifying proper ways of thinking or acting. For example, rule 2. for initial period of contact specifies that nurses should "initiate contacts with potential or actual patients in accordance with social norms, with receptiveness, and in a manner that is adjusted to patients' overtly perceptible states of health and well-being" (Orem, 1985, p. 240). What nurses do in specific nursing practice situations in their initial contacts with patients varies with the personality of the nurses and with current and prior conditions and circumstances. The quoted rule specifies a minimum set of specifications for the quality of nurse behavior in nurses' initial periods of contact with patients. This general rule, as well as all other rules in the five sets, can be made specific to college health nursing situations.

Two examples of making general rules of nursing practice (Orem, 1985) specific to college health nursing are given. The first example is for rule 2 in Set Three: Quality of Interpersonal Situations with Patients. The rule specifies that nurses should "recognize patients' degrees of socialization to their roles in the health care situation" (Orem, 1985, p. 242). The college health nurse would act to identify and describe if the student

1. is socialized to the role of self-care agent
2. is personally able to be in contact with and interact with health care professionals
3. has the words to communicate his or her health state or health care and related concerns

The second example relates to rule 1 in Set Four: Production of Nursing, which in part specifies that nurses should "engage in nursing diagnosis initially and on a continuing basis to obtain and organize data and make and verify judgments about patients' self-care abilities and limitations and their self-management capabilities within their environmental situations" (Orem, 1985, p. 243).

Adherence to the quoted portion of this rule would require that college health nurses obtain from students information about

1. Care measures they use to meet their universal self-care requisites (Orem, 1985, pp. 90–95); for example, what they always do, usually do, what they neglect to do, or special adjustments they have made
2. Problems, interests, and concerns about meeting their universal self-care requisites; for example, what they think they should do but are not sure about or what they know they should do but don't know how to do or don't have the necessary resources to do

In relation to this example, college health nurses can assume that some college students will encounter minor to major difficulties in meeting some if not all of their universal self-care requisites. Those that may be most difficult to meet include

1. Maintaining a balance between activity and rest
2. Maintaining a balance between solitude and social interaction
3. Prevention of hazards including those specific to college life and to their age group
4. Being normal, including developing and maintaining a realistic self-concept, taking action to foster specific human development, taking action to maintain and protect their structural and functional integrity, and identifying and attending to deviations from structural and functional norms

The meeting of the four named universal self-care requisites is closely associated with the basic conditioning factors of pattern of living, educational system demands, social and physical environmental conditions of daily living, and the age and developmental states of students. Some students may have difficulties in meeting other universal requisites, for example, maintenance of an adequate intake of food.

It is readily seen from these few examples that nurses who develop standards for college health nursing should be guided both by their understanding of nursing and by their knowledge of the populations to be served through nursing.

Nursing science is in a primitive state of development. In the health professions there is need on the part of practitioners for knowledge of the natural order that characterizes humankind and of the disorders that occur. But there is also need for knowledge and skills that enable the recognition of order that does not presently exist but that to some degree can be brought about through deliberate human action. Because of the undeveloped state of nursing science, it is necessary in the formulation of standards for nurses to turn to general theories of nursing, their conceptual constructs, and their models of nursing practice as a basis for (1) identifying the areas for standard setting and (2) for organizing and giving structure to findings of nursing research and the verified and reliable practices of advanced nursing practitioners.

The development of the elements and relations of elements of the self-care deficit theory of nursing contributes to its value in the formulation and expression of standards for specialty areas of nursing practice. Because of the theory's orientation to care that contributes to the continued life, health, personal development, and well-being of individuals, it is particularly suited as a guide toward formalizing not only sets of standards for the practice of college health nursing but the bodies of knowledge specific to college health nursing.

COLLEGE HEALTH NURSING

College health nursing is a nursing practice specialty by reason of (1) its place of practice, (2) the persons nursed, (3) the characteristics of the nursing required and provided (the work done), and (4) the kinds of nursing systems produced by college health nurses for and with students (the product made). From a health care perspective, nursing required and provided to college students covers the range from primary prevention to rehabilitation. Such nursing requires appropriate mixes of all five methods of helping in the attainment of nursing results—doing for, supporting, guiding and directing, teaching, and providing a developmental environment (Orem, 1985). The college health nurse and the environmental conditions created and maintained by the nurse in the health unit should be recognized for value in helping or harming students who come for care.

Nursing systems produced by college health nurses are usually supportive-educative or partly compensatory systems. In some situations and usually for short time periods nursing may be in the form of a wholly compensatory system of care (Orem, 1985).

The process of standard setting can be engaged in by college health nurses on a project basis, covering a stipulated time duration and following a designated critical path with provision for critical review and updating. Or standard setting can be an ad hoc process engaged in when college health nurses recognize either the emergence of a standard in a situation of practice or conditions and circumstances that call for standard setting. Ideally, both processes are operational.

Before undertaking the use of a general theory of nursing to guide the development or the critical review of standards, it is important that developers or reviewers understand the theory in its wholeness and be aware of the stages of development of the conceptual elements of the theory. Use of a general theory demands that college health nurses be willing to engage in mastering its constructs and in the continuing development of these constructs in relation to individual college students and populations of college students. When this commitment to mastery and development is lacking there is a tendency for nurses to use the terms in that the theory is expressed without understanding the concepts that the terms express.

College health nurses have demands to move themselves as practitioners and scholars in their chosen field. If they are to formalize and advance the field of college health nursing they must become or advance as students of a particular theoretical approach to nursing. This is essential if the specialty of college health nursing is to be given form and substance.

CHAPTER 20

Some Remarks Relevant to Nursing Practice

THEORY DEVELOPMENT

The self-care deficit theory of nursing is a general theory that descriptively explains nursing as a human health service. It should be known to nurses as it is to others who write about theories that the expression of theory assumes prior objectification on the part of the theorist. Objectification involves persons in the contemplation of their own mental processes and in giving a concrete or objective existence to a thought or a conception. Objectification in this sense involves separation of a thought or a formulated concept of something from one's mental processes.

A GENERAL THEORY OF NURSING

What Is Nursing?

Between 1959 and 1973 I formalized several definitions of nursing. They reflect the refinement of my thinking about the answer to the question "What is nursing?"

This paper was originally presented at the Columbia Veteran's Administration Hospital in Columbia, MO, on April 9, 1986.

1959   "*Nursing is* . . . the giving of direct assistance to a person, as required, because of the person's specific inabilities in self-care resulting from a situation of personal health. Care . . . may be continuous or periodic. Self-care means the care which all persons require each day. It is the personal care which adults give to themselves, including attention to ordinary health requirements, and the following of the medical directions of their physicians. Nursing may be required by persons in any age group, but it is the situation of health and not the dependencies arising from age which initiates requirements for nursing" (Orem, 1959, pp. 5–6)

1968   "*Nursing is* assistance to persons in particular life situations in the achievement of health results or a more effective way of living through continuing daily self-care based upon scientifically derived knowledge of health and disease and known effective self-care practices into which are incorporated the medical orders of the person's physician. The adult person assisted is in whole or in part unable to act for himself in self-care without assistance because of his health state or health needs. The child who requires nursing is unable to provide self-care because he is a child and because his parents or guardians are not able to care for him effectively because of his health state or needs" (Orem, 1968b, p. 17).

1970a   "*Nursing is* contributed effort toward designing, providing, and managing systems of therapeutic self-care for individuals within their environments of daily living. Nursing's health dimension is derived from its self-care focus. Self-care, if it is . . . positively therapeutic helps to sustain life processes, maintains integrated functioning, promotes normal growth and development, and prevents or controls disease and disability and their effects" (Orem, 1971, p. 41).

1970b   "As an assisting art *nursing is* the complex ability to accomplish or to contribute to the accomplishment of the patient's usual and therapeutic self-care by compensating for or aiding the patient in overcoming the conditions or disabilities that cause him (1) to be unable to act for himself, (2) to refrain from acting for himself, or (3) to act ineffectively in caring for himself" (Orem, 1971 p. 47).

1973   *Nursing is* the activation of the components of nursing agency by a legitimate nurse to deliberately control or alter the state of a legitimate patient's therapeutic self-care demand or the patient's self-care agency (NDCG, 1973, p. 71).

The 1970b and 1973 Propositions

The 1970b and the 1973 propositions are summarized diagramatically in Figure 20.1. Both propositions bring in the nurse as well as the person under nursing care. The 1970b proposition refers to the person as nurse being an agent of action in a nursing role and the person as patient being an agent of action in a patient role. These conceptualizations are refined and simplified in the 1973 proposition. This movement could occur as the underlying structure of the variables of nursing agency, therapeutic self-care demand, and self-care agency was further developed.

NURSING AND THE DISCIPLINES OF KNOWLEDGE

From the beginning my efforts have been directed toward the organization of already identified nursing knowledge and to the discovery of knowledge. My work has been guided by a concept of *practical science* or *practice discipline*. This idea of practical science was subject for many years to ridicule both within and outside of nursing circles. With the current focus on action theory and decision theory acceptance of disciplines of knowledge for the practice fields has increased.

One must live with ridicule and rejection to make progress. My belief that nursing knowledge can be structured in the form of a practice discipline led me and my colleagues to work to develop ideas about the parts of the discipline. See Table 20.1.

My firm belief that baccalaureate education for nursing should be firmly grounded in nursing developed as a discipline of knowledge that is required for practice, including the method of development of the knowledge, led me in 1974 to formulate and express twelve component parts of what I referred to as an adequate "cognitional orientation to nursing" for example, nursing content in practical nurse curriculum. The need for identification of the object of nursing and the naming of the patient or client variables in a nursing system *are reiterated*. Without these two elements of knowledge one cannot move theoretically.

Note: Often nurses work with nursing theory at a less general level; their assumptions about what nursing is (should be in a society) are often

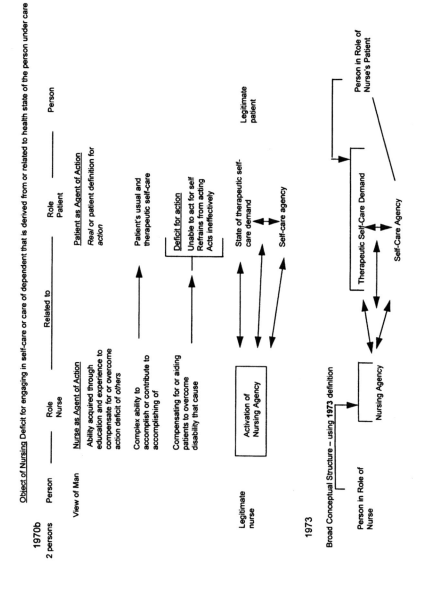

FIGURE 20.1 Relating 1970b and 1973 statements about nursing.

171

TABLE 20.1   Points of Departure for the Development of the Practice Discipline of Nursing

Starting Points	Form of the Knowledge
Formulation and expression of the object of nursing in order to (1) set limits for nursing and (2) establish an external and internal point of reference for nurses	A general concept (theory) of nursing
Formulation and expression of the general form that the practice discipline exhibits in the society	*General form*—System of action with social, interpersonal, and technological dimensions *Less general form*—A helping system *Specific form*—A nursing system
Recognition and acceptance that the practice discipline, nursing, will be comprised of (1) theoretical and (2) practical nursing knowledge	*Theoretical knowledge*—Nursing theories, hypotheses, laws, facts, problems *Practical knowledge*—Types and subtypes of nursing practice problems: technologies and rules of practice
Laying out of the specialty areas of the practice discipline of nursing	*Theoretical and practical knowledge* structured, i.e., organized by (1) types of nursing problems or (2) nursing cases or (3) situations of nursing practice

unexpressed and sometimes not formulated. Nurses in universities can do much to organize nursing. Each faculty member can work in an area of the discipline in a more secure and meaningful fashion. A general theory of nursing can help in organization.

THE SUBSTANTIVE STRUCTURE OF THE GENERAL THEORY: THE CONCEPTS UNDERLYING THE BROAD CONCEPTUAL ELEMENTS.

Analysis of the patient variables of therapeutic self-care demand and self-care analysis will reveal their substantive structure. The conceptual elements and the relationships among them together constitute a framework for understanding the patient or client variables of nursing systems (see Figure 20.2).

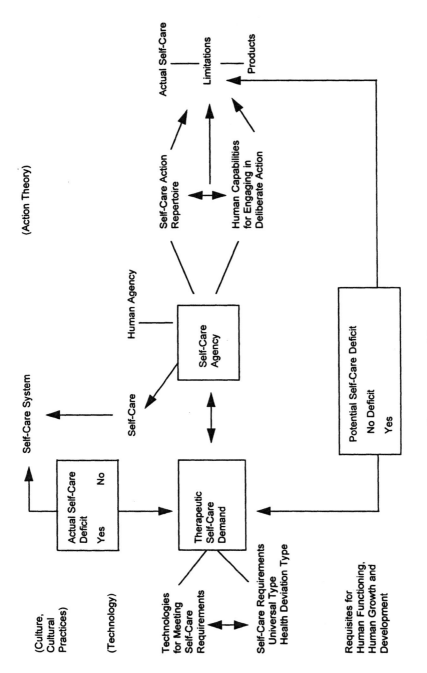

FIGURE 20.2   Substantive structure of patient variables.

173

The framework of concepts is comprised of the two concepts that express the *patient variables* and nine other concepts. The referents of these nine concepts are of importance in understanding the theory. These are the conceptual components of the theory that help us organize our knowledge, direct us in thinking nursing and guide us in attending to patients from the perspective of *nursing*. The concepts are arranged in four sets.

Set One: Self-Care and Self-Care System

Self-care is conceptualized as a product of the activation of self-care agency.

	Referents
Self-Care	Actions of individuals directed to self or environment to regulate factors or conditions in the interests of that individual's life, health, and well-being
Self-Care System	Self-care (actions) performed over time that are analyzed and arranged into coordinated systems of action
Dependent-Care System	A coordinated system of action performed over time to meet self-care requirements of a dependent person
Data descriptive of self-care	The data that is analyzed to arrive at the self-care system

Set Two: Self-Care Agency

Self-care agency is a specialized form of human agency.

	Referents
Self-Care Agency	1. Power inherent in human capabilities essential for deliberate action
	2. A self-care action repertoire
	3. Relationship between 1 and 2
Self-Care Limitation actual	Absences of an essential action or system of action from the repertoire

predicted	Absence or restriction of one of the human capabilities for engagement in deliberate action
positive/negative	The temporary or permanent or relatively permanent effect of the value of a capability on an individuals action repertoire

Set Three: Therapeutic Self-Care Demand

The therapeutic self-care demand represents the totality of action required to meet a set of self-care requirements using a set of technologies.

Self-care requirements	Formulated goals Orientations of self-care action systems Expression of input requirements for human functioning, for growth and development, for preventing, curing, or controlling disease processes.
Universal Type	Requirements that are general for all people, require adjustments to age, sex, developmental state and health state
Health Deviation Type	Requirements that have their origins in disease processes and their effects; or in medical technologies Requirements associated with developmental processes and states—pregnancy, menopause, and so on
Technologies for Meeting Requirements	Methodologies involving use of specific resources that are valid in meeting a requirement

Set Four: Self-Care Deficit

Actual self-care deficit	A descriptive statement of the relationship between the *therapeutic self-care demand* and the *self-care system* in which the actions specified by the therapeutic self-care de-

	mand are present or absent from the self-care system
Potential self-care deficit	A descriptive statement of the relationship between the therapeutic self-care demand and predicted self-care limitations

Nursing Agency

Nursing agency is the name for the human power and action repertoire associated with nursing practice. It is differentiated from the agency that marks the nursing scholar, nursing developer and nursing researcher, nursing theorist and teacher of nursing. Confusion of roles and failure to provide for the development of the skills specific to the practice field is a common omission in nursing as well as in other disciplines.

Exercise of nursing agency includes

1. Establishing the legitimacy of the relationship
2. Initial operationalization and maintaining an interpersonal system with client and with significant others
3. Diagnosis related to the two patient variables
4. Role definition as related to the assessment of self-care
5. Role definition as related to regulating the value of or exercise of self-care agency
6. Helping actions with focus on assessment of self-care
7. Helping actions with respect to *protection, enhancement* or exercise of self-care agency

Nursing System

The nursing system is the product of nursing. It is something *created.* (See Figure 20.3.) Within the nursing system there are levels of explanatory schemes related to human beings and their functioning. Professionals in the human services find themselves "at two or more levels in the hierarchy of explanatory schemes" and their acts reflect the belief that to act as if "human individuals have more value than their constituent elements . . . and this attitude, superficially at least, is not readily derivable from a reductionist philosophy" (source unknown).

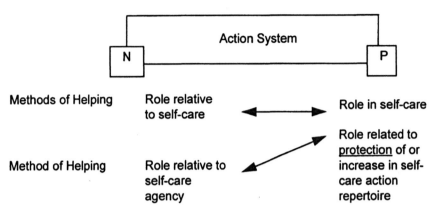

FIGURE 20.3 The nursing system.

CHAPTER 21

Nurses and Nursing Knowledge

I n communities throughout the world, nursing is supported as an institutionalized human service, including provisions for the education and training of nurses. The strength of nursing in any social group is dependent upon what nurses do to keep nursing viable and healthy as a human service and at the same time advance the frontiers of nursing knowledge. As the twentieth century draws to a close, nursing is recognized as an essential health service. It is recognized also as a knowledge-intensive service. In the 1980s, however, nursing practitioners, educators, and nursing students continue to be adversely affected by the failures of nurses during the period of modern nursing to lay out the domain and boundaries of nursing and to formalize and validate the bodies of nursing knowledge that would constitute the practical and the applied nursing sciences.

Nurses represent themselves in society as being able to help others through nursing. To do this, nurses must be able to think nursing, to communicate about nursing, to determine when and how individuals can be helped through nursing, and to design and produce nursing for individuals and groups. The unorganized state of nursing knowledge continues to be a deterrent to nursing students' development of the named capabilities. What happens to nursing in the twenty-first century is viewed as dependent on what nurses do (1) to give form and structure to nursing knowledge that is already developed and validated but scattered and unorganized and, therefore, not readily accessible, and (2) to advance the development of nursing as a field of knowledge.

This paper was originally presented at the Eighth Annual Meeting of the Spanish Association for Nursing Education, December, 1987.

In relation to the foregoing, two questions will be addressed. These are:

1. What is needed to keep nursing viable in a society?
2. How can and how do nurses proceed to develop and give form and structure to nursing as a field of knowledge, a practice discipline?

Keeping nursing viable in societies is addressed from the perspective of essential roles of nurses in social groups. The development of nursing as a field of knowledge is described in relation to the kinds of insights that accompany five stages of understanding nursing. Finally, there is an exposition of the essential concepts and central ideas of one general theory of nursing, self-care deficit theory.

KEEPING NURSING VIABLE IN A SOCIETY

Ideally, nurses direct their attention and effort to human problems that can be solved or mitigated through nursing. To do this nurses must know the following in a dynamic way:

1. What conditions and factors in persons or their environments give rise to requirements for nursing
2. What nursing meaning can be attached to these conditions and factors
3. How types of human and environmental conditions and factors affect the characteristics of, the design for, and the production of nursing for individuals and groups

Answers to these questions constitute generalizable nursing knowledge that nurses should have and should be able to use in all or some situations of practice. Nurses use this knowledge to give direction to their observations and care endeavors, to acquire empirical knowledge about concrete situations of nursing practice, to attach nursing meaning to acquired information, and to provide direction in their judgment and decision-making activities and in designing and providing nursing care.

Nursing knowledge, whatever its form and structure at specific times, is necessary not only for the work of nursing practitioners but also for nurses' fulfillment of other functional responsibilities through which nursing is maintained as an effective health service in society. The common view of what is needed to maintain nursing as an available, effective human service is the presence in communities of what this or that group perceives as an adequate number of nurses—nurses who are qualified through one or more prescribed and sanctioned forms of education and training to engage in providing nursing. Nursing leaders in the closing years of the twentieth century have more expanded and comprehensive views of what is needed to keep nursing not only viable but also effective as a human health service.

The following roles of nurses with their associated responsibilities are now recognized.

1. Nursing practitioner
2. Nursing scholar
3. Nursing theorist
4. Nursing researcher
5. Developer of nursing technologies and techniques
6. Teacher of nursing

Nurses who effectively perform in these roles contribute to the development and validation of nursing knowledge, knowledge that is necessary for nurses' use in identifying, resolving, and solving nursing practice problems and in providing nursing for populations.

The need for nurses who can function effectively in the six named roles or combinations of them must be confronted not only by the nursing community but also by the larger society. Where and how to help interested, talented, and able men and women prepare to take on and fulfill these roles are problems to which solutions need to be sought at both national and sponsoring institutional levels.

In addition to the six enumerated roles essential for keeping nursing viable in society, there are the roles of (1) nursing administrator and (2) nursing educational administrator. These two roles and their associated functional responsibilities arise not from nursing as a discipline of knowledge and practice but from organized health services and from educational institutions or agencies; the positions arise from the agencies they serve. Nursing service administrators and nursing educational administrators must know *nursing* as a discipline of knowledge and be able to use this knowledge in the fulfillment of their role functions, related respectively to ensuring the provision of nursing to populations served by the health care institution and to ensuring the provision of appropriate and valid education within university settings for nursing students who seek to fulfill particular nursing roles.

Nursing service administrators must know nursing in a dynamic way in order to ensure (1) the continuing availability and production of nursing for the population(s) served by the health service enterprise, (2) that nursing contributes to the fulfillment of the purpose or mission of the health service enterprise, and (3) that what is needed to produce nursing is provided and what is adversely affecting the continuing availability and provision of nursing is corrected. *Nursing educational administrators* must (1) be knowing about domain and boundaries of nursing as a field of knowledge, (2) understand the structure of nursing knowledge and its articulations with other fields of knowledge, (3) understand the forms of education for the occupations and professions, and (4) be able to select and organize nursing-related knowledge in a manner that is valid for specific forms of education for the occupations and professions. The nursing educational administrator understands the six roles essential for keeping nursing viable in society and ensures that educational program purposes and designs reflect preparation for fulfillment of a role or some combination of roles, for example, that of nursing practitioner and nursing scholar, or nursing scholar and nursing researcher.

Concerted effort is necessary on the part of the nursing community to provide for the recognition and acceptance of the need for nurses to function not only as practitioners but also as scholars, theorists, researchers, developers, and teachers of nursing.

Nurses are and have been in advantageous positions to contribute to constructive developments in international, national, and community-based health services. Nurses have advanced understanding of some health care problems. At times they have been in the forefront of the health professions in using new knowledge from other fields in their own practice. Two examples of this are nurses' use of emerging knowledge from the field of child growth and development in the nursing of children in the 1940s and the scholarly work on the interpersonal dimension of nursing in the 1950s and 1960s. If the work of nurses is to continue to develop and advance nursing as a human health service, the interests and talents of nurses must be directed to help them understand how each can contribute to the development, validation, and dissemination of nursing knowledge within the nursing community.

STAGES OF UNDERSTANDING NURSING

Nursing knowledge has its foundations in the concrete world of nurses and in the way that nurses deal with their world as they function in relation to the men, women, and children for whom they provide care. A first step in understanding nursing is to ask and answer the question: What condition exists when valid judgments can be made that individuals are in need of and can be helped through nursing? Investigation of this question leads nurses to conceptualize and express the *proper object* or focus of nursing. Proper object is used in the philosophic and scientific sense as that which is studied or observed, that to which action is directed to obtain information or to bring about some new conditions. Nurses often provide care for the same men, women, and children who are being cared for by physicians or other health workers. Nursing is a different form of care because the proper object of nursing differs from that of medicine or other health service (Orem, 1985a).

The ideal beginning for knowing nursing as field of knowledge and practice is to be introduced to and to develop understanding of when and why people need and can be helped through nursing. Once nursing students or nurses have such understanding they are in a position to identify and understand the features of practice situations and the relations among them. They know that nurses and patients are the human parts of nursing situations but they also know the conditions of patients that render them in need of nursing care and therefore why they become objects of nurses' attention and interest.

Two definitions of nursing that appeared in nursing publications in the United States in the 1950s explicitly express the proper object of nursing (Henderson, 1955; Orem, 1956, 1959). Both of these expressions represent that men and women ordinarily care for themselves on a daily basis to maintain life, health, and well-being, but that they can experience limitations in so doing. These limitations are associated with what individuals know how to do to care for themselves but are unable to do at particular times and with what they need to do but don't know how to do or don't want to do.

Human beings need nursing because of health-derived or health-associated limitations for engagement in required self-care. Self-care is understood as the performance by individuals of measures to regulate internal and external conditions and factors on a day-to-day basis in the interests of life, health, and well-being. In child nursing situations, it is the parents or guardians who are not able to provide the day-to-day care needed by a child because of the child's health state or health care requirements.

The conceptualization, expression, and acceptance of the proper object of nursing is an essential step for nurses in understanding nursing and in movement toward its formalization as a discipline of knowledge. The development of any science, including the practical sciences or practice disciplines, occurs in stages. A stage is understood in terms of the development of understanding about specific things. Stages are identified in relation to the kinds of data and the images involved in the development of insights, and not in terms of the times of the occurrence of particular insights.

Five stages of development of nursing are identified and expressed on the basis of experience and in relation to nursing as a practice field. They are as follows.

I   The *stage of identifying and conceptualizing* the features of patients and nurses that are invariant in nursing practice situations, naming these features, and expressing relations among them. This stage is finalized with (1) the conceptualization of nursing as an interactive interpersonal process and (2) the conceptualization of the product of nursing, namely, systems of nursing care. The results of this stage are expressed as concepts, models, and theories and may be in process at the same time in individual nurses once a reasonable degree of understanding has been achieved in Stage I.

II   The *stage of identifying and arranging* the ranges of values of the nurse/patient variables of the nursing situation. The nature and substantive structure of the conceptual elements is explored. During this stage research leads to emergence of less comprehensive theories.

III The *stage of investigation and description of concrete situations* including identifying, naming, and exploring patient variables and human and environmental factors that can condition those variables. In this stage it becomes possible to develop models and classifications of nursing cases.

IV   The *stage of developing models and general principles of nursing practice* through in-depth studying of descriptions of nursing cases and the relationships of associated variables. Practice models, rules of practice and nursing prescriptions are outcomes of this stage.

V   The *stage of formulating and validating models and rules* for the provision of nursing for populations. The work of this stage is accomplished through the identification and description of nursing cases by common features of patient variables. This stage could contribute to the development of the applied sciences of nursing economics and nursing administration.

THE SELF-CARE DEFICIT THEORY OF NURSING

Nursing, when considered either theoretically or in concrete form, is a *whole thing*, understood from its principles, concepts, and concrete conditions and action. The interest of nurses in conceptual models and theories of nursing is of importance in bringing about advances in nursing knowledge. General theories of nursing focus on the whole of nursing, including the essential human elements of nursing practice situations and the relations among the elements. Self-care deficit or self-care nursing theory is one general theory of nursing that expresses the universal principles of nursing in the form of concepts and theories. Such principles are not obvious or self-evident. They go beyond common sense and result from the insights of individuals following investigation, analyses, and syntheses. Theorists, practitioners, scholars, and researchers use this theory and contribute to its continuing development.

The self-care deficit theory of nursing provides nurses with a way of knowing, thinking, designing, and producing nursing for others and with a way of communicating about nursing. It provides teachers and educators with a nucleus of theoretical nursing knowledge that is enabling for the development of nursing-based educational programs that are designed to help nursing students to attain initial and higher-level understandings of nursing. Nurses and nursing students who become scholars of self-care nursing theory move themselves through a stage of static mastery of the concepts of the theory to a stage of dynamic knowing when they understand the theory as descriptively explanatory of the human features, the events, and the conditions and factors that are operational in concrete situations of nursing practice. This is the stage of nurses' acceptance and ownership of the theory.

THREE THEORIES

The conceptual structure of self-care deficit nursing theory is developed in relation to the two human elements of nursing situations: the nurse and the nurse's patient. The conditions and factors that legitimize individuals as nurses and nurses' patients are conceptualized and expressed as nurse and patient variables. Both nurses and patients are viewed as agents of action and as having role responsibilities within nursing situations. Nurses are characterized as having the capability to nurse others. This capability is named *nursing agency*. Patients are characterized as having (1) demands on them for action to regulate their own functioning through day-to-day personalized care and (2) developed capabilities to provide this care or a potential for development of such capabilities. Developed self-care capabilities may or may not be operational or adequate at specific times. The presence of health-derived or health-related inabilities of individuals to take action to know and meet current or projected demands for personalized care to regulate their own human functioning (self-care) results in a deficit relationship between their care demand and their capabilities to engage in care. This type of deficit relationship between the care needed (therapeutic self-care demand) and individuals' care capabilities (self-care agency) is named *self-care deficit*.

The presence of a health-derived or health-associated self-care deficit indicates a need for nursing. The theory of self-care and the theory of self-care deficit are constituent parts of the self-care deficit theory of nursing. The *central* ideas of these two patient oriented parts of the theory are expressed in the following statements.

Theory of Self-Care

The central idea of this theory explains self-care as a human regulatory function. Maturing or mature persons contribute to the regulation of their own functioning and development and to the prevention, control, or amelioration of disease and injury and their effects by performing, within the context of their day-to-day living, learned actions directed to themselves or their environments that are known or assumed to have regulatory value with respect to human functioning and development. Self-care as a human regulatory function is understood as analogous to neuroendocrine regulatory processes [Ed. Note: For further discussion of topic see Orem, 2001, p. 45 and p. 132]. Self-care also is understood as behavior, conduct, or deliberate action learned within the context of individuals' membership and interactions in social groups.

Theory of Self-Care Deficit

The central idea of this theory expresses when and why people need and can benefit from nursing. The self-care agency of mature or maturing individuals in its relation to their knowing and meeting their therapeutic self-care demands can be adversely affected by health-associated conditions and factors internal or external to such individuals that render their self-care agency wholly or partially nonoperational or qualitatively or quantitatively inadequate for knowing and meeting their therapeutic self-care demands and thus giving rise to legitimate requirements for nursing. The theory of self-care deficit expresses a relation between the two patient variables of *therapeutic self-care demand* and *self-care agency*. The presence of a deficit relationship between the self-care needed by patients and their self-care capabilities legitimizes a nurse–patient relationship.

Theory of Nursing System

This theory brings the nurse variable *nursing agency* into relationship with the two patient variables of self-care agency and therapeutic self-care demand. The theory is technologically oriented to the proper work of nurses that takes place within a framework of the interpersonal and larger social features of nurses' work.

All action systems that are *nursing systems* are produced by nurses through the exercise of their nursing agency within the context of their contractual and interpersonal relations with individuals who are characterized by health-associated self-care deficits for purposes of ensuring that their therapeutic self-care demands are known and met and their self-care agency is protected or its exercise or development is regulated. Nurses make nursing systems as they perform the process operations of nursing practice, namely, nursing diagnosis, nursing prescription, and nursing regulation. The self-care deficit theory of nursing gives focus and structure for these operations (see Orem, 1985, pp. 29–39).

A CONCEPTUAL MODEL

The essential elements of nursing expressed in the central idea of the three theoretical components of self-care deficit nursing theory form a circle of terms and relationships, a word model of nursing (see Figure 14.2). The patient variables of therapeutic self-care demand and self-care agency stand in relation one to the other. Values of self-care agency that are not equal to persons' meeting their therapeutic self-care demands bring about a deficit relationship between the two variables.

Nurses exercise their nursing agency to determine the values of the two patient variables and the relations between them. Nurses exercise their nursing agency to ensure that patients' therapeutic self-care demands are met and that the exercise of development of their self-care agency is regulated.

The values of the two patient variables and the nurse variable are affected by a number of conditions and factors external or internal to the person elements of nursing situations. The conditions and factors are collectively referred to as basic conditioning factors. These include physical environmental conditions, age, sex, developmental state, health state, family system factors, health care system factors, socioeconomic factors, culture orientations, and resources.

Nurses produce nursing care through investigative and estimative operations to determine for individuals what self-care is being produced; what self-care is required; and what patients are doing, not doing, or are not able to do with respect to knowing and meeting their requisites for functional regulation (self-care requisites) through the effective performance of care measures. Nurses also produce nursing care when they make judgments and decisions about and help patients understand (1) the care that they use and (2) how this care can be provided under existent conditions and circumstances. Finally, nurses produce nursing care when they assist individual patients or members of patients' families to know and meet the patients' day-to-day care demands and to regulate the exercise or development of patients' capabilities to meet their own care demands. Production of care by nurses for patients may be in the form of wholly or partly compensating care systems or they may be supportive-educative systems (Orem, 1985, pp. 222–240).

THE FUTURE OF NURSING

The position expressed in this paper is that the future of nursing as a profession and occupation, in countries throughout the world, is largely dependent upon what nurses do to advance the development of nursing as a discipline of knowledge with recognition of the proper object of nursing. Failure to do so will perpetuate the time-honored position that nursing is the performance of prescribed repetitive tasks, such as bathing or feeding, or structured care systems, such as postoperative care.

Nurses whose nursing knowledge is structured primarily in the form of tasks or care systems increase their knowledge by accretion through learning to perform new tasks. This is not an economical, intellectually stimulating, or satisfying approach for nurses to advance themselves in nursing. Nor is it productive of valid nursing results.

Nurses should know concrete nursing practice situations from a nursing perspective. Even a health service perspective is not adequate for the achievement of nursing results. It is essential that nurses know why and when people need and can be helped through nursing. A valid general theory of nursing can be used by nurses to give form and content to nursing as a discipline of knowledge, including both theoretically and clinically oriented knowledge. A valid generalizable theory not only provides bases for structuring nursing information, it also provides questions for investigation by scholars and researchers.

Instructional staffs, faculties of nursing, and nursing educational administrators require understanding of the kinds of insights about nursing that students preparing for specific roles must develop for purposes of effectiveness in role fulfillment. They must be able to structure and sequence nursing courses in accord with valid and available nursing knowledge. The mastery and continued development of an expressed and valid general theory of nursing is essential in doing this.

Recognition of and efforts to assist nurses and nursing students to fill the roles identified as necessary to keep nursing viable in society is important. Of equal importance is understanding that nursing is a practice field and that both theoretically practical and clinically practical knowledge must be structured and validated.

CHAPTER 22

Development and Dissemination of a General Theory of Nursing: The Past, Present, and Future

The focus of this conference is a specific general theory of nursing known as self-care deficit or self-care nursing theory. Theories attach meaning to nursing and express what theorists have objectified about their own thought processes and their developed insight about nursing. Some of you may be scholars of the self-care deficit theory of nursing as well as nursing practitioners or researchers who understand nursing according to the principles, models, and rules of this general theory of nursing. On the other hand, you may have in-depth knowledge of another theory of nursing and be interested in learning about the tenets held by nurses' awareness of the need to formalize and validate nursing knowledge, that is, to develop nursing as a discipline of knowledge central to the performances of *nurse* roles in social groups.

There is a growing industry centered around the work of nursing theorists. It includes the production of books about what theorists write, the holding of conferences, lecture series, and the making of audio and video tapes. The results of such undertakings from a professional perspective are measured in terms of cognitive and affective changes in nursing that will lead theorists to contribute to the advancement of nursing as a science, or, if you prefer, a discipline of knowledge.

This chapter consists of notes preparatory to a presentation at a self-care conference in the fall of 1987.

One task of each nurse who aspires to master, work with, and contribute to the continued development of a general theory of nursing is to consider how nursing is a science or a discipline of knowledge. For too long there have been unsubstantiated pronouncements by nurses that nursing is both a science and an art, as well as pronouncements that nursing is not and can never be a science. Regardless of which position is taken there are things about which some if not all nurses do agree.

1. Nursing is a knowledge-intensive field of practice.
2. Nursing knowledge is grounded in the nature and characteristics of human beings and their activities.
3. Nursing practice involves nurses (a) in determining *what is* in singular nursing situations, (b) in determining *what can* and *what should be brought about* in light of existent conditions, (c) with *construction of a design* and a *plan* for producing results sought, and (d) with *action to produce* the results sought in singular situations of nursing practice.

Furthermore, nurses understand that nursing theories are not concerned with the singular nursing practice situation as such. Theories are about what is common to all situations of nursing practice or to subsets of situations. It is necessary to recognize and accept that nurses may resist the abstract thinking demanded by movement to the mastery and use of theoretical formulations about nursing. Nursing students today should be helped to think nursing, to communicate nursing to others, as well as to effectively perform the operations of nursing practice. They should be helped to understand and explain to others why nursing as a discipline of knowledge is a *practical science* and a *set of applied sciences*.

In summary to this introduction two questions are suggested for investigation or reflection.

1. Can nurses develop nursing as a discipline of knowledge through common sense approaches?
2. Can a general theory of nursing contribute to the development of nursing as a discipline of knowledge? If so, how?

THE PROCESS OF DEVELOPMENT OF A THEORY

Nursing as an institutionalized component of the culture of human societies is understood by individuals from a commonsense or from a theoretical viewpoint. This conference aspires to the taking of a theoretical approach. The goal of this presentation is to bring together the events and changes that originated the self-care deficit theory of nursing and its dissemination within the profession. The approach is not properly historical because it is a bringing together of personal experiences and changes. The "data of history lie in the experiences of many" (Lonergan, 1972, p. 179). Historians, however, are concerned with what is going forward in particular places and times. If there is repetition of routines, as with the present focus on the writings of nursing theorists, the historian wants to know what started the routine. My focus is on one theory and on the events and changes directly associated with its formulation, expression, and development extending from the 1950s to the present.

During the years from 1950 to 1959, my experiences with nurses and nursing were extensive and intensive. From 1949 to 1957, I was in a position that enabled me to look at nursing service organizations and nursing practice situations objectively in the sense that I was not personally involved in their conduct as practitioner, administrator, or clinical teacher of nursing students. I came to appreciate and to understand more clearly the demands on nurses and the conditions under which they worked. I also saw their capabilities and their interest in moving nursing forward, as well as their limitations and needs, including those associated with the inadequacies of their formal preparation for nursing practice. During these years I was a nurse consultant in the Division of Hospitals and Institutional Services of the Indiana State Board of Health. The Division was concerned with both hospital licensure and hospital construction as provided for by Indiana State Law related to the Federal Hill-Burton Act. My specific area of responsibility was to work with the nurses in the Division toward the upgrading of nursing services in the general hospitals of Indiana.

These ideas about nurses and nursing were formulated as a result of events and experiences during these years.

1. Nurses accept responsibility for the presence and perpetuation of the ills prevalent in the hospital field when the burden of bearing the responsibility is placed on them by hospital administrators and physicians.
2. Nurses provide nursing but they are not able to talk about nursing to patients, members of patients' families, physicians, or hospital administrators.
3. Nurses express the results they aspire to help patients achieve in a commonsense fashion, for example, to get better and go home.

4. Specialists in rehabilitation medicine perceive nurses as unprepared and therefore unsuitable to work with patients when patients are learning to engage in the activities of daily living.
5. Nurses must have a central, organizing point of view about persons in need of nursing, some starting point if they are to proceed with planning for nursing care.
6. The offering and provision of nursing as a health service require performance of distribution, production, and financing functions common to all service enterprises.
7. Hospitals are large-scale, complex enterprises. There is little to no evidence of comprehensive designs and plans for the provision of nursing or other services, regardless of hospital size.
8. The purposes of service enterprises such as health care and educational institutions are achieved at the operational level where service is produced.
9. The hierarchical emphasis in the upgrading of nursing service organizations has neglected the operational level where nursing is produced.

During the years I spent with the Indiana State Board of Health I was offered the opportunity to read and master the then available literature in the fields of organization and administration and to attend seminars of the American Management Association. One result was the experiencing of a need for a means to give structure to my knowledge in these fields. I pursued readings in the field of social philosophy and found what I needed in philosophical expositions about *wholes composed of parts* and concepts of *order* and *relations*. Categorizations of types of wholes and Aquinas's points of order in wholes composed of parts (Niemeyer, 1951) were helpful in understanding the formation and operations of human organizations. Later, Chester Barnard's work *The Functions of the Executive* (1962) contributed to my increase in insights about human organizations.

In 1958 and 1959 I served as a consultant in the Office of Education, U.S. Department of Health, Education and Welfare, working on a national project for the upgrading of practical or vocational nurse training programs. This experience, combined with prior experiences with hospital-employed practical nurses and practical nurse education, contributed to the developing insight that practical nurse training programs lacked the qualifying characteristics of either authentic vocational training programs or low-level technical-type programs. In programs, the selection of content from sciences foundational to nursing was arbitrary. Lists of occupational tasks were the training focus. Teachers had as their teaching model the way they had been taught in hospital diploma programs.

Early in my work in this project I reached these conclusions.

1. If the worker being prepared is offered the title of nurse, there should be nursing content included in the training program.
2. The selection of nursing content for a training program requires that selectors have knowledge of the domain and boundaries of nursing as a field of knowledge and a field of practice.
3. The roles of practical nurses in nursing practice situations should afford criterion measures for the selection of nursing content.
4. Nursing content should have clear articulations with content from nursing-related fields. It is not a student's responsibility to discover these articulations.

These conclusions led in later years to the continued study of the forms of education for nursing, and the content and organization of content in nursing components of professional and technical curricula.

During the period from 1956 to 1959 I was able to formulate and express some ideas and understandings of nursing developed during the two described work experiences.

1. An essay about hospital services appended to a report of a study of nursing administration positions in one Indiana hospital (Orem, 1956)
2. A definition of nursing that contained an expression of nursing's proper object that differentiates nursing from other human services (Orem, 1956)
3. The naming of the condition that exists when judgments are made that persons are in need of and can benefit from nursing, namely, the inability to provide the amount and the quality of required self-care when the inability is associated with health state or health care requirements (Orem, 1958)
4. Beginning descriptions of nursing situations, including development of categories and classifications during 1958 and 1959:
   a. their social nature, including social complexity
   b. nursing as being within the context of daily living of nurses' patients, including the influences of the physical and social

environment on daily living
c. situations of personal health, including health deviations
d. conditions and states that affect individuals' abilities to engage in deliberate action, including self-care
e. identification of factors applicable in describing situations of nursing practice
f. operations (activity areas) of nursing practice
g. standards of assistance for adults, aged adults, infants and children, male and female patients
h. standards for assistance to help individuals meet health care requirements

The foregoing represent a primarily cognitive movement in my development. Development, however, was also affective. I felt the impact of each idea and each increase in understanding of nursing and responded with activity toward and increased hope for the development of nursing as a field of knowledge with its own domain and boundaries. Two publications were produced: *Hospital Nursing Service. An Analysis*, Indiana State Board of Health, Indianapolis, Indiana, 1956, and *Guides for Developing Curricula for the Education of Practical Nurses*, Office of Education, U.S. Department of Health, Education and Welfare, U.S. Government Printing Office, Washington, DC, 1959.

The ideas about nursing expressed in these two works are primitive. From my own perspective they primarily represent stages in my movement toward the development and use of theory in attaching meaning to nursing.

CONCEPTUALIZATION

Throughout the 1960s, I was director of the program Administration of Nursing Education at the School of Nursing, The Catholic University of America. I conducted graduate courses in this field and participated in seminars in the Administration of Nursing Services program. During the later 1960s I developed and taught core courses in Nursing and in Organizational Theory for all students enrolled in Master's Programs, as well as a course in curriculum development for technical nursing programs. I continued my solitary work toward the development and validation of *nursing* knowledge and in 1965 joined my efforts with colleagues at The Catholic University of America to work toward the development of a research model for nursing. This work is fully recounted in both the first and second editions of *Concept Formalization in Nursing: Process and Product* (Nursing Development Conference Group, 1973, 1979). I attended the first conference on nursing theory sponsored by the School of Nursing at Case Western Reserve University. I was able to compare the results of my own efforts and those of the Committee on the Nursing Model with the Conference offerings: I was satisfied that we were making progress. As in the 1950s, my experiences during the 1960s and early 1970s led me to formalize some factors and conditions that indicated the need for the development of nursing as a field of knowledge. I reached the conclusions that follow.

1. Graduate students enrolled in clinical nursing programs have no nursing basis for participating in curriculum design and development for nursing programs.
2. Works on curriculum development by nurses do not address the question of the domain and boundaries of nursing as a field of knowledge and practice.
3. The unanswered questions in nursing that require investigation are not set forth.
4. The articulations of nursing with other fields of knowledge are not established. Students are expected to determine the articulations.
5. Written descriptions of nursing courses in baccalaureate or associate degree programs do not contain explicit nursing content.
6. Some faculty members in universities cannot deal with nursing abstractly, as is necessary in analysis and theory formulation.
7. There is evidence that some nursing service administrators and hospital administrators are reluctant to have hospital populations studied from a nursing perspective.

The foregoing reinforced my convictions that nurses must be able to attach meaning to nursing, to communicate about nursing matters, and to think nursing if they are to perform effectively the operations of nursing practice or perform in other nurse roles necessary to keep nursing viable in society. The difficulties to be faced by nurses in moving from a common-sense to a theoretical position for understanding nursing were obvious.

From the perspective of the development of the self-care deficit theory of nursing, the 1960s and early 1970s were devoted to the following:

1. Accepting and developing understanding of nursing as a practical science and a set of applied sciences

2. Developing insights about deliberate action, action systems, and self-organizing systems
3. Conceptualizing understandings of the patient and nurse elements invariant in nursing practice situations, naming these elements, and expressing relations among them
4. Developing insights about the product of nursing and conceptualizing this product as a nursing system
5. Identification and description of methods of assisting or helping
6. Classifying nursing systems on the basis of nurse and patient roles associated with the methods of assisting patients used by nurses
7. Identifying the types of technologies that nurses use in nursing practice
8. A beginning organization of knowledge around the concept of self-care
9. A formalization and expression of a general concept of nursing

My work and that of my colleagues during the 1960s and early 1970s provided a basis for two publications. These are the first edition of *Nursing: Concepts of Practice* (1971) and the first edition of the Nursing Development Conference Group's *Concept Formalization in Nursing: Process and Product* (1973). The two books were developed to serve different purposes. *Nursing: Concepts of Practice*, as the title indicates, was developed as a text to introduce nursing students to nursing content to help them understand nursing as a field of practice. *Concept Formalization*, on the other hand, emphasized the need for approaches to the conceptualization of nursing elements and the beginning organization of nursing knowledge. It was used primarily in baccalaureate and graduate nursing programs. *Nursing: Concepts of Practice* was used both in baccalaureate and in technical-level programs. During the 1960s and early 1970s, the conceptualization of nursing common to both books was used by a few nursing practitioners and provided the basis for the design of the nurse-managed clinics developed at The Johns Hopkins Hospitals.

CONCEPT, MODEL, THEORY

The period of the 1970s to the present has been spent in consultation in nursing education and nursing services, conference work relative to nursing concepts and nursing theory, and continued work to contribute to the development of nursing as a discipline of knowledge. The time period is marked by three major developments on my part and that of my colleagues toward the formalization and expression of a general theory of nursing.

In November 1970, final work was done by members of the Nursing Development Conference Group in defining the creative end product of nursing as a *nursing system* and in expressing a detailed but succinct conceptualization of *nursing*. The form for both of these expressions was adopted from W. R. Ashby's description of self-organizing systems (Ashby, 1964, p. 108). The following quotation about expressed conceptualizations of nursing system and nursing are from the Nursing Development Conference Group's work (1973, pp. 70–71; 1979, p. 107).

> A *nursing system*, like other systems for the provision of personal services, is the product of a series of relations between persons who belong to different sets (classes), the set A and the set B. From a nursing perspective any member of the set A (legitimate patient) presents evidence descriptive of the complex subsets *self-care agency* and *therapeutic self-care demand* and the condition that in A demand exceeds *agency* due to health or health-related causes. Any member of the set B (legitimate nurse) presents evidence descriptive of the complex subset *nursing agency* which includes valuation of the legitimate relations between self as nurse and instances where, in A, certain values of the component phenomena of *self-care agency* and *therapeutic self-care demand* prevail.
>
> B's perceptions of the conditionality of A's subset objective *therapeutic self-care demand* on the subset *self-care agency* establishes the conditionality of changes in the states of A's two subsets on the state of and changes in the state of B's subset *nursing agency*. The activation of the components of the subset nursing agency (change in state) by B to deliberately control or alter the state of one or both of A's subsets—*therapeutic self-care demand* and *self-care agency*—is nursing. The perceived relations among the parts of the three subsets (actual system) constitute the organization. The "mapping" of the behaviors in "mathematical or behavioral terms" provides a record of the system.

The formulation of this two-paragraph statement followed concentrated work by Group members to formalize their conceptualizations of the constant and essential elements of nursing practice situations, self-care agency, therapeutic self-care demand, and nursing agency; to set forth relationships among the elements; and to place them within the context of self-care and daily living of persons in need of nursing within their environmental situations (Nursing Development Conference Group, 1979).

The movement from the formalized, theoretically conceptualized parts of nursing to general concepts of nursing and nursing system illustrate the composite mode that follows the analytical mode of proceeding in the development of knowledge in practice disciplines (Wallace, 1979).

Throughout the period of conceptualizing nursing, beginning in 1958, work was guided by the idea that the creative end product of nursing is a nursing system. Endeavor to understand and visualize the creative end product of practitioners in a practice field is essential not only in practice but in the structuring and validation of knowledge in the field. The November 1970 expressed conceptualizations of *nursing system* and *nursing* were judged by Group members to exhibit reliability and validity and as being more theoretical and scientifically useful than prior concepts used by the Group (Nursing Development Conference Group, 1979). These conceptualizations are the result of integrations of knowledge moving individuals to higher, more complex and intricate viewpoints about nursing.

The November 1970 expressed concepts of nursing system and nursing were enabling for the expression of a word model of nursing system (Orem, 1985). A word model consists of a circle of terms and relationships. The word model of a nursing system expressed in the 1970s names the patient and nurse variables of nursing systems and shows the relationships among them. The parameters of these variables from a nursing systems perspective were named *basic conditioning factors* (Nursing Development Conference Group, 1979). Basic conditioning factors that are affecting one or both of the patient variables in singular nursing practice situations would bring into consideration by the nurse knowledge organized from the perspective of one or more of the special views of man, human beings, essential in understanding nursing, namely, person, agent, symbolizer, organism (Nursing Development Conference Group, 1979).

The culmination of my movement from a commonsense to a theoretical perspective of nursing was the formulation of a general theory descriptively explanatory of nursing. The theory is constituted from the articulation of a theory of self-care with a theory of self-care deficit and the incorporation of the elements of these theories into a theory of nursing system. The three theories appear in the second (1980) edition and the third (1985) edition of *Nursing: Concepts of Practice*. The latest, refined expression of the theories are found in *Case Studies in Nursing Theory* (Winstead-Fry, 1986).

The *theory of nursing system* is descriptively explanatory of the creative end product of nursing and its production within the frame of broader interpersonal and social relationships of nurses with persons with health-derived or health-associated self-care deficits. It specifies transactions between nurse and patient variables and the transformations to be sought in the real world referents of these variables. The *theory of self-care deficit* expresses the conditionality of the capabilities of persons to regulate their own functioning on internal and external health associated conditions and factors. The *theory of self-care* explains it as a regulatory function of mature and maturing individuals.

THEORY AND THE STAGES OF UNDERSTANDING NURSING

The development of any science, including practical sciences or practice disciplines, occurs in stages. What is initially known is subjected to intricate arrangements and patterns until higher integrations of insight are reached. A stage is understood in terms of the occurrence of sets of insights about specifics. It is what the insights are all about, the kinds of data and the images involved, and not the time of occurrence that provide the basis for distinguishing and naming stages of development. Five stages of development of practical nursing science are recognized from developments that have occurred in formation of self-care deficit nursing theory.

1. The stage of describing and explaining nursing in a general theory of nursing
2. The stage of laying out the range of variation of the conceptual elements of the general theory of nursing
3. The stage of formulating and validating models and rules of nursing practice
4. The stage of describing nursing cases, including their natural history
5. The stage of formulating and validating models and rules for providing nursing for populations

The development and validation of technologies and description of their limits of effectiveness are associated with stages three, four, and five. Work was done in all of the named stages during the time period 1956 to the present. The work is unfinished but it continues. Nurses in our own country, in Canada, in South America, Europe, Asia, and Australia are contributing efforts toward development of nursing through their use of the theoretical constructs of self-care nursing theory.

CHAPTER 23

Changes in Professional Nursing Practice Associated With Nurses' Use of Orem's General Theory of Nursing

O ne result of this conference should be a view of how a general theory of nursing can serve nursing practitioners. Two preliminary questions are suggested for consideration by conference participants.

1. Do I engage in the practice of nursing?
2. Am I developing or have I developed a healthy sense of professionalism?

It is not reasonable to talk about changes in professional nursing practice without attention to these questions. Each conference participant should attend to them and be able to attach meaning to the terms *practice of nursing* and *professionalism*. Van Eron (1985) suggests that it is not a nurse's initial and subsequent forms of education for nursing, or his or her theoretical orientations or experiences that are the critical factors in selecting nurses to fill practice positions. It is what a nurse thinks about all of them in relation to self that is important.

This paper was originally presented at Le Centre Hospitalier De Gatineau, Gatineau, Quebec, Canada, May 12, 1987.

NURSING PRACTICE AND NURSING KNOWLEDGE

Nursing practice is the regular engagement in the work of nursing persons who need and can be helped through the effective provision of this health service. A nurse's style of practice is personal, but the nursing knowledge that is antecedent to practice and gives direction to it is from bodies of information that nurses formulate and structure within the boundaries of the profession's domain. Knowledge development in nursing begins with this question: When and why do people need nursing and how are they helped through its provision? The answer to the question is a beginning identification of the sector of reality that is the world of the nurse. Nurses deal with nursing's sector of reality in particular ways. Medicine and other health services are concerned with other sectors of reality and have their own specialized ways of handling matters within their sectors.

Nursing in the closing decades of the twentieth century is a knowledge-intensive service and field of practice. The work of nursing practitioners and educators is adversely affected by the fact that nurses have not formalized, structured, and validated bodies of nursing knowledge that not only specify and describe the elements or parts of nursing practice situations but also explain the relationships among the parts. Nursing knowledge continues to be scattered and fragmented. Nurses have not adequately addressed the question: Can and how can fragments of nursing knowledge be brought together to better serve nursing students and nursing practitioners to understand nursing? Knowledge specific to practice fields such as nursing is formulated, expressed, and validated to serve persons who practice within the field. Such knowledge serves practical purposes, that is, the bringing about through deliberate human effort of conditions or events that do not presently exist or have not occurred. Structured nursing knowledge, because of its practical nature, would have the forms common to other practice fields such as medicine or engineering. There would be developed

1. Practical nursing sciences in the form of
    a. theoretical nursing sciences
    b. clinical nursing sciences and
2. Sets of applied sciences of nursing—sciences developed from existent sciences that articulate with points of theory or facts from the practical nursing sciences

In all practice fields, there are interpersonal and broader social dimensions as well as technological dimensions of practice. The practical and applied nursing sciences would include areas of knowledge that are developed from questions and problems that arise with respect to the social and interpersonal aspects of nursing practice as well as its clinical and technological aspects.

Nurses today are dependent upon formulated, expressed, and developing general and less general theories of nursing to give form and structure to their practice and to organize validated but scattered and fragmented nursing knowledge. Theorists who deal with the realities of nursing practice situations in an abstract and theoretical manner in order to understand nursing provide both content and structure for the nursing sciences whenever theories describe and explain the realities of nursing practice situations. As theoretical constructs of nursing are developed, points of articulation with existent sciences are identified, providing the bases for applied sciences of nursing. General theories of nursing are the foundations of the practical science of theoretical nursing.

The laying out of the forms of nursing knowledge that can and should be developed as a base for nursing practice does not include the personal and private knowledge that nurses acquire through experience in nursing practice situations. Maritain (1959) speaks to this kind of knowledge and states that it cannot be reduced to other forms. Nurses and other health professionals recognize that they have this kind of knowledge.

Since the nursing sciences are in beginning stages of development, today's nursing practitioners must be or become scholars within a developing theoretical structure for nursing. A nurse's knowledge of nursing is a dynamic process that functions in all the process operations of nursing practice. It is enabling in observing features of nursing practice situations, in thinking nursing, in doing nursing, and in communicating nursing to others.

To give structure to nursing process nurses must master conceptual models of nursing, know their theoretical origins, and come to understand their reality bases in nursing practice situations. This need suggests additional questions to be addressed by nurses.

1. Am I a nursing scholar within the framework of a theory of nursing?
2. Do I understand the referents of the conceptual elements and relationships of this theory within concrete situations of nursing practice?

A HEALTHY PROFESSIONALISM

Professional nursing practice is a term with a number of meanings. To avoid ambiguity the phrase *practicing nursing with a healthy sense of professionalism* is used.

Nurses who practice nursing with a healthy sense of professionalism are first and foremost aware of the relationship between what they know and what they do. In the practice of nursing, as in the practice of other human services, practitioners must be able to identify and focus on the realities with which they deal as nurses and make judgments about what action can and should be taken in reality situations. It is not enough for nurses to think of themselves as nurses; it is necessary for them to know the domain and boundaries of their practice, their legitimate authority and responsibility in some range of types of nursing practice situations, their personal capabilities in nursing practice, and their stages of development as practitioners. Nurses also must ask and answer this question in every situation of nursing practice: Am I a legitimate nurse in this practice situation?

The development of a healthy professionalism by nurses can and should be fostered in both nursing education and nursing practice situations. It demands educational and nursing service situations that foster nurses' engagement in nursing practice as well as development of nurses' personal styles of practice and their continuing formation of themselves as nursing practitioners and scholars. Understanding role functions of nurses within the frame of a general theory of nursing may be a first step in the effective development of individual nurses to take on the responsibilities of professionals.

THEORETICAL ORIENTATIONS AND NURSING PRACTICE

The self-care deficit theory of nursing is a nucleus of a developing practical science of nursing. A practical science describes and explains reality situations as well as deliberate human actions of particular kinds and in particular sequences that can contribute to bringing about conditions in these reality situations that range from desirable to essential but that do not exist at the time they are sought. Self-care deficit theory is descriptive and explanatory of nursing. It is abstract. It is not concerned with singular nursing situations as such. It provides nurses with a way of knowing, thinking, doing, and communicating nursing. Nurses who make a theory their own use it in singular concrete situations of nursing practice and in organizing nursing and nursing-related knowledge in forms that facilitate teaching and learning nursing. Nurses who seek to master a general theory of nursing as their way of knowing and thinking nursing move through a stage of static mastery of its concepts to a stage of dynamic knowing. This is the stage of acceptance and ownership of the theory.

Nurses who make the self-care deficit theory of nursing their own not only use the theory but also contribute to its continuing development and refinement. The continued development of the theory requires the work of nursing researchers and scholars.

Self-care nursing theory, as it is sometimes called, has been under active development since 1958. The theory is grounded in the nature of human beings and human activity. The continued development of the theory, after the formulation and expression of some of its essential concepts, proceeded with the explicit acceptance of nursing as a form of practical endeavor that could be understood in terms of its universal principles, principles that represent the essential features and relationships of nursing practice situations. Universal principles of nursing expressed as concepts and theories are not obvious or self-evident and therefore require investigation.

The self-care deficit theory of nursing is now described as a conceptual model that sets forth the essential features and the relationships of nursing practice situations. The concepts of the model are derived from a theory of self-care, a theory of self-care deficit, and a theory of nursing system. The central ideas of the three theories that together constitute self-care deficit nursing theory are then expressed following presentation of the model. The expressed theory and its conceptual structure are accepted as parts of the practical science of theoretical nursing.

THEORETICAL NURSING

The self-care deficit theory of nursing in its fully articulated form is referred to as *theoretical nursing* because (1) it is remote from the concrete operations of nursing practice and (2) it is descriptively explanatory of human conditions and actions that are within the domain of nursing. Nursing is a product, a human service. The theory and the conceptual model express the defining characteristics of this service.

The conceptual structure of the theory is described in relation to two human agents or actors: the nurse and the nurse's patient. The term *agent* or actor is used to identify that both nurse and patient are viewed as having role responsibilities for action within nursing situations. Patients may not be able to fulfill their role responsibilities. The conceptual model is relatively simple with respect to the number of concepts and number of relationships. The concepts include the following:

1. The nurse variable *nursing agency* that refers to the power to provide nursing to others
2. Two patient variables: (a) *self-care agency*, that is, the power of individuals to meet their continuing requisites for regulating their functioning in the interests of their own life, health, and well-being and (b) *therapeutic self-care demand*, that is, the actions to be performed to meet the requisites for self-regulation of one's human functioning in the interests of one's life, health, and well-being
3. The concept *self-care deficit* has as its referent a state where self-care agency is unequal because of the conditioning effects of health or health-related factors on persons who act to know or meet their therapeutic self-care demands
4. *Self-care* refers to the regulatory actions of persons who know and expend effort to meet their therapeutic self-care demands
5. *Nursing system* refers to the product made by nurses who activate their nursing agency to know the values of patients' self-care agency, their therapeutic self-care demands, and the relationships between them, and with this knowledge act to ensure that patients' therapeutic self-care demands are met, self-care agency is protected, and the exercise or development of self-care is regulated
6. The concept *basic conditioning factors* has as its referents conditions internal or external to nurses and to nurses' patients that affect the current or future values of nurses' nursing agency and the current or future values of patients' self-care agency and therapeutic self-care demands

These six concepts are the main and essential concepts of the self-care deficit theory of nursing. Together they form a circle of terms and relationships, a conceptual model.

A conceptual model is analogous to the framework or skeleton of a nursing theory, constituted from its main conceptual elements. Theories are expressed in terms of central ideas, propositions, and presuppositions. [*Ed. Note:* The most recent description of self-care deficit nursing theory can be found in Orem, 2001, pp. 136–157.]

Nurses make nursing systems as they perform the process operations of nursing practice, namely, nursing diagnosis, nursing prescription, and nursing regulation. The self-care deficit theory of nursing gives focus and structure to these operations. The substantive or internal structure of the six main conceptual elements of the theory identify the human and environmental features of nursing practice situations to which each of the nursing process operations is directed by nurses.

The named process operations of nursing practice express the landmarks for the production of nursing for individuals or multi-person units, such as families. There is a way to reach each landmark in the form of sets of action that constitute the road leading to each. For example, nursing diagnosis as a process operation begins with observation and ends with diagnostic statements.

Process operations are not in and of themselves unique to nursing. There are process operations for every human service. It is knowledge of the domain and boundaries of nursing and mastery of theoretical nursing that enables nurses to perform the process operations of nursing.

CHANGES IN PROFESSIONAL NURSING PRACTICE

Changes in nursing practice reflect changes both in nursing practitioners and in the environments in which they practice. Individual nurses can bring about changes in themselves through introspection, mastery of authentic nursing knowledge, and skill development and skill perfection. Individual nurses in practice cannot change the environments in which they practice unless there is the active knowing and goal-oriented participation of nursing administration. It is for this reason that nursing administration must become concerned about and meet its responsibilities and demands for development and validation of models and rules for the provision of nursing to populations.

The matter of change in professional nursing practice is addressed first from the perspective of individual practicing nurses and then from the perspective of nursing administration.

Changes in Nurses and in Their Practice of Nursing

Perhaps the most comprehensive change associated with nurses' mastery and use of self-care deficit nursing theory is an increase in their sense of self-worth as nurses. The nurse who knows nurses' roles in health care situations, who thinks nursing, and has a nursing language in which to communicate facts, ideas, and questions about nursing is not apt to depreciate his or her nursing work by saying, "I am only a nurse." This nurse can do nursing, think nursing, and communicate his or her own nursing actions and patients' nursing conditions to patients, members of patients' families, other nurses, and other health workers. He or she has a positive image of self-as-nurse based on personal capabilities and not upon how someone at some time has told the nurse to think about self.

The mastery and use of self-care deficit nursing theory is enabling for nurses to view nursing practice situations comprehensively and to understand the range of possible ideal roles of nurses' patients, nurses, and members of patients' families who may have to take over or participate in meeting patients' therapeutic self-care demands. Nurses view the knowing and meeting of their patients' therapeutic self-care demands, as well as the protection and the regulation of the exercise or development of patients' self-care agency, as continuing processes in time, regardless of the location of patients. They are familiar with, talk about, and help others to monitor the accumulated stress, the energy requirements, the time requirements, the material resources, and the human actions and effort required to provide one's own self-care or to meet the therapeutic self-care demands of dependents under conditions of impaired health or human structural or functional limitations.

Positive changes in nursing practice have been noted in situations where nurses have mastered and use the self-care deficit theory as a way of knowing nursing in order to give direction and meaning to nursing practice.

1. Nurses develop their personal styles of practice within the domain and boundaries of nursing set by the theory.
2. Nurses focus on providing nursing to persons whose legitimate need for nursing is established through the criterion of the existence of health-derived or health-related self-care deficit. Stereotyping is eventually eliminated.
3. Nursing diagnoses become more valid and are expressed within a nursing frame of reference.
4. Therapeutic self-care demands and ways to protect and to regulate the exercise or development of self-care agency are determined and prescribed. Nursing care systems are designed.
5. Nursing documentation increases and improves.
6. There is an increase in and upgrading of the kind of referrals made by nurses. This includes referrals to nursing specialties.

7. There is recognition by nurses and gradual recognition by physicians of the need for nursing discharge of patients. This recognition of and increase in the practice of nursing discharge has led to
   a. patients remaining as hospital inpatients beyond the time of medical discharge
   b. the discharge of patients by hospital nurses to community health nurses or to nurses in other residence care facilities
   c. the discharge of patients to care by family members with the prior establishment of designs for the dependent-care systems that will be provided in homes with provision for nursing consultation as required
8. There is movement toward nurse-managed clinics.
9. Nurses recognize that they have a theoretical base that serves them in performing the professional function of design of systems of nursing care. The design function is retained by and specific to the professional person.
10. Nurses, through their design of systems of nursing, bring into focus their own role responsibilities and role functions as well as those of other nurses, their patients, and members of patients' families who are or are becoming dependent-care agents.

Such practice changes are most likely to occur in health service enterprises where nursing administration views self-care nursing theory as one means to aid in efforts to ensure the continuing provision of effective nursing within the health care enterprise.

Changes in Nursing Administration

Nursing administration is organization or enterprise oriented and has as its focus current or future populations to be served by the enterprise through the continuing availability and production of nursing. Nursing administrators properly perform the work of managers. Their managerial powers and responsibilities within health service enterprises are defined by (1) positional location in the enterprise, (2) the nursing orientation of their managerial powers and responsibilities, and (3) the size and characteristics of the populations to be provided with nursing now and at future times. Nursing administrators require theoretical orientations to nursing if they are to fulfill their managerial responsibilities.

Self-care nursing theory is of value in fulfillment of the managerial functions of

1. Continuous descriptions of populations in need of nursing
2. Continuous calculation of what is required to provide nursing to the populations and subpopulations described
3. Development and validation of models and rules for ensuring the availability and provision of nursing for members of the described populations

A general theory of nursing provides administrators with a way of knowing nursing that helps them focus on populations to be served through nursing and to envision what is required for the provision of nursing. This includes the requisite capabilities of nurses, the environmental conditions that permit nurses to practice nursing, the complement of nurses needed, and the interpersonal and social climate that fosters collaboration and coordination among nurses and between nurses and other health care providers. Commitment to this approach to knowing and providing nursing has facilitated the writing of statements of philosophy, the formulation of objectives, the description of positions for both practitioners and administrators, and the establishing and maintaining of conditions that facilitate nursing practice. The Horn and Swain study at the University of Michigan (Horn & Swain, 1977) demonstrates the value of this nursing orientation to measuring the quality of nursing care on an institutional basis.

The active and effective collaboration of nursing practitioners, clinical nursing specialists and nursing administrators is enabling for both the design and production of nursing according to the self-care deficit way of knowing nursing.

QUESTIONS RELATED TO THE ASSESSMENT PROCESS

1. Initially and subsequently do I obtain and use
    a. essential social and nursing-related background information about patients?
    b. interpersonally relevant background information to help me understand patient behaviors and for adjusting my own approaches in interpersonal situations?
    c. information that will help me make tentative judgments about the extent and intensity of my interactions with patients as

related to time requirements, the meaning of nursing, and the importance of nursing for patients?

2. Do I have and maintain awareness of my relationship to patients who constitute my case load?

    a.   Are the relationships contractual for nursing?

    b.   Do my interpersonal relationships give evidence of being professional? Helping? Nursing?

    c.   Do I know my role responsibilities and functions? Do my patients know theirs? Do patients' family members know theirs? Is there agreement among us?

3. Do I understand that the meeting of patients' therapeutic self-care demands is continuous in time?

    a.   Initially or at an appropriate time do I determine what is a patient's usual self-care system?

    b.   Initially do I know whether a patient's usual self-care system or components thereof can be continued or whether there is a complete change? Is there any change in components?

    c.   Initially and subsequently do patients know their nurses' roles and their own roles in meeting their therapeutic self-care demands and in protecting and regulating the exercise or development of their self-care agency?

4. Do I initially and throughout my period of contact and interaction with patients accumulate a data base for factors that have affected, are affecting, or have a potential for affecting the values of patients' self-care agency or their therapeutic self-care demands? Conditioning factors include:

    a.   age, development state, and gender

    b.   conditions of living

    c.   family system factors, sociocultural orientations, patterns of living, occupational or educational endeavors

    d.   health state and health care system factors

5. Do I engage in actions that are components of the processes of nursing diagnosis, prescription, and regulation in my initial and subsequent contacts with patients?

    5.1.   Do I organize and evaluate results of my observations as a basis for formulating and expressing?

        a.   patients' therapeutic self-care demands?

        b.   the kinds of limitations for self-care that patients are experiencing?

        c.   the presence and nature of self-care deficits?

        d.   Do I make prescriptions and reach agreements with patients or members of patients' families about the ideal or adjusted therapeutic self-care demand?

   e. Do I make prescriptions about patients refraining from engagement in self-care or for their engaging in endeavors to regulate the exercise as development of their self-care agency?

5.2. Do I design and make adjustments in designs for systems of nursing care for patients that take into consideration nurse role, patient role, and the roles of family members in

   a. the continuous meeting of patients' therapeutic self-care demands?

   b. the protection of their capacities for engaging in self-care?

   c. the regulation of the exercise or development of self-care agency?

5.3. Do I plan for the materials, the timing of actions, and so forth necessary to execute the desired action?

5.4. Do I consistently engage in the provision of health regulating care with and for patients to

   a. meet their therapeutic self-care demands?

   b. protect their powers of self-care agency?

   c. regulate the exercise of development of their capabilities to engage in self-care?

6. Do I know when and how to seek nursing consultation? Do I seek it?

7. Do I know when patients are ready for discharge from nursing with or without provision for continuing nursing consultation?

8. Do I produce effective designs so that patients and families can know and meet patients' therapeutic self-care demands and take action to overcome or compensate for patients' self-care limitations after nursing discharge?

9. Do I know when patients should be discharged from my care to the care of other nurses? Do I know how and do I proceed to make such discharges effectively to community health nurses? To nurses in resident care facilities, for example, another hospital, a nursing home?

Questions related to the Assessment Process adapted from Chapter 5, "The Practice of Nursing," *Nursing: Concepts of Practice*, 3rd edition (1985). New York: McGraw-Hill.

CHAPTER 24

Self-Care and Health Promotion: Understanding Self-Care

SELF-CARE

Human beings, like other living things, are dependent for the continuance of life on interchanges with their environments and on the compatibility of available materials and conditions with requisites for human functioning and development. Self-care is the continuous performance of sets of related actions by older children and adults that supply the materials and bring about the conditions that are regulatory of their own functioning and development. Such actions, when performed by responsible adults for socially dependent family members, are named dependent-care.

Self-care is human behavior that is self-directed and self-permitted. It is conduct or deliberate action or ego-processed behavior. It is behavior learned by children and adults within their contacts and communications as members of social groups—the family, the school, recreational groups, and so forth. The notion of self-care is implicit in expressions such as "You are not taking care of yourself" or "Mrs. B. can't take care of herself anymore." In reality situations where persons express such judgments, we assume that the judgments are based upon observed behavior of the individuals referred to over some period of time. Awareness of the requirements for continuing care is expressed in the admonition of a seriously

This paper was originally presented at the Wesley Hospital Conference, "Hospitals in the Community—A Vision," in Brisbane, Australia, June 3–5, 1987.

ill patient in a cardiac intensive care unit to his nurse: "Don't tell me one more thing; just take care of me."

Self-care requires knowledge as well as a wide range of skills. Ideally there is consistency between what a person knows and what the person does. Mr. K., 34 years old with a ten-year history of diabetes mellitus, had been taught the basics of diabetic management (Orem & Taylor, 1986). He can recall this basic information when questioned. At the time of a hospitalization, because his diabetes was out of control and because of a submandibular abscess and a high fever, he was asked by his nurse to describe his current self-care system. He made the following statements:

> I work from sunrise to sundown and I barely have time to eat a candy bar for lunch. I take my insulin usually when I have time to. I eat one meal a day. I shoot up with insulin and then eat a large meal. Sometimes I wake up at night hungry so I take some sugar. I can't see real well right now. My vision is blurry but it is getting better. Today I didn't eat breakfast 'cause I was nauseated. I don't wear an ID tag [Medic-Alert]; don't see that it matters and it gets in my way. (p. 61)

Assuming the validity of Mr. K.'s statements, it is possible to make some judgments about the quality of his self-care regimen as related to management of his diabetes.

Self-care is not the performance of this act or that act. Self-care requires the seeing of relationships among factors, for example, diet, activity, and insulin in the management of a diabetic condition. It requires the making of adjustments in care actions on a day-to-day basis or more frequently. It requires the incorporation of self-care into the pattern of daily living. It requires material resources and time, and when self-care is excessively time consuming it is not only burdensome, it may require the giving up of other things and activities.

Health professionals have given little attention to self-care and dependent-care, perhaps because they are such integral parts of the daily living of individuals and families. Nurses cannot fulfill their role responsibilities in the world today if they ignore this area of human endeavor and fail to contribute to the structuring and validation of knowledge about self-care and dependent-care.

SELF-CARE AND NURSING

I first used the term *self-care* in 1956 in formulating a definition of nursing (Orem, 1956). In describing the need for nursing I used the phrase "activities contributory to health, or its recovery (or to a peaceful death) that (an individual) would perform unaided if he had the necessary strength, will, or knowledge."

Prior to the 1950s, nurses in their writings had recognized the social dependency of their patients and had identified ways of helping or assisting them. It was the nurse's role, however, that was emphasized. Thus it was not until the 1950s in the United States that some nurses recognized and identified that persons under nursing care were self-care agents and as such bore role functions and responsibilities for self-care. The 1950s was the period of active development of rehabilitation medicine. There is no doubt that the emergence in nursing of an emphasis on the self-care role of older children and adults was stimulated, at least in part, by the rehabilitation movement.

The year 1956 marked the beginning of my efforts to understand and to conceptualize self-care and the beginning of my path toward understanding and expressing the proper object of nursing as a field of knowledge and a field of practice. My expression in 1958 of the proper object of nursing occurred as a response to the question: What condition exists in a person when that person or a family member or the attending physician or a nurse makes the judgment that the person should be under nursing care, that nurses should become a part of the health care situation? My developing understanding of why persons needed and could be helped through nursing were formulated and expressed as follows:

> . . . the inability of a person to provide continuously for self the amount and quality of required self-care because of the situation of personal health. Self-care is conceptualized as the personal care that human beings require each day and that may be modified by health care, environmental conditions [nature of/and] effects of medical care, and other factors. [Orem, 1959, personal knowledge]

The expression of the proper object of nursing further specified that in child nursing situations it is the parent or guardian who is not able to provide the amount and quality of continuing personal care required by the child because of the child's health situation. As the self-care deficit theory of nursing developed, the term *dependent-care* was introduced to include care provided for dependent family members regardless of age.

My own work and that of my colleagues during the period from 1958 to the late 1970s was concerned with validation of the concept of self-care, with increasing our understanding of this form of practical endeavor, and with structuring knowledge around the concept. A theory of self-care was expressed in 1980 as one of three theories that in their articulations constitute the self-care deficit theory of nursing. The two theories that articulate with the theory of self-care are the theory of self-care deficit and the theory of nursing system. In their articulations the three theories form a unitary theory of nursing referred to as self-care deficit nursing theory or self-care nursing theory.

SELF-CARE—A THEORY

A revised statement of the 1980 theory of self-care descriptively explains self-care as regulatory of human functioning and human development.

> Mature and maturing persons contribute to the continuing regulation of their own functioning and development and to the prevention, control and amelioration of disease, injury and their effects by performing within the context of day to day living learned sets of actions that bring about events and conditions that are known or assumed to have value in keeping or bringing human or environmental factors within norms compatible with human life, health and well-being (Orem, 1980, unpublished paper).

The theory expresses a number of elements and relationships, the study of which will lead to further insights about self-care as a form of human endeavor. The essential contribution of the theory is its highlighting of the regulatory function of self-care. Self-care as a human regulatory function is viewed as analogous to neuroendocrine regulation or autoregulation, as it is named in the science of biology. The theory also affords maturing and mature persons position and role functions and responsibilities as self-care agents, and, by extension, role functions and responsibilities as dependent-care agents. Nurses and other health professionals often ignore the self-care and dependent-care responsibilities of patients and members of their families.

This theoretical position about self-care affords nurses and others the opportunity to begin to structure and validate knowledge about these human functions. For example: What are the characteristics of self-care and dependent-care practices in various populations or sub-populations and how do self-care and dependent-care fit into their patterns of day-to-day living? Self-care and dependent-care have interpersonal as well as broader social dimensions that health professionals must be helped to understand. Both forms of care must be understood in relation to culture groups and family configurations of roles and role responsibilities. For example, within a population group in the United States, a young mother may seek to care for her infant in the way that is explained to her as most beneficial for the infant but meets with opposition from her mother, the dominant household figure.

Knowledge that is available to nurses and others about self-care is fragmented and scattered. The theory of self-care and a dynamic concept of self-care can help individual nurses and other interested persons to form the practical theoretical science and the applied science of self-care. Self-care is necessarily accepted as a form of practical endeavor through which individuals seek to bring about conditions that are desired and valued and that do not prevail at the time of taking action. Nurses must have antecedent knowledge about self-care developed in accord with its practical nature if they are to participate in helping individuals and families to design, plan for, conduct, and manage effective systems of self-care and dependent-care.

CONCEPTUALIZING SELF-CARE

In the process of the search for insights about self-care and dependent-care my colleagues and I studied individual nursing cases, categories of patients (the unconscious patient, the conscious but paralyzed patient), and films depicting nursing practice situations (Nursing Development Conference Group, 1979). Premises and propositions about self-care were developed, reviewed, and expanded, giving greater recognition to the effects of psychologic and social factors on self-care. The development by Louise Hartnett (NDCG, 1979) of a model of self-care valid for the maintenance of normal body temperature and areas for nursing assessment of action abilities of individuals related to this area of self-care contributed to making our static concepts of self-care dynamic and therefore helpful in thinking self-care and in studying it. The appropriate methods of investigation, the research methodology that we agreed upon as valid for early empirical investigation of self-care included (1) the case method, including the natural history of cases and (2) the hypothetical deductive method to identify elements within concepts and linkages between the elements. Scholarly pursuit of related fields is of great importance in the use of the hypothetical deductive method; for example, in Louise Hartnett's (NDCG, 1979) work on developing a model for maintenance of normal body temperature, her study of environmental physiology and reported research was essential to development of the final model.

Valid concepts of self-care express insight about its nature as deliberate action and its ultimate purpose as set forth in the following statement:

Self-care is the self-initiated and self-directed actions of persons to know their current and future requirements for regulating their own functioning and development and to select and use means to meet these requirements in order to sustain life and to promote health and well-being. (Orem, working papers)

My work and that of my colleagues to conceptualize our insights about self-care resulted in the identification and naming of four conceptual elements.

1. Self-care requisites
2. Self-care measures or practices (method + sets of action)
3. Self-care behaviors of individuals in reality situations
4. Self-care systems of individuals in reality situations

The closely related concepts of self-care agency and self-care agent and the concept of therapeutic self-care demand were formulated and expressed. Within the self-care deficit theory of nursing, self-care agency and therapeutic self-care demand are the two related patient variables, the values of which at this or that time determine the presence or absence of a self-care deficit. Some of the concepts named above will be described in order to lay out areas for structuring and validating knowledge about self-care and related concepts.

STRUCTURING KNOWLEDGE OF SELF-CARE

Developing areas of knowledge specific to self-care can be structured around three concepts:

1. Self-care requisites
2. Therapeutic self-care demand
3. Self-care operations

The concepts are interrelated but each will be developed separately. Self-care requisites and therapeutic self-care demand are described. Self-care operations will be addressed under "Motivating Self-Care" [Ed. Note: See chapter 25].

Self-Care Requisites

Self-care requisites are generalizations about purposes to be achieved through self-care with purposes expressed in an action frame. Consider the requisite *maintain a balance between activity and rest*. The requisite is not expressed in terms of health or well-being but in terms of action to bring about a valued or desirable relationship between persons being at rest and being active. The events and the internal states resultant from the maintenance of this balance over time would keep energy expenditures in balance with energy supplies and balance the engagement of individuals in physical work, intellectual and creative endeavors, and purely recreational pursuits. Movement from one type of activity to another is in itself restful. Three types of categories of requisites have been identified and described: universal, developmental, and health-deviation.

Universal Type Self-Care Requisites are so named because they are common to all human beings at all stages of the life cycle. Even so, they must be adjusted to age, developmental state, environmental factors, and health state of each individual, and to other conditioning factors. When such adjustments are made the requisite is said to be particularized for the individual. Eight universal self-care requisites have been described. Nursing practitioners view them as having validity. Some nurses (Patricia Underwood and her colleagues), who have promoted the use of the self-care deficit theory of nursing in one type of nursing practice situation, modify the listing. The eight universal type requisites are expressed in the third edition of *Nursing: Concepts of Practice* (Orem, 1985, pp. 90–91). Self-care or dependent-care effectively structured around particularized universal self-care requisites fosters positive health and well-being, including prevention and maintenance.

Developmental Self-Care Requisites are associated with human developmental processes, including affective and cognitive processes, during the stages of maturation, and with the self-preservation and emotional behaviors associated with severe illness, anesthesia, and impending death. Two categories of developmental self-care requisites are identified in the third edition of *Nursing: Concepts of Practice* (Orem, 1985, p. 96). The first category is concerned with the bringing about and maintenance of conditions of living that support life processes and promote human developmental processes toward higher levels of organization at each stage of the life cycle. This category of requisite is closely linked to the universal self-care requisite. The second category is concerned with action to prevent or to overcome the deleterious effects of personal deprivations, inadequacies of the social environment, and ill health and disability on development.

Nursing practitioners express that they experience difficulty in identifying the existence of, particularizing, and expressing developmental-type requisites. Nurses have a range of degrees of ability to identify and particularize such requisites for patients in various age groups. For example, one nurse identified that a patient's behavioral responses to normal everyday situations were similar to those of the self-indulgent adolescent. She went on to say that "although it can only be speculative, modification of his self-concept to accept his present health state [resultant from a cerebellar astrocytoma and treatment for same] has taken a toll on this patient's individuation process with a great need to maintain his sick role" (personal conference notes). Fear of the unknown, his future, no doubt, is affecting this young man's efforts to care for himself and is a motivating force in his seeking continuous contact with nurses and physicians.

Health-Deviation Type Self-Care Requisites are associated with disorders of human structure and functioning, active disease processes and injuries and their effects, and with the nature and effects of medical diagnostic and treatment measures. Six categories of health-deviation self-care requisites are identified in *Nursing: Concepts of Practice* (Orem, 1985, p. 99).

Nurses must be able to identify and particularize the health-deviation self-care requisites of their patients. They also must be able, under some conditions, to help patients or family members identify emerging requisites or make adjustments in existent ones. Nursing practitioners at times want to use the universal self-care requisites as their base for identifying health-deviation self-care requisites. The points of departure should be evidence indicative of the health state of the patient, including the lived experiences of the patient as well as the nature of and the expected and actual results of medical diagnostic and treatment measures.

In nursing practice it is important that nurses search out and understand existent and emerging relationships among self-care requisites. For example, the universal requisites of prevention of hazards and being normal are associated with each of the other six universal requisites. It is of great importance that nurses identify when patients' behaviors are in themselves hazards. For example, Mr. L.'s nurse asked herself: Why does this man have such an inadequate and health-destructive system of caring for himself? What additional knowledge do I need if I am to help out? What is his potential for development?

Particularization of the universal, developmental, and health-deviation self-care requisites of individuals is followed by the selection of a way or ways for meeting them. Then there is identification and setting of specifications for the sets and sequences of actions to be performed, to use a selected way or method to meet each particularized requisite. This work results in a product named the *therapeutic self-care demand.*

Therapeutic Self-Care Demand as a concept has as its referents sets of self-care measures or practices that have or are assumed to have some degree of validity and reliability in meeting particularized self-care requisites of individuals. Care measures or self-care or dependent-care practices result from investigation of questions about how self-care requisites can be met under prevailing conditions. A question about a requisite is: What is a sufficient intake of nutrients for a 10-month-old infant by time periods? If X is the quantity and quality of food and water that is sufficient for a 10-month-old infant, how can this food and water be provided to the infant?

This is a question about *method* or *means.* A question about *production operations* is: What actions must be performed using this method to provide the infant with this quality and quantity of food and water? Method and operations are combined in the term *procedure,* commonly used in nursing. In the frame of reference of self-care the preferred term is *care practices* or *care measures.*

The term *therapeutic self-care demand* has presented considerable difficulty to nurses. The formulation and expression of this concept took place over a period of three years during the 1960s, although as a notion it had been an integral theme in my own work and that of my colleagues in the validation of my concept of nursing. One difficulty noted in the beginning is the process of achieving conceptual consistency in the use of the term. This is related to the clustering of elements in the concept, which is a construction. Self-care requisites, methods of meeting them, and care measures do not concretely cluster together as a real world entity or event. The three-part cluster must be deliberately constructed by a person who seeks knowledge of what is the demand on this individual to engage in self-care. The use of the concept and the term requires a broad interpretation of the word *therapeutic* in the sense that the operations or purposive action that constitute the demand for self-care are projected as instrumentally productive of positive health results for an individual for whom the demand is computed.

From a practical action perspective, a properly constructed therapeutic self-care demand is a design for a system of self-care or dependent-care for an individual. The execution of this design with adjustments as needed by the individual's day-to-day performance of the specified measures of care, results in observable self-care or dependent care behaviors, which, in their relations to one another, reveal individual systems of self-care or dependent care. Nurses should be or become skilled in calculating therapeutic self-care demands for their patients and in helping patients to calculate or make adjustments in them.

From a health promotion perspective, it is the composition of the therapeutic self-care demand that reveals how its design is projected to contribute to the health and well-being of patients. When the design is constituted around a mix of universal and developmental self-care requisites focused on normal developmental process, prevention and maintenance, as well as promotion, are the health care foci. When the mix of requisites includes health-deviation requisites, there is added focus of movement to promote a more desirable state of health and to prevent deleterious effects on development.

The case method and the hypothetical-deductive method are useful in the empirical exploration of therapeutic self-care demands. The hypothetical-deductive method is applicable to exploration of some major influences determining therapeutic self-care demand in categories of patients. The case method is especially useful in describing the summation of self-care requisites specific to persons and self-care systems in relation to the therapeutic self-care demand.

THE WORK OF UNDERSTANDING SELF-CARE

Interest in self-care is on the increase. There are popular self-care movements, some of which are linked to notions referred to as *holistic care* and *holistic medicine*. Some of these movements negate the value of the time-honored health professions. There is the international movement within segments of the medical profession that emphasizes physicians helping patients learn to perform selected medical diagnostic and treatment measures. For example, a program titled the *Self-Activated Patient* was developed in the 1970s through the Department of Community Medicine of Georgetown University Medical School.

On a broader scale a Self-Care Institute was established in 1986 at the George Mason University School of Nursing in Fairfax, Virginia. A brochure indicates that "The . . . Institute seeks to bring together professionals from research, education, and practice to support the discovery and dissemination of knowledge for the advancement of self-care, and the understanding of health and illness from the consumer's point of view." This institute has its origin in The Center for Consumer Health Education established in 1976. Early research conducted by the Center demonstrated that a self-care program reduced physician visits, improved life style, and increased confidence in making decisions about health and medical care.

My concern is that these programs are instituted and conducted without adequate insight about the domain and boundaries of the human regulatory function named self-care and the nature of self-care as human endeavor. Nurses who accept and work with the self-care deficit theory of nursing have or should have those essential insights. Nurses in Sweden, Denmark, and Switzerland have been studying self-care with respect to the elderly patient. Nurses in Japan are interested and are embarking on a similar endeavor. Although a discipline of knowledge about self-care extends beyond nursing I see that the nursing profession can and should take the initiative in developing the theoretical, practical science of self-care and the related applied sciences. These are essential in the development of the practical and applied nursing sciences.

CHAPTER 25

Motivating Self-Care—The Reality: Persons as Self-Care Agents

INTRODUCTION

Self-care is action deliberately engaged in by men, women, and older children. It is activity learned through interpersonal relations and communications. Self-care is practical endeavor and as such is concerned with bringing about events and conditions that do not exist at the time when self-care actions are initiated. Actions produce events in time. When a specific action is completed what remains is the effect or result it produced. When specific actions are performed in sets and sequences to bring about events and results related to the production of some desired goal(s) reference is made to an action system. In this context self-care systems of individuals can be conceptualized.

The terms *self-care measures* or *self-care practices* have reference to all the sets of actions required in order for a specific self-care requisite to be met. For example, all the specific actions that must be performed in ordered relationships, one to another, to maintain fluid intake at a certain quantitative level, or the actions that must be performed to prevent the supplemental oxygen being provided to a person from being a hazard to the person's life and health, are self-care practices.

This paper was originally presented at the Wesley Hospital Conference, "Hospitals in the Community—A Vision," in Brisbane, Australia, June 3–5, 1987.

Nurses thus must have knowledge of the concrete actions that do and should constitute the self-care of individuals. They must know not only patients' usual self-care systems but also the self-care measures that are equal to the effective meeting of particularized self-care requisites, using one or a combination of methodologies: for example, meeting the requisite for maintenance of a sufficient intake of air by the breathing of environmental air supplemented when necessary by breathing an air-oxygen mixture.

Nurses who engage in nursing practice perform actions to bring about nursing results, namely, to ensure that patients' therapeutic self-care demands are met, that their capabilities to engage in self-care are protected, and that the exercise or development of their capabilities to engage in self-care is regulated. The term *nursing agency* is used to refer to capabilities needed by nurses if nursing results are to be attained for and with patients. Nurses must be knowledgeable and perceptive, not only about their individual patients as active or potential self-care agents, but also about themselves as active practitioners of nursing.

The topic "motivating self-care" must be understood and addressed within the broader frame of reference of human action. One psychologist, O'Doherty (1965), suggests that the concept of motivation is the most complex section of the whole of psychology. Allport (1960) and Arnold (1960) both developed lengthy and detailed analyses of theories of motivation. Motivation for these psychologists is linked to personality. In the context of nursing, motivation is addressed from the human perspective of individuals who consciously engage in action to bring about conditions in themselves, in their dependents, or in their environments that are or will be regulatory of their own or their dependents' functioning or development. Before proceeding to discuss motivational problems relative to self-care and dependent-care, I will present some assumptions and positions about motives and motivation.

MOTIVES AND MOTIVATION

Arnold (1960), in addressing motivation, raises two questions: Why does a living being act at all? and Why does he act as he does? She rejects the notion that living beings are "passive reactive systems" and postulates, on the basis of physiological data, that there is inherent activity in the "living organism as a whole, as well as within various organ systems," activity that is not initiated by sensory stimulation and ceases only with death.

Starting with the assumption of inherent activity rather than passivity or strict reactivity, Arnold seeks an explanation of how a specific action is initiated in any given case. Her position is that motives that arouse, sustain, and direct action are over and above internal.

Allport (1960) associates human motivation with intention, that is, with what the individual is trying to do, intention often taking the form of a self-image. He cites the example of the reformed thumb sucker, who, having adopted a concept of what he wants to be, is constrained to make good in the role he assumed. He associates specific goals set by persons for accomplishment with their long-range intentions and to dependable and desirable sets of values that they hold.

O'Doherty (1965) places motives within the frame of reference of human action and the causality inherent in it. He describes a motive as any thing, any event, or any process that contributes in any manner whatsoever to bring about a piece of behavior that can be observed. Thus the person's purposes, goals, and intentions; imagery, emotion, and instincts; long-range goals that impose form on specific behaviors; as well as the person's use of his or her functional capabilities, operate simultaneously as motives.

O'Doherty (1965) and Arnold (1960) indicate that every act of every human being is motivated and that there is no such thing as an unmotivated act. If nurses accept this position as well as the position that self-care and dependent-care are forms of human action directed to attain practical results in relation to the continuance of life, health, and well-being, then nurses must do two things:

1. Work from a model of deliberate goal seeking action for self-care, dependent-care, and nursing
2. Relate a theory or model of motivation to the model of deliberate action

These two tasks of nurses will now be addressed.

Models of Action and Motivation

In approaching the question of models of action and motivation it is necessary to take a position about human intelligence and understanding. The following ideas are adopted from Lonergan's 1967 work titled *Insight*.

Factual Insight

First, there are insights or understandings that are *factual* or *speculative*. For example, I see a person and make the judgment that the person is at least 80 years of age. I also see that the person is in a wheelchair. I then ask what is the *relation*, if any, between the age of the individual and the person being in a wheelchair? This is a question for investigation and I will need additional data to answer it. When I have the needed data I must give a *yes* or *no* answer to the question: Does the age of the person correlate with or govern the person's being in a wheelchair? There are two questions here: the question for investigation and the question for reflection.

Practical Insight

Second, there are insights or understandings that are *practical*. These understandings result from investigations that reveal the unities and relations of possible courses of action to bring about events and conditions in concrete situations, such as situations of nursing practice, that do not presently exist: for example, how to help Mrs. B. maintain an upright position. Insights about a possible course of action may give rise to further questions and should not lead blindly to performance of action. Reflection occurs and raises concerns *about the reasons* for taking this or that course of action and may reach the conclusion that the proposed action is "concretely possible, clearly effective, highly agreeable, quite useful, morally obligatory," and so on (Lonergan, 1967, p. 611).

Practical insight and reflection result in knowing what could be done in some concrete situation to change it and some or all of the reasons for doing these things. Reflection can go on and on and on, for there is no internal terminus to stop it. That which stops reflection (knowing) is the decision to do and the doing of the action. Lonergan (1967) suggests that reflection about things to be done occurs because as rationally self-conscious human beings we demand knowledge of what we propose to do and our reasons for doing it. He states that the normal duration of reflection is "the length of time needed to learn, the object [the goal] of the proposed act and to persuade oneself to willingness to perform the act" (p. 612). According to Lonergan, the normal duration (of reflection) is a variable that is inverse to one's antecedent knowledge and willingness. With a person's decision to act and as long as the person remains decided, the proposed course of action "has begun to be an actuality" (p. 612).

A Model of Deliberate Action

Any model of human action is schematic and does not reflect the complexity of a person taking action to achieve some foreseen end or goal. A number of models of deliberate action were developed or selected and used during the process of conceptualization and expression of the self-care deficit theory of nursing. Louise Hartnett's basic physiologic models of action reproduced in *Concept Formalization in Nursing: Process and Product* (second edition, NDCG, 1979, pp. 134–149) aided in the formalization of the concept of self-care agency. Talcott Parson's (1964) structural model of the unit act was adapted to nursing (see NDCG, 1979, p. 158). Arnold's model of deliberate action is useful for nursing purposes because it is a functional model. It includes knowing and appraising an object sought, wanting to know, wanting to do something, wanting to do this when something is appraised as good for action or when appraised as bad, resulting in inhibition of action (see Arnold, 1960, Vol. II, pp. 193–201, especially p. 201).

Concept Formalization in Nursing (NDCG, 1979, pp. 192–193) as well as *Nursing: Concepts of Practice* (Orem, 1980, pp. 68–69 and Orem, 1985, pp. 115–128) contain word models of deliberate action that are described in terms of phases of action and the operations associated with each phase. *Phase* is used in the sense of unfolding, a manifestation. *Operation* is used in the sense of a series of procedures to accomplish results specific to the phases of action. Self-care conceptualized as deliberate action is described as having three phases requiring performance of three separate sets of operations, one set for each phase.

The phases and operations of self-care are described.

Phase One—Estimative Type Operations—Product is Knowledge

- Investigation of internal and external conditions and factors significant for self-care
- Investigation of the meaning of these conditions for life, health, and well-being, and the importance of their regulation
- Investigation of the question: Can and how can existent conditions be changed or maintained?
- Reflection to determine the desirability of changing or maintaining conditions

Phase Two—Transitional Type Operations—Product is Decision

- Reflection to determine which course of self-care should be followed
- Deciding what will be done

Phase Three—Productive Type Operations—Product is Self-Care

- Preparation of self, materials, and the environment for performance of self-care measures
- Performance of regulatory care measures including monitoring during performance
- Monitoring for effects and results
- Reflection to determine adequacy of results and if action should be continued

The descriptions of self-care operations in *Nursing: Concepts of Practice* (Orem, 1980) combine the operations described for phases two and three into a single phase.

A Model of Motivation

Arnold's concept of motivation is an integral part of her model of deliberate action. Motivation is associated with reflection and is identified as the appraising of an action impulse (one's own) as desirable, that is, good. The process is described as moving from something appraised as good, for example, an object, a proposal, and so on, to a decision to act or to refrain from action. Arnold conceptualizes motivation within an action process.

First, there is the appraising of something as good or beneficial, for example, water or food, a cooler environment. This appraisal precedes movement toward the thing appraised. *Second,* there is the experiencing of an action impulse (a want) that is appraised as good—a good way to act, to drink, or eat. This experiencing of an action impulse, a wanting, requires that what we want to do be formed as an idea or that it is imagined before we decide to do it. The appraisal that it is desirable, good to act in this way, is the motivation that channels action in a particular way. *Finally,* there are decision and action to obtain what was appraised as good or beneficial and inhibit action toward what was appraised as bad, as disliked.

It is well known that men, women, and children take action to reach goals that have practical value but are not pleasurable. Strong desires for pleasurable goals are sacrificed for the sake of more important motives or wantings. Appraisals that result in such decisions about engagement in self-care at times mean discomfort and even hardship. According to Arnold, persons' awareness that they want something and their reflective judgment that their impulse to action is good together arouse both an emotion and a volitional tendency. She refers to these together as an *appetitive function* since they combine affective and desiring or striving (conative) aspects. Arnold's model of motivation thus combines the cognitive functions of knowing and judging with the described appetitive function.

This model of motivation is useful for nursing purposes when it is placed and understood within the larger configuration of action sequences needed to achieve results specific to self-care and to nursing. To make deliberate goal-attaining action sequences manageable, we deal with them in terms of operations. As nurses, to help patients make intelligent and reasonable decisions to meet or not meet their self-care requisites, we must help them make realistic appraisals and engage in reflection. Nurses' failures to help patients acquire knowledge and engage in reflection may result in failures of motivation on the part of patients. Sometimes patients are more able and more aware of such matters than are their nurses.

Conditions and Practices for Motivating Self-Care

The foregoing exposition of motivation leads us to stipulate that motivation is operational in all the stages of deliberate action—estimative, transitional, and productive. It is most clear-cut in the transitional phase where persons make decisions to practice specific forms of self-care to meet particularized self-care requisites or to take action to regulate the exercise or development of their self-care agency. Special assistance may be needed by persons under nursing care in any one or all of the stages. For example, a woman chooses to follow a diabetic management regimen. In assessing patient progress the nurse finds that the woman substitutes cake for bread. Six conditions that may encourage action tendencies for self-care are presented. These reflect the elements of Arnold's model of motivation. They are reproduced in the list that follows. Given acceptance of these conditions by nurses, rules of practice as well as technologies can be developed.

1. Persons must have available to them the knowledge that is necessary to distinguish something as good or desirable or bad and undesirable and to reflect upon its desirability or undesirability. The goal and ways to achieve it must be conceptualized or imagined.

2. Reasons for selection of ways of action to attain what has been appraised as good or desirable and afforded the tentative status of a goal should be known.

3. Time as well as knowledge is required in order for persons to form ideas about this or that way of action or to form images of each way of action as related to the goal.

4. Reflection should be directed to the questions: Is this way of acting good or desirable. Is it more desirable or less desirable than other ways of acting to achieve the goal?

5. Reflection about choosing a way of action could go on forever; therefore, it should be brought to a close with a decision when the ways of action have been conceived as clear ideas or clear images are formed.

6. A person owns his or her appraisal of possible ways of action to attain a goal and his or her decision to act according to one or a combination of these ways, when this way of acting is formalized and incorporated into the person's self-image or self-concept.

Self-Care Decisions

Insights about motivation can be derived from case materials accumulated by nurses in practice situations. The following examples of decisions made by a 68-year-old man, R., are taken from a retrospective study done by an acute care nursing specialist at a hospital in Columbia, Missouri, while R. was hospitalized for a second myocardial infarction that occurred within six weeks after the first episode (McEwan, 1986). The data descriptive of the decisions made were obtained by an interview that was focused on R.'s meeting of his health-deviation self-care requisites. Prior to the interview and after reading the chart, the acute care nursing specialist wrote, "I came away with the impression that R. was noncompliant. He was lacking in motivation or ability to learn to deal with his health state and possibly was a bit contrary." After the interview the nurse wrote, "All of the above was in error. R. was indeed very creative in dealing with his health state through self-care."

Decision 1: R. was in the waiting room of the garage where he was having his car tuned when he started having substernal chest pain with nausea, vomiting, and radiation of pain down both arms. He was diaphoretic and felt weak after the pain. He had the garage clerk call the ambulance to take him to the hospital.

Decision 2:   R. verbalized to the nurse, "My lungs are bad, don't pick up oxygen. My heart doesn't get enough oxygen which causes it to die. The last time I was here I pushed the doctor to release me. Now I'm going to stay until he says go."

Decision 3:   Early during R.'s prior hospital stay, on his physician's order he started the physical therapy part of the cardiac rehabilitation program. Nursing had assessed his readiness for rehabilitation and had found that he was not ready. Because of failures in communication he entered the program. The physiotherapist made the notation, eight days after R. entered the program, that "patient was not motivated to progress in the rehabilitation program," and ten days later the notation "patient declines further rehabilitation." R. said that he stopped the program because "they wanted me to do more than I've been able to do for the last 5–6 years 'cause of my lungs. I knew that I wasn't going to do that much at home."

Decision 4:   During hospitalization for the first heart attack R. had dietary consults. A dietitian made the following notation: R. "needs convincing that diet will help him." R. said that when he got home his neighbor, a dietitian, talked with him about his diet. "She made me go to two classes in town and she cooked for two days for me. I stopped the classes; they didn't tell me anything different from the books I had from the hospital. I stopped having her bring me food. She didn't use the salt right. You have to cook it into the food and you have to have it just right or it tastes bitter sure enough."

Decision 5:   R. has a small riding tractor that he uses to go fishing and go around for short distances. He has used this for many years because of his "breathing problem." When oxygen home therapy was approved for his use he planned to fix a place for his oxygen in the wagon he pulls behind his tractor so he could take it with him when he goes fishing.

The critical care nurse specialist, in a series of concluding statements, indicated that the effective use of the constructs of the self-care deficit theory of nursing by nurses caring for R. would have facilitated the development of an individualized plan of care that would have decreased R.'s stress during hospitalization and after hospital discharge, and provided essential information for physiotherapists and diet therapists and for his neighbor, the dietitian. R.'s need for maintenance of a balance between activity and rest would have been properly represented and planned for.

Examination of R.'s decisions and the appraisal of desirable and undesirable ways of action perhaps can be helped by reference to a philosophical exposition of the good and/or the desirable. Lonergan (1967), the Canadian philosopher and theologian, recently deceased, in his work titled *Insight* suggests that there are three levels of the good or the desirable. These are:

1. The elementary level of the good where what is good is the object of desire. At this level the good is coupled with its opposite, the bad. For example, to be cured of cancer is a good; if attained it is pleasant, enjoyable, satisfying.
2. The second level or aspect of the good is good of order, where the unique desire of human beings to know leads through understanding to the ordering of desires and adversions in concrete situations, formulations, and proposals, reaching agreements about them, and putting them into execution. The good of order is a function of human intersubjectivity. "A single order . . . constitutes the link between conditioning action and conditioning results" (p. 213).
3. The third level or aspect of the good is value as worth. This aspect emerges on the level of reflection and with deliberation and rational choice. Values are the object of choice and values are hierarchic. They must therefore be placed in an intelligible order by individuals.

Considering R.'s self-care decisions in relation to aspects of the desirable, the good allows us to formulate additional conditions for motivating self-care. Four conditions are added to the six already mentioned.

1. Persons should organize their knowledge about their particularized self-care requisites and the meaning of meeting these requisites for life, health, and well-being.
2. Persons should lay out the sets of actions and their proper sequences for meeting each particularized self-care requisite and attach to each the essential materials and environmental conditions, the times of performance, the duration of performance, and the labor required.
3. Persons should be able to estimate the discomfort or pain and the stress associated with prescribed courses of self-care.
4. Persons should be able to locate prescribed self-care within their hierarchies of values.

Motivation and Nursing Cases

Within the self-care deficit theory of nursing, motivating self-care can be viewed from two perspectives. The first is the performance of the estimative, transitional, and productive operations of self-care to meet therapeutic self-care demands. The second relates to actions persons engage in to develop or refine their capabilities to perform self-care operations.

Perspectives

These perspectives are illustrated by a nurse's description of the primarily white male population she worked with over a period of two years as hospital inpatients and as outpatients in her nursing clinic and by telephone (Robinson, 1986).

With respect to self-care operations it was identified that the majority of the patients needed to modify or change their management systems related to elimination and skin integrity. This often involved major modifications and the patients needed to learn a completely new system of managing. These types of demands are associated with (1) the pathology and treatment of cancer of the Gl or GU systems, or perforated diverticulum or fistula requiring a diversion or (2) wounds and drains requiring continuous management after hospital discharge and (3) skin breakdowns secondary to pressure. All patients required assistance in order for them to move to change their body image and to incorporate the changed ways into their self-concept.

Patients were generally highly motivated. They wanted to learn and to acquire the requisite knowledge and skills for performing the operations of self-care so that they could return to their homes. Most patients were from rural areas and were used to working with their hands as farmers, mechanics, and carpenters and hence had good manipulative skills. Patients usually had a support person—wife, other family member, or friend who was able to act as a dependent-care agent if needed.

This nurse identified a number of problems that she faced in practice but they were not related to absence of action tendencies to engage in self-care or dependent-care. The problems were related to energy levels of patients and dependent-care agents that permitted for learning and availability of systems to help patients manage chronic pain.

Types of Cases

In working with an adult ambulatory population Backscheider (1973) identified four major determiners of the amount and type of nursing required by members of the population. One determiner identified was that of motivational-emotional deficits. She indicates that such deficits may arise from the type of household, the environment, from which the patient comes. Two potentially detrimental type environments were identified.

1. High-stress, high demand households: The self-care limitation here is the amount of available energy the patient is free to direct to himself or herself. In this situation the important factor is the patient's position in the household in relation to management of the crisis.
2. Environmental situations where there is limited emotional input to the persons who are patients: The deficit here is in the area of reinforcement to the patient of his or her own value and support in maintaining consistency of the self-care regimen.

Another identified determiner that brings motivating self-care to the forefront was *major deficits in health with orientation combined with lack of time and prior orientation*. Backscheider identified this as a serious deficit when a patient's state results from the cultural environment and when the patient is dependent on orientation to this environment.

In cases of motivational-emotional deficits, there was a suggestion for compensatory actions on the part of nurses, ranging from recommendations for environmental changes to establishing ongoing systems of supportive nursing to the individual under care and of teaching and support for the family. In cases of major deficits in health orientation in situations where there is evidence of capacity and willingness to change, educative measures directed to the patient's significant others and an extensive educative-supportive nursing system for the patient were suggested.

SUMMARY

Motivating self-care is a matter internal to persons who are confronted with self-care requisites to be understood and met and with the development of the requisite knowledge and skills. Nurses should be aware of factors and events that may condition what patients can and do judge as desirable or undesirable action impulses preceding decisions to act in this way or that way. Some factors, events, and conditions are summarized.

1. Goals set by others for patient achievement are known by the patient to be unattainable.
2. Prescribed self-care measures are judged as irrelevant because the patient does not own a self that has need for such measures or own a self with particular structured or functional alteration of health state.
3. Overriding interests and concerns interfere with patients' attaining knowledge of a proposed or prescribed self-care regimen.
4. The complexity of the therapeutic self-care demand and the time and resource requirements for meeting it are overwhelming and cannot be handled.
5. Unrestrained pursuit of one self-care or self-management goal interferes with attention to other parts of the self-care regimen.
6. Inadequate knowledge results in invalid judgments about desirability of action tendencies.
7. Inability to ask questions occurs because of lack of sufficient knowledge about a self-care situation.
8. Patients are being pressured to make a decision.
9. There is an absence of environmental conditions that permit for reflection and for needed consultation about the desirability or undesirability of choices that are open to patients.

The approach taken in this paper to motivating self-care indicates its relationship to as well as its separation from decision making that precedes action. When persons are under health care from physicians or nurses, they are owed by the professionals (1) the nature of the diagnosis or the assessment that has been made, (2) authoritative information about the courses of action open to them, (3) detailed descriptions of any course of action that is complex and stress producing, (4) time and opportunities for reflection as well as the availability of consultation during this period, (5) assistance as needed to judge the validity of and to organize their concepts and images about particular courses of action, and (6) support to help them bring their reflections to closure. Knowledge, interests, and concerns of patients need to be distinguished from knowledge, interests, and concerns of nurses and physicians.

Persons with disabling conditions that appear or occur suddenly may not be ready to deal with the larger questions of what can and should be done. They have not lived with their condition and their lived experiences are novel. Their body images need to be rehabilitated and incorporated into their self-concepts and the distance of their self-concept from their self-ideal must be confronted. Slowly developing conditions provide greater time for adjustment of the self-concept and role learning.

Concrete impulses to action are associated with emotions but they also are formed through learning. When provided with a developmental type environment and effective nursing, patients with severe disability conditions, such as cardiac myopathy, learn how to monitor themselves and know the quality and amount of data needed to make valid judgments and decisions. They may not be able to perform the productive operations for self-care for long periods of time but they form ideas and images of what this care should be. The two perspectives from which nurses should examine "motivating self-care" can be dealt with by patients while under the care of nurses who respect patients' roles as self-care agents even when patients have limitations in role performance.

The matter of habit has not been addressed. Being motivated to act in a particular way does not require that our judgments and decisions remain in consciousness while we engage in action to reach a goal.

CHAPTER 26

The Profession and Nursing Science

The provision of nursing for individuals and groups is a complex undertaking, the features of which are poorly understood by members of the nursing professions, by physicians, by health service administrators, and by the public. Crisis situations come and go in nursing. There is the current nursing shortage. In the August 1988 issue of the *Nation's Health, The Official Newspaper of the American Public Health Association* under "State Health Reports," Richard Merritt (p. 12) sets forth issues relative to the nursing shortage. These he identifies as:

1. Internal problems within the nursing profession as it continues to struggle with its identity
2. Problems of standardization of an educational process that has four different paths leading to licensure as a nurse
3. Historically weak political representation
4. Mounting job pressures—increasingly high technology environments
5. Inadequate staffing
6. The continuing problem of the public's misconception of nursing's work

The problem of shortage of nurses and its resultant impact on society cannot be solved by the setting forth of issues, although this is important, or by the addition of new workers under medical control. The problem of

This paper was originally part of a consultation at the Veterans Administration Hospital in Fresno, California in September, 1988.

shortages and related issues demands that the nursing profession look at itself with understanding and a large measure of creativity. Nursing will continue to lose practicing nurses as well as potential nursing students if the profession fails to examine the nature and complexity of its societal responsibility, if it fails to initiate means to bring stability to nursing as a practice field and at the same time to extend and develop the frontiers of nursing practice and nursing education.

TASKS OF THE PROFESSION

Nurses have not been educated to think and communicate nursing, to know and to protect the domain and boundaries of nursing as a practice field, to be responsible for and contribute actively to the development and verification of nursing as a discipline of knowledge. Above all nurses must know the domain and boundaries of nursing and maintain willingness to bear the responsibilities for nursing as professional persons and as skilled technicians in practice settings. Nurses have not learned or are unwilling to accept that all arts and all sciences have a proper object that defines their domain of concern. If nurses are unknowing about why nursing has been institutionalized as a human service within societies, it is not difficult to grasp why nursing has not been developed as a discipline of knowledge and why nurses struggle with problems of identity in the health field.

To fulfill and maintain its societal position as an institutionalized human health service, the nursing profession, from my perspective, is confronted with at least three major tasks. These are:

1. To stabilize the nursing components of programs of nursing education and ensure that nursing courses are constituted from nursing content and not from content from other fields
2. To stabilize and continuously develop the frontiers of nursing practice within the domain and boundaries of nursing as a human health service supported by developed and developing nursing sciences
3. To formally confront the need for the continuing development of the practical science of nursing and the applied nursing sciences; to devise practical approaches toward these developments and in this way help to ensure the formalization of nursing as a discipline of knowledge

These are interrelated tasks that demand not only consideration and action but also the taking of positions about the nature and the placement of nursing in the world of man and human affairs.

Some nurses in various countries of the world, individually and in groups, have been and continue to be engaged in work contributing to resolving and solving problems of education, practice, and knowledge formalization. These efforts at times are unrecognized and at times are vigorously attacked within the profession. At times it is difficult for me to accept our failures to move nursing in a more positive direction. The work of resolving problems of nursing education and partial solutions to them that were addressed in the 1940s, 1950s, and 1960s go unrecognized.

Nursing is again into its oft-repeated cycle of failure to look at what kind of education will ensure the preparation and advancements of nurses (1) as functionally effective professionals and (2) as actively knowing and skilled nursing technicians. In the 1920s and 1930s, there was the proliferation of hospital diploma schools; in the 1940s, 1950s, and 1960s, there was the proliferation of vocational or practical nurse programs; in the 1960s and 1970s, there was real advancement in the quality of baccalaureate programs, but in these same years a proliferation of associate degree programs; in the 1980s, there is evidence of a decrease in the quality of baccalaureate programs and a continuing increase in master's programs, as well as a proliferation of doctoral programs in nursing with the question of whether the degree offered should be a Doctor of Nursing Science Degree or a Doctor of Philosophy Degree. Some of these movements in nursing education have contributed and continue to contribute to improved conditions in nursing practice that are found here and there and throughout our country. However, when taken together, they have been disruptive to advancing the provision of nursing in social groups. Perhaps the most disheartening thing about nursing education is the failure of nursing educators, both administrators and teachers, to recognize that nursing is undeveloped as a discipline of knowledge and their failure to act within the profession to change the situation.

Perhaps the first thing to do as individuals is to ask and answer the question *What has been done?* Some good work is under way; some work has been done already toward task accomplishment. In 1988, as the decade and this century draw to a close, we should look for the judgments, decisions, and practical endeavors that make nursing an effective force in social groups as well as those judgments, decisions, and endeavors that continue to detract from the good that can be accomplished through nursing.

The tasks are interrelated but at the same time must be separate and apart. They must be understood by nurses both in their independence and their dependence. In the professions, the critical factor is the knowledge that members of the profession have accumulated, verified, and made available for other practitioners and for nursing students. The critical factor of nursing knowledge should be the first focus of our attention.

THE PRACTICAL SCIENCE OF NURSING

The practice fields of medicine, engineering, and architecture have developed bodies of knowledge in the form of applied sciences and practical sciences, including the technologies of each field. In nursing we are not so fortunate since nursing knowledge, for the most part, is scattered and unstructured. Why is this so? In large part, as I see it, the profession has never accepted the responsibility for the formalization and structuring of nursing knowledge, or for the quality of nursing provided. It would benefit each one of us to read Esther Lucille Brown's 1948 publication *Nursing for the Future*, especially its last page, from which the following quotation is taken.

> By every means at its disposal the nursing profession, collectively and individually, must take a positive position concerning itself and the significance of its function. It must be unquestionably in that position as are the medical and legal professions which assume that their existence—on a progressively higher level of competence—is a "social necessity and act accordingly." [p. 198]

Today, when I hear expressions from nurse leaders such as "nurses are doing their own thing," or "nurses are no longer handmaidens to physicians," I wonder why these leaders do not speak to nursing's function, its proper service to members of society, the reasons such service is needed, and how the service that is nursing relates to the service that is medicine. Professionals should be able to think nursing, to produce nursing, and to communicate nursing to their patients and patients' families, to other nurses, to physicians, and to other health professionals. To do this, nurses must know nursing as a practical science and as a set of applied sciences. Movement toward this goal has begun. One beginning is in nurses' interest in understanding nursing within the frame of reference of the self-care deficit theory of nursing, or self-care nursing theory, as it is referred to by some nurses.

ONE GENERAL THEORY OF NURSING

Self-care deficit nursing theory is a descriptive explanation of nursing that holds in all situations of nursing practice. For this reason it is referred to as a general theory. It is properly referred to as a theory because it descriptively explains the relationships between nurses and persons who can be helped through nursing in terms of their characterizing qualities. The theory is constituted from three articulated theories: the theory of nursing system, which articulates with the theory of self-care deficit and the theory of self-care. The theory of nursing system is descriptively explanatory of what nurses produce as they nurse, the objective focus and the results of their activities. The theory of self-care deficit is explanatory of why persons require and can be helped through nursing. The theory of self-care explains self-care as a human regulatory function, that is, it is essential for continued life and functioning, as well as growth and development and demands continuous production. These theories were formulated in 1986 and are expressed in Orem and Taylor (1986). [Ed. Note: The theory is also explained in some detail in Chapter 7 of Nursing Concepts of Practice, sixth edition.]

The general theory of nursing is understood in its relation to five underlying assumptions (Orem, 1985). These assumptions focus on (1) self-care and dependent care as regulatory functions essential for life; (2) the learned ability to act for self and others with respect to self-care; (3) limitations of and exercise of self-care agency and dependent care agency; (4) the institutionalization of dependent care; and (5) nursing in social groups.

The history of the development of self-care deficit nursing theory is recounted in Nursing: Concepts of Practice (Orem, 1985, pp. 18–22 and pp. 30–34), and in Concept Formalization in Nursing: Process and Product (NDCG, 1979, pp. 129–180), in the chapter titled "Dynamics of Concept Development." The figure, "Stages of Understanding Nursing" (Orem, 2001, p. 171), is helpful in understanding what has been done and what needs to be done in the continuing development of the practical science of nursing, using the conceptualizations and other constructs of self-care deficit nursing theory. It is evident from the figure that theorists, scholars, and nursing practitioners have a large role in this development. The role of the nursing administrator is also evident.

PROFESSIONAL NURSING PRACTICE

The deliberate and planned use of self-care deficit nursing theory to give direction to nursing practice has been ongoing since the late 1980s. Nurses make, that is, produce, nursing systems as they perform the process operations of nursing practice: nursing diagnosis, nursing prescription, and nursing regulation. The component elements of self-care deficit nursing give focus and structure to these operations. Process operations are not in and of themselves unique to nursing. Every human service has process operations. It is nurses' knowledge of the domain and boundaries of nursing and nurses' mastery of theoretically and clinically practical nursing that is enabling for the production of nursing. [*Ed. Note:* For a description of changes associated with mastery and use of self-care deficit nursing theory and changes in administration with use of the theory, see chapter 23, "Changes in Professional Nursing Practice Associated with Nurses' Use of Orem's General Theory of Nursing." Excerpts from that paper were included in this paper when it was originally delivered.]

THE SCIENTIFIC AND THE PRACTICAL
IN NURSING PRACTICE

There is a problem in the profession that demands concerted attention. This is the problem of nursing practitioners, educators, and researchers understanding both the practical and the scientific aspects of nursing. A laying out of the practical aspects of nursing is helpful. These aspects are taken for granted and their meaning and importance for nursing science is not addressed. We should consider and reflect upon each of the following practical features of nursing (Lonergan, 1958, pp. 609–624).

1. Nursing is provided in concrete nursing practice situations where prevailing conditions are specific to each situation of practice and where the events that occur are situation specific.
2. Nurses inquire, discern, and make concrete judgments about events that occur and conditions that prevail in each specific nursing practice situation and attach nursing meaning to them (speculative or factual insight about situations, concrete judgments of fact).
3. Nurses inquire, discern, and make judgments about possible causes of action within the domain of nursing that would bring about desirable but presently nonexistent conditions and events (practical insights, judgments about what unities and correlations can be brought about).
   Note: Practiced insight can be formulated in a proposition of the

type: Under such and such circumstances the intelligent thing to do is to make such and such a decision (Lonergan, 1958).

4. Nurses reflect about the courses of action that would bring about desirable conditions and events, scrutinize the objects of action, investigate motives for possible cause of action, and terminate reflection with decisions about what will be done.

5. Nurse act to bring about desirable conditions and events through which nursing results are achieved.

If we accept the foregoing characteristics of nursing practice we must admit that nurses must have antecedent knowledge if they are to be knowing in factual and practical ways about concrete nursing practice situations where individuals or groups are under their care. This antecedent knowledge must enable nurses to attend to nursing practice situations from the perspective of nursing, to make accurate factual and practical judgments, and to make decisions that are not arbitrary but are selections of "intelligible, intelligent, and reasonable courses of action" (Lonergan, 1958, p. 621).

Essential antecedent knowledge for nursing practice includes the accepted components of the professional or the high level technical forms of education for the occupations and professions.

Courses specific to the field of practice
Foundational science courses
Basic science courses
Liberal arts and humanities
Continuing education courses

From the beginning of university education for nursing, educators have verbalized the existence of the undeveloped nursing science. At the same time they focused their attention on the sciences foundational to nursing, sciences that are enabling for understanding courses in the professional field, and on liberal arts and humanities courses. For example, in 1939, a dean of a university school of nursing wrote as a foreword to a symposium the following:

Nursing education is a new science in the university family; as a profession nursing is undergoing rapid change. As yet from the broad fields of philosophy and science, nurse educators have not been able to select the content which may be sharply defined as in the nursing field or delete that which does not belong to it. Consequently nurse students either need to become specialists in a number

of fields of knowledge beside their own, or be content with a superficial selection
of knowledge which is helpful in the practice of the nursing arts and sciences.
[*Ed. Note:* source unknown]

Reading this quotation brings to our attention the principle that insights
about the practical science of nursing and its conceptual framework provide
the basis for the selection of the sciences foundational to understanding the
scientific developments in the practice field. For example, the conceptual
elements of self-care deficit nursing theory demand that nursing students
have knowledge of anatomy, physiology, psychology, deliberate action,
and action systems. The theoretical concept of therapeutic self-care demand
also sets up requirements from a practice perspective of the kinds of skills
and experiences that will enable nurses to be conscious of the relationship
between what they know and what they do.

The message to the profession is that scientific bodies of knowledge,
nursing sciences, developed and verified by nurses, must serve them with
respect to understanding fulfillment of the five previously named features
of nursing practice. This means that nursing science as science is necessarily
theoretical in form but practical in intent. If we accept and understand
conceptualizations of practice disciplines and practical science we know
that these scientific developments range from purely theoretical constructs
that are descriptive and explanatory of practice to those that are more
practical in that they describe and explain what is and what can be done
in some narrow segment of the practice field. "The Form of Nursing
Science" (Orem, 1988) provides a background for understanding the practical science of nursing. Understanding is represented as occurring in stages
that are not sequential but are interlocking as students of nursing move
through these five stages of

1. Describing and explaining nursing in the form of a general theory
   of nursing
2. Laying out the range of variation of the broad conceptual elements
   of the general theory of nursing based upon concrete conditions
   and factors associated with the variations
3. Development and validation of models and rules of nursing practice
4. Development of descriptions of nursing cases, including their natural history
5. Development and validation of models and rules for the provision
   of nursing to populations

Development of the technologies of nursing practice would be concurrent with the five stages of development of practical nursing science.

The self-care deficit theory of nursing, as it has been developed, and continues to be developed, is a bringing together of the scientific and practical in nursing. Through its development we have a structure for the continued development, organization, and verification of nursing knowledge. Points of theory in nursing that articulate with points of theory or facts in other fields provide the basis for development of applied nursing sciences.

Nursing science and nursing art, like all sciences and arts, begin with objectification. Objectification is the separation out of one's conceptualization of the focus or what is dealt with by the science or art and affording it an objective existence so that one can deal with it as object. My insight and conceptualization of the reason people can be helped through nursing led me in 1958 to express the proper object of nursing. For me this was a first step toward the development of theoretically and clinically practical nursing knowledge.

PRESERVICE NURSING EDUCATION

The form of education for nursing has been and continues to be a major problem for the nursing profession. One wonders if the problems of 2088 will be similar to those of 1988. Positions taken about forms of education preparatory for nursing should be based upon both enduring and changing needs of populations for nursing as well as upon what is needed to ensure the survival and advancement of nursing as a profession that truly serves society. No profession develops, survives, and advances without professionally prepared members who function as practitioners, scholars, theorists, researchers, developers, and teachers in university programs. These persons who bear the professional responsibility for stabilizing and extending the frontier of practice and for the sciences and the technologies of nursing should have university-level education. Initial and subsequent degrees, career pathways, and entry to practice should be investigated and firm decisions made about suitable courses of action.

The enduring and changing needs of members of populations for nursing and the advances made in the formalization of the combinations of technologies essential for use in producing nursing for various types of nursing cases are indicators of the feasibility of preparing persons through high-level technical education or vocational-technical type preparation. In any practice field where the knowledge essential for use in practice is scattered and relatively unstructured, persons can be educated to structure the required knowledge. If this is not done, one is left with the task approach.

Since the late 1960s, self-care deficit nursing theory and the theories from other fields related to it have been used to identify essential content for nursing courses. The main components of the theory have been used as content organizers. The theory formed within a practice frame of reference is useful in giving meaning and form to the process operations of nursing. Nursing components of preservice curricula, when designed with understanding of and around the substantive content of self-care deficit nursing theory, may need adjustments, but the need for substantial revisions is eliminated.

In the high-level technical form of occupational education and in the generic professional form at whichever level offered, there is necessarily an emphasis on the technologies essential for use in nursing practice that have demonstrated validity and reliability. In the late 1960s I developed a listing of types of nursing technologies with the understanding that some of them would have their foundations in other fields or would be taken from other health services for use within a nursing context. The technologies were identified and published in a paper titled "Levels of Nursing Education and Practice," in the *Alumnae Magazine of the Johns Hopkins Hospital School of Nursing* (Orem, 1969). A modified version of them is on p. 4 of the first edition of *Nursing: Concepts of Practice* (Orem, 1971). The technologies were identified as:

1. The technologies through which interpersonal, intergroup, and intragroup relations are in existence and maintenance as long as such relations are essential for achievement of nursing and nursing-related goals in specific nursing situations
2. The technologies of human assistance through which help or service is rendered by one person to another
3. The technologies of individual personal care that is self-administered by adults or administered by them to infants and children (culturally derived, affected or unaffected by scientific knowledge)
4. The technologies for appraising and regulating man's integrated functioning with emphasis on physiologic and psychologic modes of functioning in health and disease
5. Processes that bind persons together in therapeutic relationships

6. Technologies for bringing about and controlling the position and movement of persons in a physical environment
7. Processes, including methods and techniques of research, for formalizing and establishing the validity and reliability of the above-named technologies

A part of the development of nursing as a body of knowledge is the formal structuring of technologies that will bring about the unities or correlations understood, through the practical insights of nurses about nursing cases, to be possible as well as desirable.

Nursing education will advance in effectiveness to the degree that the profession moves to advance the development of nursing sciences, and ensures that nursing education produces nurses who can think as well as do nursing, and who function as beginning, advancing, or advanced professional nursing practitioners or as nurses qualified by high-level technical education to be creative and inventive in nursing situations that require the use of validated and reliable technologies.

A profession that overlooks or does not deal with and control the nursing practice roles of persons prepared in the educational programs approved by the profession does not serve society. Before change can come about in nursing, the profession must ensure that nursing within the health care system of the country is under the control of responsible nurses and not under the control of non-nurses, regardless of their fields or their positions.

CHAPTER 27

Theory Development in Nursing

P URPOSE: To provide the student with a basis for understanding theory construction and the role that theory plays in providing the scientific basis for practice fields.

Historically, or from a time perspective, I have been involved with questions about the domain and boundaries of nursing as a field of knowledge and a field of practice since my days as a graduate student in the 1940s.

1. In writing definitions—as a graduate student, as a staff worker, or for the current project, and in 1956 when I felt the need to express how I understood nursing (see chapters 1 and 2)
2. 1958—Need to know the domain and boundaries of nursing for purposes of curriculum development
   a. What condition exists when decisions are made that individuals are in need of nursing? Why do people need or benefit from nursing?
   b. Concept of self-care; concept of self-care limitations
   c. Concept of nursing
3. Development of a Conceptual Model
   a. Understanding elements and relationship in nursing practice systems (see Figures 27.1, 27.2, 27.3)
      Formulation and expression of concepts and relation
   b. Gradual development of substantial structure of a concept
4. Formulation and expression of a concept or a theory of nursing system

---

This paper consisting of notes prepared for presentation to students in 1988 presents the process of theory development in outline form.

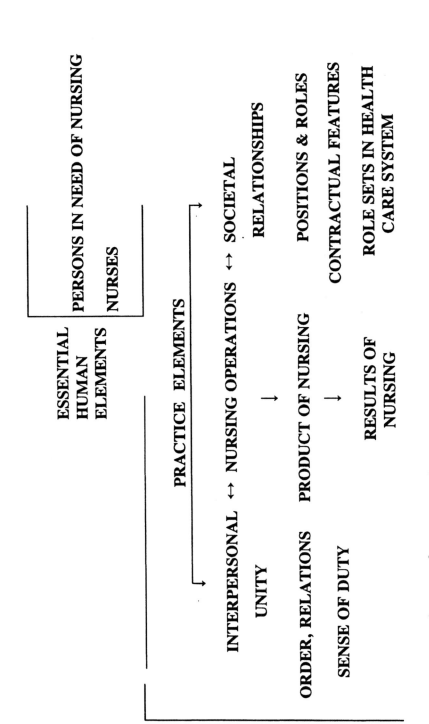

FIGURE 27.1   Elements of nursing practice.

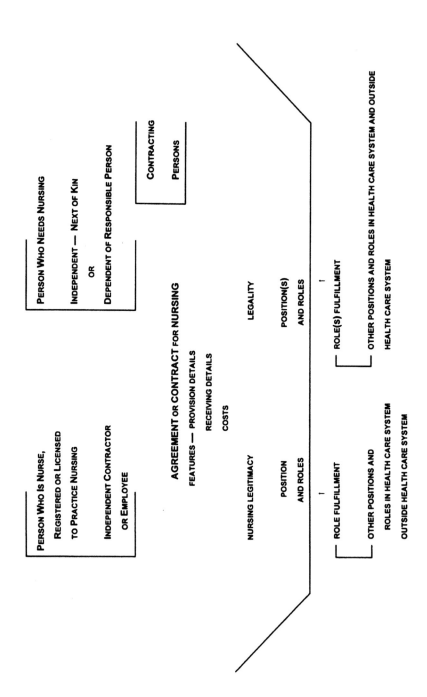

FIGURE 27.2 The societal situation.

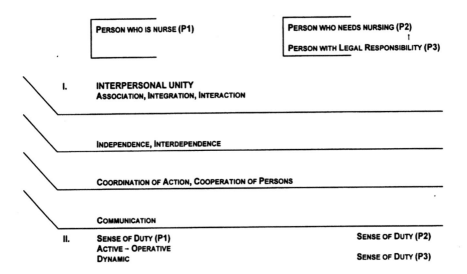

FIGURE 27.3 The interpersonal situation.

Refer: development of the concept of nursing system (see Figures 27.4, 27.5)

Basic Positions

a. nursing is a social instrument
b. practice field
c. bodies of knowledge about nurses and nursing
d. practical science and a set of applied science

The practical science of nursing

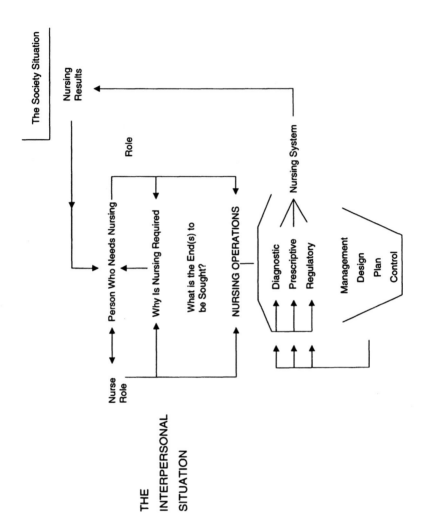

FIGURE 27.4   The focal nursing situation.

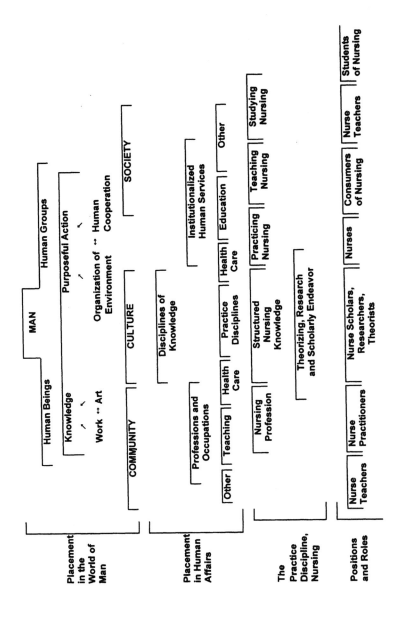

FIGURE 27.5   The placement of nursing in the world of man and human affairs.

253

The Development of the Self-Care Deficit Theory of Nursing: Events and Circumstances

This general theory of nursing, considered as a way of understanding and guiding nursing practice, has served and continues to serve as a nucleus for the development of the theoretically and clinically practical nursing sciences. The cumulative nursing insights of nurses using and developing the theory, and their reflections and judgments about their insights, constitute a well-defined system of nursing knowledge, subject throughout to checking and verification. Since I am a contemporary of these developments what I can recount about the initial and subsequent stages of theory development is autobiographical rather than historical. My experiences, my insights about the complex entity named nursing, my thoughts, and my reflections and judgments form the bases for my approach to the topic.

The presentation is in two parts. The first part identifies what I have named *positions about nursing*, mental points of view or ways of regarding ·nursing. The second part recounts events and circumstances in the development of the self-care deficit theory of nursing as the basis for development of systems of nursing knowledge. System is used in the sense of structured, interrelated knowledge components. The taking of positions about nursing and the development of the theory and its constituent elements overlap

This paper was originally prepared in August of 1988 for presentation at the University of Missouri-Columbia Conference in St. Louis, November 1988.

in time. I shall not attempt to explore the relationship between them. Some relationships are self-evident.

POSITIONS AND POSITION TAKING

Position, as previously indicated, is used in the sense of a mental point of view about nursing. My awareness of taking positions about nursing extends from the late 1930s to the present.

Taking of positions about nursing or other matters involves recognition of and attending to a question or an issue, investigation, development of insights, reflection, and finally a judgment about an answer to the question or the side of an issue that is relatively unconditioned and can, therefore, be accepted as a point of view. The taking of this or that position about nursing has a beginning. As a point of view a position, if not discarded, may develop over time. For example, in 1938 I had the insight that nursing and nursing education are distinguished by the different *consumers* of the two services, namely, persons in need of nursing and persons who aspire to work as nurses. In the 1950s, within the frame of reference of the products of organized enterprises, I developed the idea of nursing as a consumer service and the ideas of nursing education as a producer service. These ideas were formally expressed in a paper developed in the late 1960s titled "Nursing and Nursing Education: The Problem of Relations" (see chapter 10).

Position taking, as indicated, always involves choice and decision making. Choice and decision, as well as the maintenance and development of a position, require knowledge of the foundations for or the basis of the position.

Eight positions about nursing are identified as expressing my point of view about nursing as a field of practice and a field of knowledge.

1. Nursing has been introduced into and institutionalized by societies as a human service in order to meet recognized action limitations of members of these societies or social groups with respect to care of self and care of dependents. Nursing is not a naturally existent entity; it is made or produced.
2. The human service of nursing and the practice of its provision is a consumer service. Nursing education is a producer service making available to interested persons a way to qualify themselves to provide the human service of nursing.

3. Nursing as a human service is a form of practical endeavor to bring about conditions that do not exist at the time deliberate result-producing action is begun.
4. Nursing is a practice field. When developed as a field of knowledge, nursing would be descriptive and explanatory of the practice field.
5. Nursing practice involves nurses in interpersonal and contractual relationships with their patients and others.
6. Nursing as a discipline of knowledge would have the form of a practical science and a set of applied nursing sciences.
7. Applied nursing sciences are formed as facts, and points of theory from developed sciences are used to explain nursing facts and nursing points of theory and give form to nursing technologies.
8. Applied nursing sciences are differentiated from bodies of knowledge that are specialties within other fields such as philosophy, history, or law. Examples include nursing ethics, nursing history, and nursing jurisprudence.

In the nursing profession, there is a tendency to overlook the confusion that continues to exist among nurses about where we, as nurses, fit within the world of men, women, and children, and in human affairs. The taking of positions about nursing is an essential step for nursing practitioners, scholars, teachers, theorists, researchers, and developers as they fulfill their essential roles in the provision of nursing, in the preparation of nurses, and in the development and verification of nursing knowledge.

A SYSTEM OF NURSING KNOWLEDGE

Developments—1940 to 1960

My movement from a commonsense approach to knowing nursing to a scientific approach had its beginnings in 1958 when I understood and conceptualized why people need and can be helped through nursing. I had insights about the answer to this question in 1956 but it was not until 1958 that I had this knowledge in a way that was essentially a part of me and formed a basis for progressive and coalescing insights about the world of the nurse and what nurses do within this world. Prior experiences in nursing, in nursing education, and in other areas of interest, as well as a number of events that led me to focus on *nursing as knowledge,* contributed to my movement to describe and explain nursing. Three events prior to 1958 are identified.

In the early 1940s I was confronted, along with other graduate students in a curriculum development class, with the task of formulating a definition of nursing. In 1948, as a staff member of a committee to explore the redesigning of a baccalaureate program for registered nurses, I was involved again in the task of defining nursing. The results of both of these efforts placed nursing within the context of the levels of preventive health care and viewed patients of nurses as persons who functioned biologically, rationally, and spiritually. Reflection on the definition produced for the 1948 curriculum project led to judgments about the essential nature and the desirable extent and depth of the liberal arts and humanities component of the baccalaureate curriculum, and confirmed the importance of foundational science and public health science content. Nursing results were identified in terms of levels of preventive health care but there was no movement to change the content of the traditionally accepted practice areas of nursing.

A definitive movement toward my working with nursing as a field of knowledge as well as a field of practice occurred in the 1950s as I functioned as a consultant with the Division of Hospital and Institutional Services of the Indiana State Board of Health. During the period 1949 to 1957 I had intensive involvement with nurses and their practice of nursing in general hospitals in Indiana. My contacts with nurses impressed upon me their interests in nursing—their desire for progress, as well as the absence of knowing leaders in nursing. I became aware of and somewhat overwhelmed by the inability of nurses to communicate nursing to their patients, to other nurses, to physicians, to hospital administrators, and to members of hospital boards of trustees. During this time I was involved in working with Martha O'Malley, M.D., the Director of the Division, and with Robert Rogers and Carl Heinz, hospital administrators, in laying out the functions and operations of general hospitals—the patient care function, the distribution of service function, and the financing function. I also worked with Ann Poorman on studies of factors that condition the provision of nursing in general hospitals. Studies were focused on the organizational structure of nursing services, number of admissions and discharges of patients by time periods, length of patient stay, and so on. There was a one-year study of the characteristics of a population of a 600-bed hospital by admitting physician, length of patient stay, admitting and discharge medical diagnoses, and the age and sex of persons admitted. I was firmly convinced at this time and am still convinced about the importance of population studies as one basis for the design and management of nursing services.

In 1956, I completed a study of administrative positions within the nursing service of one Indiana hospital. The 1956 report of this study, titled *Hospital Nursing Service: An Analysis,* included two appended chapters titled "The Art of Nursing" (see chapter 2) and "Essential Requirements for the Practice of Nursing" (see chapter 1). After completion of the study report, I felt a need to record my thoughts about nursing. The two named chapters are the result. The named sections of these two chapters indicate the nature of the content and its organization. The definition of nursing in the chapter "The Art of Nursing" is relevant to our topic. It reads as follows:

> Nursing is an art through which the nurse, the practitioner of nursing, gives specialized assistance to persons with disabilities of such a character that more than ordinary assistance is necessary to meet daily needs for self-care and to intelligently participate in the medical care they are receiving from the physician. The art of nursing is practiced by doing for the person with the disability, by helping him do for himself and/or by helping him learn to do for himself. Nursing is also practiced by helping a capable person from the patient's family or a friend of the patient to learn how to do for the patient. Nursing the patient is thus a practical and a didactic art. [Orem, 1956, p. 85]

This 1956 definition of nursing can be contrasted with statements about nursing that appear in the 1959 U.S. Government Printing Office Publication *Guides for the Developing Curricula for the Education of Practical Nurses* (Orem, 1959).

> Nursing is for persons who need direct continuing assistance in self-care because of a health situation; requirements for assistance may relate to needs common to all people regardless of health state as well as to needs which exist only because of present state of health. [p. 2]

> The initial and the continuing development of nursing and the continued spread of nursing practice rests on the inabilities of people to care for themselves at times when they need assistance because of their states of personal health. [p. 5]

> Nursing is perhaps best described as the giving of direct assistance to a person . . . because of the person's specific inabilities in self-care resulting from a situation of personal health. Care as required may be continuous or periodic. Self-care means the care that all persons require each day. It is the personal care which

adults give to themselves, including attention to ordinary health requirements, and the following of the medical directives of their physicians. Nursing may be required by persons in any age group, but it is the situation of health and not the dependencies arising from age which initiates requirements for nursing. Requirements for nursing are modified and eventually eliminated when there is progressive favorable change in the health state of the individual, or when he learns to be self-directing in daily self-care. [pp. 5–6]

Also of interest is Chapter 59 in the *Guides* titled "Nursing Situations." Insights expressed in this chapter are later refined and coalesced to yield the guiding insights and concepts expressed in the first edition of *Nursing: Concepts of Practice* (1971) and *Concept Formalization in Nursing: Process and Product* (NDCG, 1973). What is evident in the *Guides* is my focus on inabilities in self-care due to a situation of personal health, the beginning development of the concept of self-care limitations, and the concept of self-care requisites. This focus and related concepts resulted from my 1958 insight about the proper object of nursing.

The formation of categories and classifications occupied a central position in the *Guides*. In this work I sought to lay out the domain and boundaries of nursing in order to identify an educationally justifiable nursing component for a vocational-type nursing curriculum. Prior to this time the nursing component of vocational-type curricula was identified in the form of lists of tasks.

During my tenure with the Indiana State Board of Health I was given the opportunity to become familiar with authoritative works and journals in the fields of organization and administration, to attend seminars of The American Management Association, and to have contact with a nationally recognized management consultant. I read in the fields of social philosophy and also became interested in Pitirim Sorokin's *Social and Cultural Dynamics* (1957) in four volumes. Reading in social philosophy enabled me to fit what I had learned about organization into the larger scheme of things and to develop understanding of order and relations and of organizations as created entities. Sorokin's work was generally illuminating and practically helpful in understanding the whole area of relationships. His developments of contractual, familial, and coercive relationships and his treatment of social interaction were particularly helpful. Interest in both fields continued and increased.

During the period of the 1940s to the 1960s, I accepted that nursing and self-care were forms of deliberate human action. I trace my attention to the idea of deliberate action back to my exposures to lectures in general ethics and the distinction between acts of man (involuntary acts) and human acts (voluntary acts). I became interested in and pursued the treatment of human action in the *Summa Theologica* of Thomas Aquinas (1974) and in Aristotle's Book II, Chapter 3 of *Nicomachean Ethics*. I was impressed with Talcott Parsons' expressed concept of the unit act and his analysis of its elements and the relationships among the elements expressed in his early work, *The Social System* (1951). In one of his later works he states: "By conceiving the processes of the social system as action processes, in the technical sense . . . it becomes possible to articulate with the established knowledge of motivation which has been developed in modern psychology and thereby as it were, to tap an enormous reservoir of knowledge" (Parsons, 1964, p. 20). He continues by stating that the act is the unit of any system of action. "The act becomes a unit of a social system so far as it is a process of interaction between its author and other actors" (p. 24). Parsons clearly distinguishes his use of the term *actor* or *agent*: "the actor is himself a social unit, the organized system of all the statuses and roles referable to him as a social object and as the author of a system of role activities" (p. 25). The differentiation of the meaning Parsons attributes to the term actor or agent from the meaning attributed to it in self-care deficit nursing theory, namely a person who performs a specific kind of action, is mentioned at this time because of published references to the influences of Talcott Parsons on my work. My interest in human action and action theory continued into the next period of theory development from 1960 to 1970. One of the matters that was faced during this period was the need within nursing to clearly distinguish action in interpersonal situations from action in the broader societal perspective. It was Eamon O'Doherty, a behavioral scientist, who helped me and my colleagues in making this distinction.

Developments—1960 to 1970

The most appropriate title for this period is the conceptualization of the end product of nursing. My work and the work of my colleagues had a basis and a point of departure in the concepts of nursing and the concepts of self-care expressed and published in the 1959 *Guides for Developing Curricula for the Education of Practical Nurses* and in further ideas I expressed during the period 1959 to 1965.

From 1959 to 1970, I taught and worked with graduate students at The Catholic University of America in the School of Nursing's program in

Administration of Nursing Education. From the perspective of teaching and scholarship, it was for me both an enlightening and a somewhat overwhelming experience, since three practice fields had to be brought together—the practice field *education* and to be articulated with the practice field *nursing* and then with the practice field *administration*. I also contributed to the teaching of core courses for graduate students, courses focused on organization and on nursing. During the entire period of the 1960s I continued to develop insights about nursing and to coalesce them into concepts and conceptual structures. The results of this effort are found in the first edition of *Nursing: Concepts of Practice* (1971). The nursing practice content in this work appeared in manuscript form in the 1960s and was used as a basis for curriculum development in the nursing component of one associate degree program at Morris Harvey College in Charleston, West Virginia. The manuscript was made available for use by nursing students enrolled in the program. During this period McGraw-Hill was interested in my development of a textbook on nursing as part of a series of textbooks for practical or vocational nursing students. As my insights about nursing increased, I saw their importance for all levels of nursing education. I knew that it would be impossible for me to write a book developing a conceptual structure for nursing that could be kept within the domain of work of the practical nurse. Finally, the McGraw-Hill editor, Joseph Breem, saw the worth of my efforts and made the decision to publish *Nursing: Concepts of Practice* in 1971. During this period I became a member of a faculty committee of the School of Nursing of The Catholic University of America named the Nursing Model Committee. The history of the work of this committee is recounted in both editions of *Concept Formalization in Nursing: Process and Product* in 1973 and 1979. The overall concern of this committee and its successor, The Nursing Development Conference Group, as expressed in 1965, was the development of a research model in the art of nursing, The position was taken that such a model is a "model for *a creative end product* and the end product is the test of the research" (Nursing Development Conference Group, 1979, p. 105). This expressed purpose led to the frequent asking of two questions by Committee and Group members: What do nurses make when they nurse? What is the product of nursing? There was agreement that insights about the end product of nursing would be put to two tests;

1. Can existent realities in nursing practice situations be shaped in conformity with the conceptualized product of nursing?

2. Does the result conform to the conceptualization of the product of nursing?

My interest and concerns and those of my colleagues were focused on finding the order in nursing as well as on describing and explaining nursing's end product. Early in our work (1965) we accepted that a body of nursing knowledge would have the form of a set of applied nursing sciences and a practical science of nursing. We accepted that practical science was one of action, behavior, conduct. It says how we ought to behave and includes development of a method. Our combined work has contributed primarily to the development of the practical science of nursing. Points of articulation of nursing theory with other sciences continue to develop.

By 1968 the elements of my 1958–1959 expressed concept of nursing had been verified by me and my colleagues through analysis of nursing cases. New insights enabled me and other group members at a three-day work session to formulate and express the now well-known concepts of therapeutic self-care demand, self-care agency, and nursing agency. These concepts were incorporated into the concept of nursing system expressed in 1968. These conceptualized characteristics of persons in need of nursing and of persons who are nurses and the dynamics among the attributed characteristics were expressed as dependent upon the dynamics of the persons involved. This general concept of nursing system had implicit in it the *idea* of self-care deficit but did not name it. The expression of the concept of nursing system marked the beginning of the accomplishment of the 1965 purpose of development of a research model for the art of nursing.

Reflection on the accomplishments of the years 1965 to 1968 leads one to question how so much progress was made in such a limited time period. For me the answer rests in the members of the group, their identified abilities and interests, and their willingness to work with both freedom and responsibility. One factor that I see as important was the keeping of detailed minutes of each session. Minutes served to keep the members of the group oriented to the work at hand, to the questions to be investigated, to the results of investigation, and to judgments made. Another factor was the differences in clinical nursing specialty areas represented by group members, their backgrounds in both nursing practice and nursing education, their positions in practice and education, and the variety of scholarly achievements of individual members.

Prior pursuit of courses in epistemology, formal logic, and metaphysics enabled members of the Nursing Model Committee to profit from the lectures of William A. Wallace, philosopher of science, on the forms of knowledge in practice fields, and from the efforts of Eamon O'Doherty, a behavioral scientist, to help us to (1) differentiate the interpersonal from the sociological aspects of nursing, (2) develop insights about the stages of development of the sciences, and (3) deal with the logic of nursing. Dr. O'Doherty respected the intellectual capacities of nurses and saw clearly the deleterious effects of the then common attitude *I am only a nurse.*

Another development in this period is my 1968 expression of seven types of technologies that are essential in the practice of nursing. The types of technologies are named in a paper titled "Levels of Nursing Education and Practice" (Orem, 1969) published in the *Alumnae Magazine* of the Johns Hopkins School of Nursing (see chapter 6). A modified version of them is on page 4 of the first edition of *Nursing: Concepts of Practice* (Orem, 1971). The technologies were perceived as important by Joan Backscheider and other members of the Center for Experimentation and Development in Nursing of The Johns Hopkins Institutions. For example, minutes of an October 12, 1969 Center meeting, in which I participated as a consultant, include an analysis of a nursing approach to use of technologies with emphasis on the requirement that someone have a mental picture of the whole; some assumptions about patients; a detailed analysis of the technology for bringing about and maintaining interpersonal, intergroup, and intragroup relationship with respect to both patient and nurse; and a detailed analysis of technology five sustaining and maintaining life processes. Joan Backscheider developed a set of *Rules Pertaining to Technologies* in April of 1969. During this period and into the 1970s she did a clinically focused study of communication demands placed on patients in health care settings.

This work on technologies has not but should become an integral part of developing bodies of nursing knowledge organized around self-care deficit nursing theory.

Developments—1970 to 1986

The last year of the 1960s and the beginning years of the 1970s were devoted to the work involved in the publication of *Nursing: Concepts of Practice* and *Concept Formalization in Nursing: Process and Product.* This period was marked by the tragic deaths of Joan Backscheider and Mary

Collins in 1972. Joan Backscheider was a member of the Nursing Model Committee and the Conference Group from their inception. Her chapter "Dynamics of Concept Development" in *Concept Formalization* (Backscheider, 1973) attests to her involvement with and her insights into what had transpired within the Committee and Group. Her use of Committee and Group minutes in developing the chapter is evident. Mary Collins became a member of the Group when she filled a position in the Center for Experimentation and Development in Nursing, initiated by Sarah Allison at the Johns Hopkins Hospital. There, Mary Collins contributed in a significant way to the development and operation of the Diabetic Nurse Management Clinic and to other Center endeavors. She was an experienced clinician and teacher.

From the perspective of the developing theory of nursing and theoretically practical nursing science, the 1970s were devoted to the explication of the substantive conceptual structure of the three broad elements of the concept of nursing system, namely, the concepts *therapeutic self-care demand, self-care agency,* and *nursing agency.* From the perspective of clinically practical nursing science, the focus was on the development of models of nursing systems for populations (see *Concept Formalization,* 1979, pp. 171–211 for more). Work also continued on what was developing into a construct named *basic conditioning factors.* Insights about these factors identified in my early work (1958–1959) continued to develop. The greatest amount of work was devoted to health state and its conditioning effects on therapeutic self-care demand and self-care agency. By 1978, eight conditioning factors were named, with the consideration that other factors could be added as they were identified. During the 1970s, some Group members worked on a major baccalaureate curriculum project at Georgetown University School of Nursing. Joan Backscheider's work to bring together a body of knowledge about the operational knowing capabilities of freshman college students fed into her study of operational knowing capabilities of patients in the Diabetic Nurse Management Clinic at the Johns Hopkins Hospital who were not progressing in knowing and meeting their therapeutic self-care demands (see *Concept Formalization in Nursing,* 1979, pp. 218–231).

The work of the 1970s was brought to a close with the 1979 publication of the second edition of *Concept Formalization in Nursing: Process and Product* and with the preparation for publication of the second edition of *Nursing: Concepts of Practice* in 1980.

Developments in the 1980s

This is the period of the formalization of my insights about nursing in a way that continues the development of the scientific approach to nursing initiated by the 1968 conceptualization of nursing system. The commonsense approach asks the question: How do things relate to me? The scientific approach asks the question: How do things relate to one another? The 1968 concept of nursing system expressed relationships between different individuals and between their characterizing qualities from a nursing perspective. The relationship between patient characteristics that generated a requirement for nursing was formulated as the theory of self-care deficit, which articulated with the theory of self-care. Both of these theories articulated with the theory of nursing system. The central ideas of the three theories were expressed along with sets of propositions and presuppositions for each in the 1980 edition of *Nursing: Concepts of Practice*. In the 1985 edition of the same publication, five assumptions underlying this general theory of nursing constituted from three articulated theories were published. The assumptions had been formulated in 1973 and presented in a paper at a Marquette University seminar. The central ideas of the three theories were refined for the Winstead-Fry publication *Case Studies in Nursing Theory* (Orem & Taylor, 1986).

Other work in the 1980s includes my work with Janet Fitzwater, started in the late 1970s, to identify factors that interfere with the meeting of the universal self-care requisites. Our concern was not with factors that indicated the particular values at which requisites should be but with factors that affected if and how they could be met. Such factors set up demands for the use of technologies that would surmount the interferences. We developed a tentative listing of factors for each of the universal-type self-care requisites. We developed and validated a classification of factors that interfere with meeting the requisite for maintaining an adequate intake of air and a classification of factors that interfere with the maintenance of a sufficient intake of water and food. Evelyn Vardiman participated in the development of the classification on water and food, contributing an important psychologic and neurophysiologic perspective. The work on interferences should be continued and articulated with work on technologies. [*Ed. Note:* This work is included in Appendix C, Orem, 2001.]

During the 1980s I was involved with Susan Taylor in analyzing the nursing operation diagnosis, including the nature of and the modes for expressing diagnoses. Considerable work was done during this period in formalizing approaches to multiperson units of service in nursing practice with Susan Taylor and others.

I was involved during the 1980s in clarifying and becoming able to express my judgments about nursing as a practical science. I developed a number of working papers on nursing science. One result of this effort appears in the third edition of *Nursing: Concepts of Practice* (1985) in the section titled "An Overview of the Practice Discipline Nursing."

A part of the development of nursing as a body of knowledge is the formal structuring of technologies that will bring about the unities or correlations, understood through the practical insights of nurses about nursing cases, to be possible as well as desirable.

Nursing education will advance in effectiveness to the degree that the profession moves to advance the development of nursing sciences, and ensures that nursing education produces nurses who can think as well as do nursing and who function as beginning, advancing, or advanced professional nursing practitioners, or as nurses qualified by high-level technical education.

During the 1970s and 1980s, I endeavored to master some of the ideas of Bernard Lonergan as expressed in his work *Insight* (1978). Through trying to gain insight about my own insights, I have come to know nursing as a field of theoretical and clinically practiced knowledge that is essential for the designing and doing of nursing in nursing practice situations of all types in all environmental settings.

CHAPTER 29

A Perspective on Theory-Based Nursing

W e have come together at this conference because of our work with one general theory of nursing. The perspective that I express is confined to this theory. It was developed by looking at self-care deficit nursing theory with respect to its content, its structure, and the processes involved in its initial and continuing development. Nurses who do critiques of the theory identify it as a systems theory, a needs theory, or a philosophy of nursing. These identifications indicate lack of understanding of the theory as a theory. It is clear to me that self-care deficit nursing theory constituted from the theory of nursing system, the theory of self-care deficit, and the theory of self-care is a *practice theory*. I suggest that we should not hesitate to state the basis for this categorization. The results of my examination of the structure and the content of the theory and its process of development justify self-care deficit nursing theory as a *practice theory*.

ESSENTIAL QUALITIES OF PRACTICE THEORIES

Nursing as a profession remains in that stage of development where members must clarify for themselves, the public, and other professionals what nursing is, what nursing can be and should be, and how nursing is produced. Because of this, general theories that describe and explain nursing as a practice field are needed if nursing is to be moved to its stature as a

---

This paper was originally presented at the Seventh Annual Self-Care Deficit Theory Conference, University of Missouri, in St. Louis, MO in November 1988.

professional field. Otherwise, it will remain a task-oriented occupation. General theories disappear with the development of the practical sciences and applied sciences of a practice field.

Practice theories that are general, that hold for all situations of practice in a field, express the essential characteristics of practice fields including architecture, engineering, and medicine.

These include the following:

1. A name for what is designed and produced within the field—the product
2. The purpose, the results sought, and the limits of use or value of the product
3. The concrete conditions and factors to be taken into account in product design and in the production operation of the field
4. The meaning of identified conditions and factors in the processes of design and production as they relate to purpose, means, effects, and results of action taken by designers and producers
5. The characterizing qualities of persons who are competent designers and producers within the practice field

In practice fields that are direct human services, like nursing or medicine, other essential characteristics are added to the foregoing five.

1. At least two agents or actors are specified for process operations of the field. One of these agents requires the service; the other bears responsibility for its design and production.
2. There is a basis for differentiation and specification of roles and role change.
3. The practical focus, action to be taken, is some condition or combination of factors in the person seeking or in need of the human service that (a) specify conditions that do not presently exist and that should be brought about and (b) limit what the person in need of the service can do to bring about the desired conditions.

A look at the three articulated theories that comprise the self-care deficit nursing theory reveals these practice-oriented features. For example, the theory of nursing system that sets forth the form of nursing as a practice field expresses in general terms the practical and technical features of nursing and identifies the product as a nursing system and its means of production. The first idea within my perspective of theory-based nursing is that *self-care deficit nursing theory is a practice theory.*

CONTINUED AND INCREASING USE OF SELF-CARE DEFICIT NURSING THEORY

The second idea within my perspective of theory-based nursing is that nurses select and use self-care deficit nursing theory in practice, education, and research because (1) self-care deficit nursing theory is a practice theory and (2) the main conceptual elements within the theory have been formulated, expressed, and validated and have had their substantive structure developed to the degree that their structures are useful in dealing with concrete conditions and factors in real nursing situations. The development of the substantive structure of self-care agency is an example of this. Theory-based nursing is difficult with self-care deficit nursing theory. It is more difficult, if not impossible, if the nursing theory is not a practice theory, if it is only a part of a practice theory, or its conceptual elements are not set forth and developed. One must already have conceptualized nursing to work with what is proposed as a nursing theory.

INITIAL AND CONTINUED DEVELOPMENT OF SELF-CARE DEFICIT NURSING THEORY

The developers of the self-care deficit nursing model and the formulators of the three theories that describe and explain what nursing is were guided by two principles or, if you prefer, assumptions. The first is that nursing is a social institution. The second is that there is an explanation or a reason for when and why men, women, and children need and can be helped through nursing. The existence of nursing as a human service is placed within the structure of particular social groups and societies. We accept that social institutions become part of the fabric of societies because of conditions of living and characterizing features of persons who make up the social group that warrant the initial introduction as well as the continued availability of particular services. Self-care deficit nursing theory had its beginnings in the acceptance of nursing as an existent human service and in the results of investigation of the question: When and why can people be helped through nursing?

The answer to the question brought into the focus of the developers the concepts of *self-care* and *limitation for engagement in self-care.* Limitation for engagement in self-care provided the basis for the assisting or helping actions of nurses as these related to the overcoming of limitations and the meeting of requirements for self-care. The conceptual model was developed by movement from these initial concepts. The conceptual model was first; the expression of the theory of nursing system was second. This was initially referred to as a concept of nursing system. The theories of self-care deficit and self-care were developed later.

The practice theory, known as the self-care deficit theory of nursing, is compositive in mode. Its development was based on insights into concrete nursing situations, conceptualization, hypothetico-deductive reasoning, and analysis. If we accept this theory, our proper work is to continue its development. To do this we must address the processes involved in the development and validation of knowledge in practice fields. This is a matter that is somewhat or entirely neglected in university schools of nursing. I suggest that we look to and plan for the day when teaching in this general theory of nursing is replaced by making available to students the practical and applied nursing sciences that are developments of the elements of the theory. I suggest the convening of work groups comprised of practitioners, educators, and researchers to consider this matter. You understand that *Nursing: Concepts of Practice* and *Concept Formalization* do contain elements of the practical and applied nursing sciences.

CHAPTER 30

Multiple Roles of Nurses

N ursing as a human health service can remain viable and progress in a society only when there are nurses engaged in the fulfilling of professional role responsibilities in nursing. Six roles that are essential for the existence and development of nursing are identified.

1. Practitioner of nursing
2. Nursing theorist
3. Nursing researcher
4. Nursing scholar
5. Developer of nursing technologies and techniques
6. Teacher of nursing or practitioner of nursing education

These six roles are specified as essential because nursing is a distinct health service with its field of knowledge as well as its field of practice, with needs for adequate numbers of persons qualified to practice nursing and fill the other essential roles. Since the administrator roles in nursing services and nursing education are enterprise-derived roles they are not included in this listing of essential professional nursing roles.

Role is used in the sense of kinds of obligations and demands associated with certain social positions or statuses. Some positions, for example, that of university professor, carry with them a number of associated roles, namely, the roles of teacher, scholar, researcher. Another example of multiple roles is that of the high-level technician in a field who is a master of the technology, who keeps up with the latest developments in the sciences underlying it and at the same time is creative and innovative with respect to development of new features of the technology.

This is a working paper prepared circa 1988 as part of extensive consulting being done at the time.

Multiple roles, in the sense just described, must be differentiated from the idea of role set, which relates to a single role, for example, that of nursing practitioner. A nursing practitioner may have obligations and relationships associated with a number of individuals: the person under nursing care, that person's family, the physician, and so on. Each role of persons fulfilling multiple roles will have its own role set.

It is necessary that nurses know the work operations and responsibilities associated with each of the six roles essential for keeping nursing viable in a society. It is important that nurses know their own talents and interests as related to these roles and their developed and developing competencies for role performance. Each of the six identified roles is named with the word *nursing*. This places the burden on each nurse who takes on and accepts the responsibilities for one or a combination of roles from the essential set of six to maintain a central orientation to nursing as a developing field of theoretical and practical knowledge essential for use in nursing practice (Nursing Development Conference Group, 1979).

THE PROBLEM OF ROLE DISTINCTIONS AND ROLE DIFFERENTIATIONS

In nursing, as in other professional fields, the need for and the distinctions between roles gradually emerge. This is followed by persons in the field developing insight about the particular characteristics of each role. My initial and early interest in role distinctions was associated with the need for answers to two questions.

1. How does nursing practice differ from nursing education?
2. How does nursing practice differ from nursing service in the institution or agency sense?

The first question arose because of the practice in the United States of using nursing students as a means of introducing nursing into hospitals, and the protracted use of nursing students in the provision of nursing in hospitals, and in homes in the communities. This question was answered at the time it arose by differentiating the *material objects* of the two fields. The material object of nursing practice is persons who can be helped through nursing, whereas the material object of nursing education is persons who seek to prepare themselves to practice nursing. The second question was associated with the emphasis in the 1930s and 1940s on providing nursing to hospital populations or to a population served by a public health or visiting nurse agency. The answer to this question emerged with understanding that the health care agency perspective has to be differentiated from the nursing practice perspective of individual nurses.

Interest in role distinctions continued. In 1971 the Nursing Development Conference Group formulated and expressed the concept *nursing agency*. This concept was based on the insight that nursing practitioners' knowing of nursing, their skills, their orientations, and their convictions and attitudes formed a core of capabilities that was enabling for nursing practice if these capabilities were activated (see Nursing Development Conference Group, 1979, pp. 120–122). The concept *nursing agency* is specific to nurses' practice of nursing and does not extend to other essential roles. Some nurses who work with self-care deficit nursing theory tend to use the more general term *nurse agency* rather than the specific term *nursing agency*. Nurses often have a variety of types of agency. The core of capabilities necessary for role fulfillment differs for each of the six essential roles; therefore, the term *nurse agency* is not a distinguishing term.

Another personal effort to identify and clarify roles within the nursing profession was initiated in 1974 and completed in 1978. This effort involved the expression of nursing's placement or fit in the "world of man and human affairs." Nursing's placement was identified in three frames moving (1) from man generically considered to community, culture, and society, (2) to fields of knowledge and human endeavor expressed in the three areas of professions and service occupations, practice disciplines, and institutionalized human services, and (3) finally to the third frame, nursing. The six essential roles for keeping nursing viable in a society are identified in the third frame. The roles of nursing scholar, theorist, researcher, and developer are related to nursing as a practice discipline; the roles of nursing practitioner and teacher of nursing are related to institutionalized human services and to professions and service operations. (For a representation of the results of this analysis see Nursing Development Conference Group, 1979, p. 22; see also Orem, 2001, p. 75.)

There is need for continuing attention on the part of nurses to the broad cultural and societal scheme within which nursing fits. The foregoing representation is considered as an attempt to place nursing and the six associated professional roles within the broad picture of human affairs in social groups.

ROLE OBLIGATIONS AND DEMANDS

Continued work with nursing roles was done in conjunction with a federally funded study identified as the *Organization of Nursing Faculty Responsi-*

bility (Georgetown University School of Nursing, 1976). The study was conducted in a university school of nursing within the larger structure of the university's medical center. The project was designed in two phases. The first phase addressed two questions:

1. What kinds of work operations and cost centers are associated with the activities of nursing faculty in the education of nursing students enrolled in the baccalaureate program?
2. What are nursing faculty members prepared for, interested in, and concerned about with respect to nursing faculty functioning?

Answers to these questions were viewed as essential for designing and conducting the proposed second phase that was to address designs for role combinations and planning for faculty members' taking on of multiple roles. The first phase was completed but not the second.

As a part of this project activity systems or work operations, or tasks or duties associated with the six professional nursing roles were identified and consensual validation sought and obtained.

In and of themselves, listings of work operations associated with essential professional roles in nursing have little value. Their value rests in the use to which they are put. The past and continued emphasis on nurses taking on multiple roles in nursing both in university schools of nursing and health care centers demands that nurses and administrators understand the obligation and demands of specific roles and role combinations. For this reason listings of role-associated work operations have considerable value in helping individuals gain understanding of role obligations, demands, and possible incompatibilities of some role combinations for individuals. Role-associated work operations also lead to insights about time requirements and resources needed for effective fulfillment of role responsibilities.

The types of work operations for fulfillment of the obligations and demands of two essential professional nursing roles are presented. They are presented in a summary fashion by naming the sets into which essential work operations or activity systems are grouped. Within the sets there are subsets and sub-subsets of essential operations. The sets for each role are named according to the characteristics of the operations or activity systems within the sets. The two roles presented are practitioner of nursing education and nursing scholar.

PRACTITIONER OF NURSING EDUCATION

In the Project on nursing faculty responsibilities the essential role of *teacher of nursing* was expanded to that of *practitioner of nursing education*. This was done because it was an assumption of the Project that "the course is the unit of organization and production in institutions of higher education." Following initial development and validation the revision resulted in nine sets of work operations for the practitioner of nursing education with a range of four to seven subsets for the nine sets (Georgetown University School of Nursing, 1976). The members of the nine sets, as well as the names of the sets, are course oriented. The sets are as follows:

Set 1: Course Design and Development
Set 2: General Planning over Time to Formalize and Operationalize the Major Content Areas and Experiential Areas of the Course
Set 3: Short-Term Planning to Put a Course into Operation
Set 4: Distribution of Opportunities to Students for Enrollment in the Course
Set 5: Planning, Preparing for, Conducting, and Regulating Course Experiences of Students in Class or Small Group Sessions
Set 6: Planning, Preparing for, Conducting, and Regulating Institutional Experience of Students in Health Care or Other Personal Service-Type Agencies
Set 7: Planning, Preparing for, Guiding, and Regulating Experiences of Students in Personalized Systems of Instruction
Set 8: Evaluation of Students' Activities and Progress in the Course
Set 9: Course-, Program-, and Career-Focused Educational Guidance of Students

Experienced practitioners of nursing education understand and accept the foregoing role obligations and demands. Understanding will not have been reached by neophyte teachers. In some situations educational administrators evidence little understanding of what is involved when faculty members are developing, revising, or conducting courses.

The sets of work operations for the practice of nursing education is revealing about the ways of knowing, the skills, the orientations, and the attitudes and interests of nurses who can function effectively in this role in accord with their developmental state as teachers of nursing. It is necessary that practitioners of nursing education view themselves realistically with respect to education and nursing. They are teachers of nursing, and in the role of teachers they at times take on the role of practitioner of nursing. They must also be scholars, not only in the field of nursing within one or more areas of nursing with their related foundational sciences, but also in the field of education, with a special focus on education, for the occupations and professions.

The sets of role obligations and demands for the practitioner of nursing education illustrate quite clearly not only role obligations and demands but also how essential professional roles combine within a single role. The suggested types of work operation illustrate that *practitioners of nursing education* must not only be scholars in the field of nursing and the field of education, but also practitioners of education and at times of nursing. These are heavy demands that are often combined with demands for engagement in nursing research and nursing practice outside the teaching role.

There is no doubt that there is need for definitive design, planning, and negotiations for nurses' taking on of multiple roles. The time-honored system of academic rank in universities was one design for dealing with multiple roles. The instructor and assistant professor were the academic ranks primarily focused on teaching, while the rank of full professor was focused on research and the teaching of graduate students engaged in research. Instructors and assistant professors were expected to continue to develop themselves as scholars, with associated movement into research endeavors and the rank of associate professor. The nursing community must face the problem of multiple roles on the part of its members in universities and colleges as well as in health care settings.

NURSING SCHOLAR

The role of nursing scholar is associated with each of the other five essential professional roles in the sense that one must fulfill the obligations and demands of this role before the obligations and demands of the other five roles can be adequately fulfilled. The term *scholar* is used in the sense of one who, through pursuit of systematic study, has gained a mastery of knowledge in a field as well as accuracy and skill in investigation and the abilities for critical analysis and interpretation of knowledge. There is a critical need in nursing for promotion of understanding about the work of and the need for nursing scholars. Since nursing is so poorly structured as a field of knowledge, the work of nursing scholars is fraught with difficulties that are not found in highly structured fields.

The approach to identification of the work operations of nursing scholars was general and not specific to nursing. It was assumed that the types of work operations of scholars would be the same, regardless of field. This, of course, could be assumed for other essential roles but not to the degree that it can be assumed for scholars.

In 1979 the original listing of work operations of nursing scholars was revised, organized into eight sets, and names attached to the sets (Faculty Participants, 1979). The named sets are as follows:

Set 1: Defining the Domain of Concern
Set 2: Investigating Sources of Information
Set 3: Building Knowledge
Set 4: Achieving Understanding
Set 5: Achieving an Authoritative List of Sources of Information
Set 6: Constructing a Framework for Investigation of a Domain
Set 7: Elaborating and Communicating the Framework
Set 8: Formalizing the Domain of Concern

The sets express movement and mastery on the part of scholars. To express these dynamics work operations or activity systems for sets one and four are presented. [*Ed. Note:* See chapter 15 for complete description.]

Set One: Defining the Domain of Concern

This set includes operations to identify the area(s) of a field of knowledge to be investigated. These operations are accompanied or followed by operations to identify or to posit points of articulation of the area(s) with other fields of knowledge. Aspects of the real world that areas of knowledge describe or explain are identified. Movement from this initial position is reflected in operations of Set IV.

Set Four: Achieving Understanding

The operations of this set are directed toward the clarification and synthesis of knowledge through discussions with colleagues, identification of key ideas, and expression of the real-world entities being dealt with. There are also the operations of formulating and expressing in speech or writing developed insights, perceived issues, and unanswered questions. Evaluating oneself for consistently correct use of terms is another obligation.

The laying out of sets of work operations for the scholar role or any other role does not specify a linear progression. Individuals may be engaged during a particular time period with operations in more than one set. In fact it may be necessary as a scholar to engage in operations of Sets 2 and 3 before completing operations in Set 1. These sets, as do those for the practitioner of nursing education, represent activity or functional areas that define role obligations and demands.

RELATIONS OF ROLES

The six essential professional roles can be viewed in their separateness but they must also be viewed in their relatedness. As previously indicated, filling some positions, such as that of university professor, demands the taking on of multiple roles, or a single role may involve a multiplicity of roles. In situations such as these the matter of role relatedness is an important consideration. It is especially important in the health professions where clinical practice is an essential professional role.

Individual nurses as well as the nursing community have the task of working through what is feasible with respect to multiple role expectations for already existent positions or positions under development in nursing education. Some professional groups have done this with a considerable degree of success. Success, however, is dependent upon understanding of the time and energy expenditure demands, the conditions, and resource requirements for effective fulfillment of role obligations, and the intellectual demands of fulfilling role obligations.

Scholarly advancement within nursing and in related fields is a necessary condition for fulfillment of other roles. For this reason undergraduate nursing students in educational programs of professional caliber should be preparing themselves to function both as nursing scholars and as nursing practitioners. In high-level technical-type programs nursing students should be preparing themselves to continue as students in nursing, in foundational science fields, and in particular technologies of nursing.

The nursing community must learn to put a premium on scholarship in nursing. It is necessary for nurses in positions of leadership to give priority to endeavors for the development of the practical and the applied nursing sciences. This will help ensure that teachers and practitioners of nursing have available to them structured bodies of nursing knowledge, and that nursing knowledge generated and validated in role performance by theorists, researchers, and developers will be recognized as elements of nursing science.

CHAPTER 31

Nursing Systems

olitical systems, social systems, organizational systems, health care systems, the solar system are familiar terms that are used freely in everyday conversations or in professional discussions. We understand the word *system* in terms of sets of things or objects, together with relationships between the things or objects in the sets and between their properties or attributes. The things or objects in the set(s) behave together as a whole, and changes in any part, including changes in the properties of the parts, affect the whole. Although the word *system* connotes things in relationships, the tendency is to focus on the functioning of the whole that is the system.

When existent systems do not function at all or are not functioning according to expectations, interest turns to the things that constitute the parts, the properties, or attributes of these things and to the relationships among them. To find out why an existent system does not work or to understand an existent system it is necessary to engage in analysis. To produce or make a system the producer must engage in synthesis to select and to bring appropriate parts together in functional relationships. To identify the parts that can and should be brought together, the producer engages in analysis of the situation(s) of action to determine the presence of essential parts in time–space localizations, and the properties of parts or the absence of parts, but the producer must also have practical insight

This paper was originally presented at Newark Beth Israel Medical Center, Newark, N.J. April 10, 1989.
[*Ed. Note:* The content included in the sections titled "An Analysis of the Theory of Nursing Systems" and "Results of Nursing" is taken in part from the paper "A Nursing Practice Theory in Three Parts, 1956–1989," presented on April 8, 1989, in Miami, Florida, at the First South Florida Nursing Theorist Conference, Cedars Medical Center, Education Department. See Orem, 1990 in references.]

about changes in the parts or their relationships that can be brought about, and have a mental image, a design, for bringing the parts together for synthesizing them into a functional unity.

Some functional unities that can be characterized and understood as systems are naturally existent, such as the solar system or the various described systems of living organisms that are useful to us in understanding the functioning of living things. Nursing systems are not naturally existent; they are artificial or humanly produced systems. As systems they can be described and understood as (1) practical, deliberate result-seeking systems of action, (2) systems of action in the nature of direct personal service or care, and (3) self-organizing systems in Ashby's sense of systems "that exist when and for the duration that there are self-connecting links between the behavior or state of independent parts or subjects, the connection occurring at some point of conditionality between them" (NDCG, 1979, p. 125).

The independent parts of nursing systems are persons with properties or attributes that distinguish them one from another. The order of the parts in nursing systems can be understood within the frame of reference of points of order in functional unities with distinguishable parts. These are (1) the order of each part to its own operation, (2) the order of each part to other parts, (3) the order of the parts to the operation of the whole, the unity, and (4) the operation of the whole with respect to some extrinsic end (Niemeyer, 1951). These points of order are useful to nurses who seek understanding of nursing systems, as is Ashby's concept of self-organizing systems (Ashby, 1964).

EXPRESSED CONCEPTS OF NURSING SYSTEMS

The term *nursing system* came into use by members of the Nursing Development Conference Group in the late 1960s. "The notion that the creative end product of nursing is a nursing system" emerged during the Group's work of "identifying the dimensions of nursing as a practical science" (NDCG, 1979, p. 106). The time frame was the middle 1960s to the early 1970s, when there was a major focus in academic circles on systems theory, cybernetics, and adaptation. In Nursing Development Conference Group deliberations and in private discussions among members the question: *What do nurses make when they nurse?* would arise. The question required an answer because of Group members' acceptance (1) that nursing is a form of practical endeavor and (2) that practical endeavor brings into existence something that did not exist before the practical activities were begun, a creative end product.

The Nursing Development Conference Group accepted and worked with an expressed conceptualization of nursing system in 1968 and with a refined conceptualization from 1970. Both conceptualizations appear in the 1973 and 1979 editions of *Concept Formalization in Nursing: Process and Product*. The 1968 expression identifies a nursing system as a complex action system, sets forth its method of formation as involving one or a combination of ways of assisting, and specifies what nursing systems are designed to achieve (NDCG, 1979). The 1970 conceptualization (NDCG, 1973) is a descriptive explanation of the parts and the relationships between and among the parts of nursing systems. This conceptualization is expressed in systems language and in the form of Ashby's (1964) concept of self-organizing systems. It is essentially a *theory* because (1) its focus is on things in relationship one to the other, and (2) the variables of the systems are expressed through the use of theoretical rather than concrete concepts. It is recognized that this 1970 expression of the theory of nursing system lays out the domain and boundaries of the practical science of nursing.

The 1970 detailed expression of the theory of nursing systems provided the conceptual elements and the language used to structure the familiar word model of nursing expressed as a circle of terms and relationships and referred to as a conceptual framework. The following is a succinct expression of the central idea of the theory of nursing system.

> All action systems that are nursing systems are produced by nurses through the exercise of their nursing agency within the context of their contractual and interpersonal relations with individuals who are characterized by health associated self-care deficits for purposes of ensuring that their therapeutic self-care demands are known and met and their self-care agency is protected and its exercise or development is regulated. [Orem & Taylor, 1986, p. 44]

The theory of nursing system does not and cannot stand alone. It is understood in its relationship to the theory of self-care deficit and to the theory of self-care. Together the three theories constitute a general theory of nursing. The theory of nursing system is the central part, the core of the self-care deficit theory of nursing.

AN ANALYSIS OF THE THEORY OF NURSING SYSTEMS

The theory of nursing systems is expressed in part through the use of the conceptual elements of the theory of self-care deficit and the theory of self-care. The theory of nursing system is a descriptive explanation of how persons with health-derived or health-related self-care or dependent-care deficits can be helped through the production of nursing by nurses so that their own or their dependent's therapeutic self-care demands are known and met, the property of self-care agency protected, and the exercise or development of self-care or dependent-care agency regulated. In a sense the conceptual structure of the theory of nursing system subsumes and relates the conceptual elements of the theory of self-care deficit with elements of the theory of self-care.

Each of the three theories within the self-care deficit theory of nursing expresses four categories of conceptualizations, all of which are required because of the practical action orientation. The categories of conceptualizations are

1. The conceptualized entity, person, or persons in a space–time localization
2. Properties or attributes
3. Motion or change
4. Effects or results, what is produced

These four categories will be used as a basis for analysis of the theory of nursing system.

The Conceptualized Entity

The entity conceptualized in the theory of nursing system is an *interpersonal unity*. The human dimension is we, not you and me, as in the theory of self-care deficit, or not the self, the *I*, as in the theory of self-care. This interpersonal unity is formed by nurses in their associations and interactions with persons with health-derived or health-related self-care deficits who enter into agreements to accept and participate in nursing and with relatives or persons who bear responsibility for individuals requiring nursing. The unity must be continuously maintained by communication, by the coordination of the actions of persons forming the unity, and by their cooperative relationships. Each person within the unity ideally recognizes the independence as well as the interdependence of the cooperating individuals, and each person ideally maintains an active operative sense of duty.

The ages, the sex, the culture, the life experiences, the self-concepts, and the interests, concerns, and expectations of members of the nursing unity will have a conditioning influence on both the quality and number of their actions and their interactions. The health state and the developmental state of persons who require nursing will condition the extent and intensity of interactions between and among persons who constitute the interpersonal unity.

Attributes or Properties

Attributes or properties are attributed to both the interpersonal unity and to persons who form it. The attributes conceptualized for the interpersonal unity are societal in their perspective. The unity must include a nurse who is qualified and registered or licensed to practice nursing within the jurisdiction where nursing is being provided. The agreement or contract must specify the provision of the service of nursing. From a nursing perspective the interpersonal unity must exhibit nursing legitimacy. This means that there is evidence of (1) existent, emerging or potential self-care deficits (or dependent-care deficits) on the part of persons who seek nursing and (2) on the part of providers of nursing (nurses) there is evidence of the developed capabilities and experiential knowledge specific to the provisions of nursing for the particular type of nursing case in one or in changing time–space localizations.

The attributes or properties are attributed both to persons who require and seek nursing and persons who provide nursing. These attributes afford them the position of nurse and nurse's patient or client within the interpersonal unity. Nurses' patients or clients are conceptualized as having therapeutic self-care demands to be known and met and as having inadequate capabilities (self-care or dependent-care agency) for knowing and meeting their demand for care of a therapeutic quality. Nurses are conceptualized as having the property of nursing agency, namely, the developed and operational capabilities to perform the essential operations of nursing practice—nursing diagnosis, nursing prescription, nursing regulation—for and with persons who require nursing. The theory of nursing system specifies conditionality between the therapeutic self-care demands and the self-care agency of persons who are nurses' patients, as well as conditionality between the nursing agency of the nurse and the therapeutic self-care demands and self-care agency of persons who require nursing. There are relationships to be understood, not only between the persons who form and maintain the interpersonal unity but also between and among their distinguishing attributes.

Other attributes or properties of persons who require nursing and those who produce it include their present interests and concerns that interfere with or facilitate their acceptance and fulfillment of roles and responsibilities within the interpersonal unity. The self-concepts of persons who are nurses or nurses' patients also are properties that can have a positive or negative influence on what these persons do within the interpersonal unity to maintain it and keep it operational.

Motion or Change

Motion or change is conceptualized for the interpersonal unity, the persons forming it, and the properties and attributes.

Communication between and among members of the unity and the time and place and conditions and circumstances of its occurrence is motion or change that contributes to the maintenance of the unity. The unity is functional as a nursing unity when nurses activate their powers of nursing agency in order to know and meet the therapeutic self-care demands of the persons who require nursing and to protect and regulate the exercise or development of their self-care agency. More specific changes include increases or decreases in dependence, independence, and interdependence of persons within the interpersonal unity and changes in role responsibilities.

With respect to persons and properties, persons requiring nursing may have increases or decreases in the number and kind of self-care capabilities and limitations, increase or decrease in willingness to participate in nursing, increase or decrease in the number and kinds of self-care requisites or changes in available means of meeting them, increase or decrease in engagement in self-care or in regulation of the exercise or development of self-care agency. Persons who are nurses are conceptualized as moving from the performance of one nursing practice operation to performance of another operation, from use of one method of helping or some combination of methods to the use of other methods of helping, from movement including willingness to maintain the nursing relationship to movement to end it (Orem, 1990).

Products

The actions and interactions of persons forming an interpersonal unity, when seen in their relatedness, can be conceptualized as a system, as a whole thing. Nursing systems so conceptualized are created over some time duration and in a place or places. Nursing systems are structured from specific action sequences and interactions of members of the nursing unity. They have form that derives from the method or methods of helping in use by nurses and from the allocation and performance of role functions by persons who form the nursing unity. Nursing systems so conceptualized can be categorized according to methods of helping and associated role functions as wholly compensatory, partly compensatory, and supportive-educative for persons who are nurses' patients or clients.

The whole thing that is a nursing system cannot be generated without products that are developed in relation to properties and attributes of members of the interpersonal unity. Ten products are identified without reference to the process of production in the following list of products of a nursing system.

1. A body of information descriptive of existent or past self-care or dependent-care systems of persons who require nursing, the quality of such systems, and their producers' judgments about them
2. The calculated therapeutic self-care demand or specified components thereof for persons requiring nursing
3. A body of information descriptive of self-care capabilities and limitations of persons requiring nursing
4. A selection of the ways of helping that are valid and appropriate to the nature and extent of the self-care limitations of persons requiring nursing and to the immediate and continued meeting of the components of their therapeutic self-care demands
5. An establishment and allocation of role functions of members of the interpersonal unity and a design for their performance in a time–place matrix in order to have continuous information about and continuously meet components of nurses' patients' therapeutic

self-care demands and to protect or regulate the exercise or development of their self-care agency

6. Emergence of stable or changing nursing systems as allocated role functions are performed
7. A body of information about the adequacy of nursing agency of nurses within the interpersonal unity
8. Having requested nursing consultation
9. Having nurse replacements or additional nurse members of the interpersonal unity to ensure the adequate and timely performance of nursing; diagnostic, prescriptive and production operations
10. A body of information about the adequacy and effectiveness of nurse management of the case and the results being produced for persons who require nursing

The products conceptualized within the theory of nursing system differ in number and kind through the period of existence of interpersonal unities formed under agreements to provide nursing. The products depend upon the practical insights of nurses and of persons who require nursing and upon the effectiveness of their investigative, decision-making, and productive functions.

Results of Nursing

The results of nursing are understood and expressed within the theory of nursing system in relation to the two patient or client variables, namely, their therapeutic self-care demands and their self-care agency. Results of nursing include (1) persons within the nursing unity having knowledge of the components of therapeutic self-care demands and the regulatory value of each component as related to human functioning and development, (2) the effective meeting of components of therapeutic self-care demands in time specific sequences, (3) regulation of the exercise and development of self-care or dependent-care agency, and (4) nurses' knowledge and judgments about the need to alter the form of the nursing system, to continue it, or to move to a dependent-care or self-care system.

It is the validity and the reliability of the technologies selected to meet particularized self-care requisites as well as the accuracy of the identification and particularization of requisites that determine whether or not desirable levels of regulation of human functioning and human development are achieved. Such results may or may not be immediately perceptible to members of the nursing unity. When self-care requisites exist but cannot be met because of absence of valid or reliable technologies, when the use of technologies to meet one requisite interferes with the meeting of other requisites, when there is reluctance or refusal to use certain technologies and when structural or functional conditions do not permit for regulatory action then the nursing system and the results expected from it must be adjusted to existent conditions (Orem, 1990, pp. 56–57).

The results of nursing, as well as the characteristics of nursing system, are affected and conditioned positively or negatively by factors both extrinsic and intrinsic to the interpersonal unity and the persons who form it. This includes the governmental system and the health care system within which nursing systems are formed. These systems exert influence on the nursing system in the form of opportunities or constraints. A major influence on the production and maintenance of nursing systems is the other systems of health care in which nurses, patients, or clients are concurrently participating, most commonly medical care systems.

SUMMARY

The theory of nursing system constitutes a frame of reference for nursing practitioners in their practice of nursing as well as for researchers and scholars. As a theory it subsumes and articulates with conceptual elements of the theories of self-care deficit and self-care. The use of this broad nursing frame of reference requires that nurses have knowledge of various human sciences that serve as more narrow frames of reference. The use of frames within frames is characteristic of nursing, as of all practice fields.

CHAPTER 32

Perception of Theory Application Around the World

This paper is written on the basis of my experiences and my knowledge of events related to the use of self-care deficit nursing theory around the world. Some generalizations offered in the paper are relevant to the use of any theory. The writing of this paper was deferred in order to complete other pressing work. When I was ready to write, a health problem interfered. For these reasons the paper lacks detail about dates and other matters, which I am sure some of you can supply. Perhaps the paper will be a stimulus to pursue the ideas presented and for dinner guests to make contributions.

Application is understood as putting something to practical use. Theory refers to self-care deficit nursing theory with its constituent theories of self-care, self-care deficit, and nursing system. It also refers to the conceptual constructs within the general theory and the early conceptual model of nursing. Perceptions of theory application around the world can be expressed in terms of three stages of applications:

1. The stage of dissemination of the theory to potential users
2. The stage of becoming a user
3. The stage of use of the theory in nursing practice, nursing research, continued theory development and theory refinement, development of nursing technologies, and nursing education

---

This chapter consists of preliminary notes preparatory to a self-care conference presentation in Toronto, Canada, in June 1990.

THE STAGE OF DISSEMINATION

Each stage has a number of prerequisite conditions. For the first stage these include (1) a formulated and expressed theory, (2) nurses who qualify as potential users, and (3) ways and means for dissemination of the theory. Nurses active in the profession in the United States and Canada have progressed through this stage to the stage of self-preparation to the stage of use. The stage of dissemination remains in process or has not begun for some nursing students and licensed nurses.

The language in which the theory is expressed is a critical factor in dissemination as is the language of potential users. Principal sources of self-care nursing deficit theory are expressed in the English language and have been available since the late 1960s. (*Nursing: Concepts of Practice* was available in a prepublication version before its 1971 publication.) Primarily English-speaking countries—the United States, Canada, Great Britain, and Australia—vary in terms of movement into or through this stage, with Australia and Great Britain trailing.

Translations of the English-language sources are in Japanese, Spanish, French, Dutch, and Portuguese, which is still in process, to my knowledge. Norwegian nurses did a selective translation from the first edition of *Nursing: Concepts of Practice*. Some translations are identified as "poor." There are problems associated with translations, including (1) getting an interested publisher, (2) securing foreign rights, (3) selection of a competent translator, and (4) all the problems associated with translation: for example, the need for language experts as consultants, ensuring that the translator knows the theory and its nuances, and that publishers do not take over to give the translation a European or some other flavor. There are also problems in countries in obtaining the English-language work. Long delays occur because of distances and other factors.

Other ways of dissemination of self-care deficit nursing theory used in the United States and Canada are the local, regional, national, and international conferences. These conferences have been successful and effective in dissemination. The Nurse Educators Theory Conference held in New York City was a turning point in dissemination for American nurses. In Europe and Australia dissemination has been through theorists' visits and conferences, research conferences, and, in Great Britain, at times through the efforts of Canadian nurses enrolled in British universities.

Dissemination of theory in countries when English is not the first language is related to graduate education in nursing in the United States, nurses' abilities to work with English-language sources, and conferences with English-speaking nurses versed in the theory.

THE STAGE OF BECOMING A USER

The preconditions for stage two are conditions of nurses who move themselves from being potential users to users of theory. They include (1) willingness to work with abstract material and generalizations, (2) ideas about results they will seek to bring about through use of the theory, and (3) willingness and ability to work alone or as a member of a group to understand the theory, its uses, and its application to concrete situations of nursing research, practice, education, and so on. In this precondition, *application* is used in the sense of fixing one's attention and exercising diligence and studied and unremitting work. It involves becoming a scholar of the theory and learning to model its use to achieve results to be sought. Nurses may not have the interest or be willing to spend time to fulfill this third precondition and may seek to move directly to immediate use.

Some nurses do not believe in working with abstractions and generalizations because they insist every nursing practice situation is unique. These nurses prefer to think within only concrete frames of reference and some may not be able to deal with abstract material. Nurses progressing in stage two have available to them as tutors or consultants nurses who understand the theory and who can aid them in resolving their problems and in answering their questions, as well as nurses who understand the use to which the theory is to be put. Monica Lovgren of Sweden, who used constructs of the theory in her doctoral research with a focus on bringing about conditions enabling for the active participation of elderly patients, visited Margrethe Lorenson's Geriatric Center in Copenhagen, Denmark. She visited the United States and stayed with me a week reading the third edition of *Nursing: Concepts of Practice* and *Concept Formalization in Nursing: Process and Product*, with morning and afternoon discussions with me. She read work done by other nurses and was objectively critical. On her return to Sweden she worked in a nursing research unit at the hospital in Orebro, teaching nurses and physicians the self-care deficit theory of nursing and using it in clinical practice to develop individualized nursing care programs toward the active participation of the elderly in their care. Research was ongoing.

There are numerous examples of these stage two approaches in the United States and Canada for individual nurses as well as for numbers of nurses in nursing services and nursing education. The University of Missouri Summer Institute and Fall Conference and the Self-Care Deficit Theory Study Group at Wayne State University are doing excellent work.

THE STAGE OF USE

The theory is in more extensive use in the United States and Canada than in other countries of the world. Prerequisite conditions for use include (1) the freedom of nurses to be innovative and to be leaders, (2) the interest of nurses in the development of the profession and occupation, and (3) nurses' interest in personal growth within nursing. French-Canadian nurses showed early interest in the use of the theory in education and clinical practice and in preparing themselves to use the theory. They were instrumental, after a prolonged effort, in securing a French publisher for their translation of the third edition of *Nursing: Concepts of Practice*. We are familiar with how the theory is used in our countries so I will not elaborate. We are also aware of what some nurses in other countries have done following graduate education in America.

Australian nurses use the theory in education and some nurses use it in their own clinical practice; for example, Dennis Cowell has modeled the application of self-care deficit theory to psychiatric nursing practice.

Holland and Spain are actively contributing to the use of the theory and in translation of the forthcoming fourth edition of *Nursing: Concepts of Practice*. Germany lags behind, but nurses are presently working to get German translations of the original work of various theorists. I have little knowledge of use of the theory in Great Britain and in Africa. We are all familiar with the work of Patricia Underwood in Japan and Israel.

The theory continues to be disseminated. There is a political governmental focus on the use of the theory in Europe and in Japan. One Japanese nurse writes, "A law passed the diet with concern for an increase in self-care toward the health of senior citizens." The introduction of theory courses into schools of nursing has had a great influence on dissemination. The use and translation of secondary sources is open to question.

As the pattern of nursing education changes in Europe (movement to place both graduate and undergraduate education in the universities) we shall see the continued dissemination and use of theory.

CHAPTER 33

Some Considerations in the Use of One General Theory of Nursing to Formalize the Provision of Nursing at Crawford Long Hospital

INITIAL REMARKS ABOUT THE THEORY

The theory and conceptual model you have selected to give structure to nurses' practice of nursing and to aid in the design and planning for the production of nursing for present and future populations of persons to be served has been under development since 1958. The three-part theory, named self-care deficit nursing theory, had its beginning in 1958 in my observations over time of the realities of nursing practice situations, specifically in an insight about when and why individuals, human beings, are in need of nursing. This insight was expressed as the inability of a maturing and mature person to provide for self the amount and quality of self-care required on a continuing basis because of the person's health state or the nature of the person's health care requirements. For children, the reason was expressed as the inability of parents or guardians to provide care required by the child because of the child's health situation. This expression of the *proper object* of nursing gradually and naturally led, over a period of years, to the formalization, expression, and validation of the concepts

This paper was originally presented at Crawford Long Hospital, Atlanta, GA, November 11, 1992.

of self-care, therapeutic self-care demand, self-care agency, self-care system, nursing agency and nursing system and basic conditioning factors. These concepts provided the boundaries of nursing and points of articulation with other fields of knowledge.

The self-care deficit theory of nursing is expressed as three related theories: a theory of self-care, self-care deficit, and nursing system. The theory of nursing system is the theory that organizes and subsumes the other two theories. Each theory is expressed in terms of its central idea, its presuppositions, and its propositions. Before these theories were expressed we worked with a conceptual model (Orem, 2001). Prior to the emergence of the conceptual model I had developed a model of a framework for nursing action. The model and the theories serve nurses in nursing practice, research, development, education, and further theorizing. These theories do not exhaust what is involved in nursing practice. They formalize what is the proper work of nurses and provide points of articulation of nursing with other fields of knowledge and practice. For example, the concept of health deviation self-care requisite provides points of articulation with medical knowledge and practice. The universal requisite to maintain a balance between activity and rest provides a base for articulation with understanding of knowledge about energy expenditure and so on, and raises the question of how energy expenditure can and should be balanced with rest.

In theorizing about nursing and in concept formalization and expression, four categories of conceptualization were used (1) entities, *persons* in space-time localization—nurses' patient and nurse, (2) *properties or attributes* of these persons—for nurse's patient, the property of self-care agency and therapeutic self-care demand, for nurse, the property of nursing agency, (3) *motion or change*, either in the *operations* of persons or in the *attributes or properties*, and (4) *products*—for example, the production of self-care through activation of the person's self-care agency, and the production of nursing through nurses' activation of nursing agency.

The critical concept of self-care deficit does not fall in any one of the four categories since the concept expresses a relationship between two patient properties: self-care agency and therapeutic self-care demand. The existence of such a deficit relationship should not be thought of as a property of a person. Lack of this understanding causes some nurses difficulty. We can identify a fifth category of conceptualization: nature of relationships, therapeutic self-care demand, self-care relationships, and nurse–patient legality of relationship.

The work of development of nursing's frame of reference in the form of a conceptual model included the idea that patient properties could change in value when factors such as health state, developmental state, and so forth took on certain values. These factors were identified and named basic conditioning factors—age, gender, developmental state, health state, family system factors, health care system factors, environmental factors, sociocultural and economic factors, and resources. These factors may be stable, may be actively producing change, or may be indicators of needed change in the values of the patient variables of self-care agency and therapeutic self-care demand.

From the beginning, members of the Nursing Development Conference Group perceived the value of a general theory of nursing with its inherent conceptual model. Eight functions of the self-care deficit theory of nursing are expressed in the fourth edition of *Nursing: Concepts of Practice* (Orem, 1991, p. 74). I shall read six of eight.

> To set forth the key concepts of nursing that express insights about the unity existent in all nursing practice when nursing is considered as a field of knowledge and practice and to establish a system of symbols or language. The key concepts provide a frame of reference for nursing science and nursing practice.
>
> To set limits on and orient thinking and practical endeavor in nursing practice, research, development (experimental) and education for nursing.
>
> To reduce cognitive load by providing [conceptual] subsumers for incoming data and for attaching meaning to data and to enable persons who understand the theory to categorize and form concepts from related insights about features of concrete nursing situations.
>
> To allow inferences to be made about articulations of nursing with other fields of human service and with patterns of human living of individuals and families in communities.
>
> To generate in nurses and nursing students a style of thinking and communicating nursing.
>
> To bring nurses together as communities of scholars engaged in continuing the structuring and validation of nursing knowledge.

The theory functions in accomplishment of the specified ends. It is used in the United States, Canada (both English- and French-speaking), South American countries, European countries, Australia, and some Asian countries.

INTRODUCTION AND CONTINUAL USE OF THE GENERAL THEORY OF NURSING IN A NURSING DIVISION OR DEPARTMENT

Nursing theory takes on significance as it describes, explains, and directs nurses in the practice of nursing and enables administrators of nursing,

nursing practitioners, and designers of health care systems to have a common understanding of nursing for the populations served. There are some tasks common to all that each person must perform. These include the following common tasks.

1. Admit that nursing has a *proper object*; come to understand this object in concrete situations of nursing practice and reflect upon its meaning for patients and for nurses.
2. Admit that nursing, like other health services, has boundaries established by its proper object and its frame of reference.
3. Accept that nursing is a mode or form of help and a mode or form of caring for others. Understand the features of each and their relevance to nursing but admit that neither helping nor caring for explains when and why persons individually or in groups need and can be helped through nursing.
4. Learn to use the elements and relationships expressed in the theory to direct and hold attention on patients, on environmental conditions, and on selves as reasonable nurses. These responsibilities are for ensuring that nursing can be provided for populations served, that this or that person or group is provided with nursing—the therapeutic self-care demand is known and met and self-care agency is developed or its exercise is regulated, or that an explicit design for nursing is incorporated into a larger design for a system of health care.
5. Accept that *design* is an integral function of nursing practice and that *design* is the proper *function* of professionals. Design may be in the mind of the professional or it may be an expressed design to be communicated to others. Without design, there is no evidence of professional-level practice. [*Ed. Note:* The elements of nursing design are presented in chapter 5 of *Nursing: Concepts of Practice* (Orem, 1995). "The Functions of Design in Nursing Process" are in a case example given on pp. 215–226. Six design units with their elements are identified with the assumptions underlying them on pp. 103–116.]
6. Make the concepts and the relationships among them your own. Come to understand them in reality situations. Memorized definitions will not serve you. It is your personal insights into reality situations that you can conceptualize and express and communicate to others.

You are engaged in a movement to ensure that both administrators and clinicians have a well-defined view of nursing. It is helpful within the same organization when views are philosophically and conceptually congruent. A shared vision of nursing, a shared language, and an organizing framework enable a nursing department or division to fulfill its own mission within the framework of the purposes and functions of the agency as a whole. To be able to talk about nursing and about what nurses and nursing contribute is an essential quality for nursing administrators and nursing practitioners. None of the above is possible without the deliberate selection and use of a general theory of nursing and commitment to its use. If this is your goal, how do you proceed? The first step has been taken so work can begin by administrators and practitioners. This work should be understood, and the amount of time and effort required should not be underestimated. All parts of the nursing organization will be affected. This should be recognized from the beginning. I will not talk about all the work that needs to be done. A laying out of the process of implementation at the administrative and practice level is essential, as is a nurse who is a master of the theory to serve as a coordinator or as a consultant to a less knowledgeable coordinator. There will be no success unless there is commitment and support by the nursing executive of the position of project coordinator and an executive committee.

I am not an expert in these areas so I shall confine my time to talking about one of the common tasks, namely, making the *concepts of the theory and the relationship among them* your own in a way that serves you in producing nursing or in ensuring that nursing will be provided for populations served. I suggest that we begin with accepting that

1. Nursing is a practical endeavor that is associated with cognitive, intellectual work. The reality is that the conceptual elements of the theory must be dealt with in the nursing process.
2. The use of self-care deficit theory of nursing does not preclude but demands the use of other theories, namely interpersonal interactive theory, as well as societal facts and theories. It is a practice theory put to use with an interpersonal and larger societal framework. Nursing has societal and interpersonal dimensions as well as that which nurses do for patients.

I would suggest that you reflect on the ideas that broad concepts have meaning and signify entities, properties, and change, but each broad concept has a substantive structure and it is this substantive structure that leads us to understand reality situations. Concepts to be considered include the following:

1. Self-care is action regulatory of one's human functioning and development. Its substantive structure consists of estimative operations, decision-making operations, and production operations, all directed to knowing and meeting one or more components of the therapeutic self-care demand.
2. Therapeutic self-care demand, which is constructed in the particular health care situation and references all of the actions to be taken to accomplish self-care. The substantive structure includes specific self-care requisites particularized for individuals, means for meeting them including overcoming of obstacles, and the set of care measures specific to the technology to meet the requisite.
3. Self-care agency, which is the complex ability to perform self-care. The substantive structure includes the ability to perform self-care operations in a specific context, the enabling power components, and the foundational capabilities and dispositions.

CHAPTER 34

Work to Be Done

S elf-care deficit nursing theory, from a philosophy of science perspective, is knowledge that is both theoretical and practical. This knowledge is a part of and foundational for continuing development of the practical science of nursing. The theory's conceptual constructs articulate with facts and points of theory from other fields, thus indicating areas of need for development of applied nursing sciences.

The knowledge expressed in the articulated theories of nursing system, self-care deficit, and self-care is descriptively explanatory of the end products and the results that nurses seek to make and achieve for and with persons under their care, the proper objects of nurses' attention and actions, and the structure of nurses' actions to make the products and achieve the human results proper to nursing. The usefulness of self-care deficit nursing theory is recognized by nurses who have mastered the formalized concepts and relationships of the theory and have made them dynamic in concrete singular situations of nursing practice. Usefulness is also recognized by teachers of nursing and curriculum developers who have used the theory in the development of nursing courses and in the selection of and negotiating for courses foundational to the nursing curricula. Researchers have been concerned with the validity of the conceptual structure of self-care deficit nursing theory and with the values of the constructs by populations and types of cases.

There is work to be done if self-care deficit nursing theory is to be used in further development of the practical science of nursing and in the structuring of nursing knowledge. Some broad suggestions are made.

1. Compilation and consideration of unanswered questions of nurses using the theory

---

This paper was originally prepared for a self-care study group and was written September 23, 1993.

2. Continuing identification and validation of variations in the values of real world referents of the theory's concepts by types of cases and populations, with attention to relationships and values of basic conditioning factors
3. Continuing explication of the substantive structure and referents of the concepts of self-care agency and nursing agency with a focus on operations and relationships
4. Investigation of human processes and pathways in the development of self-care agency
5. Further explication of the human regulatory functions of universal self-care requisites
6. Identification and description of self-care practices and self-care systems of individuals and groups within a community's prevailing culture and its subcultures and within the cultures of new entrants to the community
7. Study of technologies of care in current use by nurses in relationship to the three types of self-care requisites

Cooperation and coordination of effort and mechanisms for communicating results are essential.

CHAPTER 35

The World of the Nurse

INTRODUCTION

My work of seeking to understand the nature and structure of nursing during the years 1959 to the present has been concerned with two questions: What do nurses encounter in their worlds as they design and produce nursing for others? What meaning can and should nurses attach to persons, things, events, conditions, and circumstances they encounter?

Over the years, three theories have been developed to answer two questions that must have answers if we are to understand what nurses encounter and what they do as nurses.

The first question is: Why do people need nursing, or what human condition brings about a need for nursing? The theories of self-care and the theory of self-care deficit provide hypothesized answers.

The second question is: What is nursing? What is the *structure* of the entity, the service that we refer to as nursing? The theory of nursing system provides a hypothesized answer.

SCIENTIFIC KNOWLEDGE AND THEORIES

My work in theory development has focused on the beginning development of scientific knowledge in the field of nursing. Harre (1970) states that scientific knowledge consists of two main kinds of information:

This paper is reprinted with permission from the *International Orem Society Newsletter* (1996) 4(1), 2–7.

1. Knowledge of the internal structure, constitution, or nature of enti-
    ties and materials (for these are what persist), and
2. Knowledge of the statistics of events, of the behavior of persisting
    entities and materials. In this way patterns of events are discerned
    and how the discerned patterns are produced by persisting struc-
    tures is explained.

Harre (1970) identifies a theory as a "statement-picture" complex that
supplies an account of the constitution and behavior of these entities whose
interactions with each other are responsible for the manifested patterns of
behavior. A theory very often fills in a gap in available knowledge. A theorist
conceives a model, an analogue, for the presently unknown structures and
constitutions of things. Harre states, " . . . the model is itself modelled on
things and materials and processes which we do understand" (p. 35). For
example, the theory of self-care is expressed in terms of its being a deliberately brought-about human regulatory function. One basis of this is knowledge of other human regulatory functions, for example, those of the
endocrine and neurological systems. The theory of self-care also is based
upon knowledge and models of deliberate human action. The statements
within the statement-picture complex that expresses a theory will (1)
describe the phenomena for which the theory is devised (persons performing self-care actions), (2) describe the central idea of the model (self-
care as deliberately brought-about human regulatory function), and (3)
describe the material on which the central model is based (models of
human regulatory functions and of deliberate action [Harre, 1970]).

The theory of self-care is both descriptive and explanatory. It describes
actions and events that are recognized as self-care. It identifies the relation
of performed self-care actions to human functioning and development.

Today I shall not recount the formal expressions of the self-care deficit
theory of nursing and the three theories explanatory of it. My approach
is to lay out some of the ideas and thought processes involved in reaching
understandings expressed in the self-care deficit theory of nursing. I shall
address two topics.

1. Human beings and their self-regulation of their own human func-
    tioning and development in time and place frames of reference
2. The existence of a population of human beings in time and place
    frames of reference with health-associated or health-derived inca-
    pacities to engage in the self-regulation of their own functioning

and human development and how nurses can, do, and should relate to and help members of this population

As we proceed, please endeavor to understand the need for picturing, using analogies, modeling, and expressing conditional statements. For example, picturing individuals in intensive care units as contrasted with individuals in an ambulatory care clinic; using analogies, such as, Mr. X. is like a newborn, awake but not able to care for himself; forming models, for example, of what individuals under specified conditions should do or what individuals with specific action incapacities are and are not able to do for themselves; and expressing if-then statements, for example, if persons in this described condition of health are not helped, then this or that can occur.

SELF-CARE AND HUMAN FUNCTIONING AND DEVELOPMENT

If human life is to continue and development proceed there must be continuing inputs of materials and the provision or maintenance of conditions that support life, physical and psychic functioning, and developmental processes. Inputs of required materials and provision of needed conditions when deliberately made or sought by persons for themselves is named and referred to as *self-care*; when made by others for persons dependent on them it is referred to as *dependent-care*; when made by nurses for individuals with health-derived or health-associated incapacities for self-care, it is an aspect of *nursing*.

The inputs of materials and the conditions that are known or presumed to support and regulate human functioning and development are identified within three categories:

1. Those that are universally required by all individuals at each stage of the life cycle
2. Those that are specific in supporting and regulating human developmental processes
3. Those that arise from impaired or disordered physical or psychic aspects of human functioning and from measures to prevent, diagnose, or treat impaired or disordered functioning

Requirements for inputs of specific materials or specific conditions are named *self-care requisites*, for example, the requisite maintain a sufficient intake of water. What is sufficient must be determined (particularized) for individuals in relation to prevailing internal and external conditions in some time and place frame of reference. This requisite is placed within the *universally* required category. It is a universal type of self-care requisite (Orem, 1995).

An example of a developmental-type requisite is: supply and maintain conditions that permit and foster sensory-motor development in infancy. A health deviation type is: monitor individuals for signs and symptoms of bleeding and for changes in vital processes following x-type abdominal surgical procedure performed under general anesthesia.

Nurses are or should be aware that they will not find in the nursing literature or in that of other disciplines already formulated self-care requisites. Nurses must perform this task using nursing knowledge and knowledge from related disciplines.

A THEORY OF SELF-CARE

From a perspective of nursing science we must ask the question: Is *self-care* a feature of the world of man and human affairs? Does it exist? My answer is yes. But are there criteria that point to specific actions of individuals and cause me or you to judge that the action is or is not self-care? For example, we see an adult pedestrian stopping at a crosswalk when the traffic light is red and proceeding when the light turns green, after determining that motor traffic has ceased within the crosswalk. We can identify this sequence of actions as a following of pedestrian traffic rules. We also identify it as an instance of self-care. The pedestrian may see the behavior as something he or she always does; it is a habit. But it can be judged by pedestrian and observer as an instance of self-protection, an instance of self-care to meet the universal type requisite of prevention of hazards.

As nurses we must learn to differentiate self-care from other forms of behavior or other actions of individuals, as well as to understand that some behaviors, as in the example, fulfill more than one purpose. We theorize about self-care in order to be knowing about what it is and what it is not. In the development of the theory of self-care, its nature as deliberate human action was first accepted. This nature is expressed by the following statements: self-care is conduct; it is deliberate action; it is learned behavior; it is ego-processed behavior; but self-care is also work and self-care requires the expenditure of energy. Self-care is action that I perform for myself, for my own sake, for my life, health, and well-being.

Since all action is for an end, we must ask: What ends, what results are sought through self-care? Or: Why are these events and patterns of behavior that we call self-care the way they are? The answer is to supply materials and conditions that human beings require to maintain and support life, health, and well-being. We then move to formalize the theory, which hypothesizes that self-care is a human regulatory function that individuals must perform with deliberation (or have performed for them) to supply materials and conditions to maintain life, and to keep physical and psychic functioning within norms that are compatible with life and with the integrity of human functioning and development (Orem, 1995). The theory is *explanatory of self-care* because it sets forth the relationships between self-care actions and continued human life and human functioning and development. Explanations set forth relationships among entities; in this situation it is the relation of the actions performed by individuals to supply required materials and conditions and their continued human existence and functioning.

Self-Care as Process

Self-care as it is performed by individuals in time and over time is a process, series and sequences of actions and events. When performed over time self-care of individuals can be viewed as systems of care activities. So we speak of self-care systems. As persons seeking scientific knowledge we cannot be satisfied with knowing that self-care is a process in time. We want to understand its structure. To do this we first accept that even processes have a structure.

The structure of the process of self-care is viewed as those enduring elements that characterize the meeting of each and every self-care requisite, regardless of the kinds of materials or conditions being supplied or the results sought. This structure is hypothesized to consist of three types of operations—estimative operations, transitional operations, and production operations. An operation is a process or action that is part of some work to be done. In this situation the work is knowing and meeting each existent self-care requisite.

Estimative self-care operations investigate existent relevant human and environmental conditions in a time-place frame of reference. They investigate the meaning of conditions for the lives, health, and well-being of individuals. Determinations are made about what can and what should be regulated through the meeting of specific, particularized self-care requisites and the methods of technologies for meeting each requisite.

Transitional operations include selection of and appraisal of the results achieved through performance of estimative operations, making judgments about what can and should be done, and making decisions about what will be done in meeting specific, particularized self-care requisites.

Production operations are actions to secure needed resources, to bring about necessary conditions in self and environment, and to perform the measures of care associated with using specific methods in meeting each particularized self-care requisite. They are also actions to monitor for effects and results, desired and untoward. They include reflection and appraisal to determine evidence of adequacy of performance and results. Production operations also include making judgments about their continuation and about needs for a resumption of estimative operations.

This structure of operations is a part of each instance of self-care. When features of self-care have become habitual practices, the estimative and transitional operations do not require the attention and thought that must be given to new and emerging self-care requisites. This hypothesized structure of self-care as process is modeled on the structural elements of deliberate human action. A model of deliberate action is shown in *Nursing: Concepts of Practice*, Figure 3 (Orem, 1995, p. 165).

This operational model of the structure of self-care as process identifies self-care as practical endeavor, endeavor to bring about requisite human or environmental conditions that do not presently exist in individuals or their environments. The model also identifies speculative endeavors focused on knowing and reasoning, judging and arriving at decisions. The estimative and transitional operations are largely speculative.

Children are taught and learn to perform the productive operations of self-care and time and place of their performance before they master estimative and transitional operations. When adults or adolescents are confronted with new, emerging self-care requisites, time is required not only for learning how to perform care measures but also in determining what is and what can and should be done under present conditions and in deciding what they will do. Nurses should know the structure of the process of self-care and know what action demand this structure places on individuals. They should know each patient's capabilities for performing each of the three operations of self-care. For example, in a nurse-managed diabetic clinic some adults with arrested cognitive development who thought concretely were instructed about and became able to recognize the occurrence of untoward conditions. They were instructed to call the nurse if they perceived the occurrence of the conditions. The patients would then be instructed by the nurse about what to do.

Self-Care and Daily Living

Self-care is one of many result-seeking endeavors in the lives of individuals. There are two, often unrecognized, very personal endeavors that affects the performance of all other endeavors. These are self-appraisal and self-management. Children provide us with good examples of the developmental pathways toward being able to look at and manage self within the context of daily living in time and place frames of reference. The effectiveness of self-appraisal and self-management affects the performance of other types of endeavors in which persons engage, for example, occupational, educational, household, self-care, participation in family life, and care and guidance of dependent family members and others.

Nurses focus on the self-care requisites and self-care endeavors of persons under their care. At the same time nurses must understand and become able to view self-care within the context of the daily lives of individuals. The need for such understanding was expressed by a woman when a doctor and a nurse were representing to her a new and complex regimen of care. The woman, in great consternation, said to them: "How do you expect me to do all these things and continue to live my own life?" Final decisions about the components of persons' self-care demands should take into consideration persons' situations of daily living.

Populations Requiring Nursing

In any society or social group there are persons whose lives or health or well-being is endangered because their powers to provide their own self-care are not qualitatively or quantitatively equal to knowing or meeting their therapeutic self-care demands or specific component parts. When limitations for performing self-care have their origins in the health states of individuals or in the nature of their health care requirements, nursing is the required health service. The proper object or focus of nursing is not health, disease, or care. The object or focus of nursing is human beings with health-derived or health-associated self-care deficits.

Self-care deficits are understood in terms of the relationship between the amount and kind of required self-care (therapeutic self-care demand) and the action capabilities and action limitations of individuals for knowing what care is needed and producing this care. When individuals' action capabilities are not adequate to know and meet their therapeutic self-care demands, a deficit relationship exists. Nurses not only must become and be knowing about self-care, self-care requisites, and therapeutic self-care demands, but also about the human power named *self-care agency.*

Self-Care Agency, a Human Power

Persons who engage in self-care or dependent-care are referred to as agents, performers, or doers of care. To provide self-care, individuals must have the power, the capabilities to do so. This power is named *self-care agency.* According to Harre (1970), saying that someone or something has a *power* is to say what it *does* or *can do*, not just because of existent stimuli or conditions but in some measure because of its nature or constitution. When powers are ascribed to people, *can* and not *will* is the proper word to use. What a person *will do* is up to him or her regardless of what the person *can do.*

In developing insights about human powers it is important to recognize that there are *enabling conditions* that ensure a state of readiness for persons to exercise a power, and *stimulus conditions* that bring about a response if *enabling conditions* are present and operational. Harre states that power is a notion particularly associated with agency, with the initiation of trains of events, with activity.

Capabilities stand for powers that can be developed or lost without a change in the nature or constitution of the person, thing, or material. What persons can do in knowing and meeting their own self-care requisites is properly referred to as *capabilities.* Self-care agency is the name assigned to the internal enabling conditions of human beings that make it possible for them to perform the estimative, transitional, and productive operations through which self-care is effected. In the development of self-care deficit nursing theory these internal enabling conditions were identified during a search for understanding of the underlying structure of the theoretical concept of self-care agency. Three types of enabling conditions are identified.

Type 1

Foundational capabilities and dispositions (Table 35.1) include (1) three sets of physiologically or psychologically described capabilities prerequisite for learning to or engaging in deliberate action, speculative or practical, including self-care, (2) two sets of dispositions and orientations of individuals prerequisite for performing deliberate actions, including self-care in time-place frames of reference.

Type 2

Capabilities that are enabling for the initiating and performing of self-care operations in time-place frames of reference for durations of time. These were identified as power components of self-care agency because without their development and operational readiness no self-care operation could be performed. Ten power components were identified by the Nursing Development Conference Group (1979):

1. Ability to maintain attention and exercise requisite vigilance with respect to (a) self as self-care agent and (b) internal and external conditions and factors significant for self-care.
2. Controlled use of available physical energy that is sufficient for the initiation and continuation of self-care operations.
3. Ability to control the position of the body and its parts in the execution of the movements required for the initiation and completion of self-care operations.
4. Ability to reason within a self-care frame of reference.
5. Motivation (i.e., goal orientations for self-care that are in accord with its characteristics and its meaning for life, health, and well-being).
6. Ability to make decisions about care of self and to operationalize these decisions.
7. Ability to acquire technical knowledge about self-care from authoritative sources, to retain it and operationalize it.
8. A repertoire of cognitive, perceptual, manipulative, communication, and interpersonal skills adapted to the performance of self-care operations.

TABLE 35.1 Human Capabilities and Dispositions Foundational for Self-Care Agency

Conditioning factors and states[a]	Capabilities and dispositions				
	Selected basic capabilities		Knowing and doing capabilities	Dispositions affecting goals sought	Significant orientative capabilities and dispositions
	I	II			
Genetic and constitutional factors	Sensation Proprioception Exteroception	Attention	Rational agency	Self-understanding Self-awareness Self-concept Self-image	Orientations to: Time Health Other persons Events, objects
Arousal state	Learning	Perception	Operational knowing	Self-value	Priority system or value hierarchy Moral Economic Aesthetic Material Social

TABLE 35.1 (*continued*)

| Conditioning factors and states[a] | Selected basic capabilities | | Knowing and doing capabilities | Dispositions affecting goals sought | Significant orientative capabilities and dispositions |
	I	II			
Social organization	Exercise or work	Memory	Learned skills Reading Counting Writing Verbal Perceptual Manual Reasoning	Self-acceptance Self-concern Acceptance of bodily functions Willingness to meet needs of self	Interest and concerns Habits Ability to work with the body and its parts
Culture Experience	Regulation of the position and movement of the body and its parts	Central regulation of motivational emotional processes	Self-consistency in knowing and doing	Future directions	Ability to manage self and personal affairs

The table header "Capabilities and dispositions" spans the columns: Selected basic capabilities (I, II), Knowing and doing capabilities, Dispositions affecting goals sought, Significant orientative capabilities and dispositions.

From: Nursing Development Conference Group. (1979). *Concept Formalization: Process and Product*, D. Orem (Ed.), Boston: Little Brown, p. 212.

9. Ability to order discrete self-care or action systems into relationships with prior and subsequent actions toward the final achievement of regulatory goals of self-care.
10. Ability to consistently perform self-care operations, integrating them with relevant aspects of personal, family and community living (NDCG, 1979, pp. 195–196).

Type 3

Capabilities to initiate and conduct in time-place frames of reference the estimative, transitional, and productive operations in order to know, particularize, and meet existent and projected self-care requisites were also developed by the Nursing Development Conference Group (1979) (Table 35.2).

These three types of enabling conditions constitute a model of the structure of self-care agency. Self-care agency develops and operates as a power of individual human beings. It is the presence and readiness of the enabling conditions that permit human beings to exercise self-care agency as a power as they function as unitary beings. The identified enabling conditions, that is, the structure of self-care agency, provide a framework for the identification and recognition of types of limitations of self-care agency. Three types of limitations have been identified and described. These are limitations of knowing, limitations for making judgments and decisions about components of the therapeutic self-care demand, and limitations for performing result-achieving courses of action to produce self-care (Orem, 1995). Limitations are indicators of what persons are unable or probably unable to do in self-care.

Nursing requires nurses' identification and description of individuals' self-care agency limitations, including causes of the limitations. This knowledge enables nurses to make judgments about the nature and degree of persons' action limitations. But nursing also requires nurses' determination of the adequacy of individuals' powers of self-care agency for knowing and meeting their existent or projected therapeutic self-care demands. From this measuring of adequacy, determinations of the presence or absence of self-care deficits are made.

Self-care deficits are described as complete or partial. They can also be described in terms of the absence of enabling conditions or the state of readiness of enabling conditions. An unconscious person has a complete

TABLE 35.2   Capabilities Related to Self-Care Operations

OPERATIONS	RESULTS
Estimative Type	
1. Investigation of internal and external conditions and factors significant for self-care	Empirical knowledge of self and environment
2. Investigation of the meaning of characterized conditions and factors and their regulation	Experiential knowing (based in part on acquired technical knowledge) of the meaning of the existent conditions and factors for life, health, and well-being
3. Investigation of the question: How can existent conditions and factors be regulated (i.e., changed or maintained)?	Technical knowledge of what can be regulated and the means available for effective regulation
Transitional Type	
4. Reflection to determine which course of self-care should be followed	An affirming judgment that one course of self-care is preferred, or that a series of courses is preferred, or that none should be pursued
5. Deciding what to do with respect to self-care	A decision to engage in or not engage in specific regulatory self-care operations
Productive Type	
6. Preparation of self, materials, or environmental settings for the performance of a regulatory-type self-care operation	Conditions of readiness for performing self-care operations for regulatory purposes
7a. Performance of productive self-care operations with specific regulatory purposes within a time period	Knowledge that regulatory measures are in process or are complicated
7b. Determining presence of and monitoring, during performance, conditions know to affect effectiveness or performance and results	Information that conditions and factors affecting performance and results are, are not present
8. Monitoring for evidence of effects and results a. desired b. untoward	Information about events indicating that regulation is or is not being achieved
9. Reflection to determine and confirm evidence of adequacy of performance and presence of regulatory results	An affirming judgment as related to specific self-care regulatory operations should continue, should be discontinued, should be resumed at a future time

(continued)

TABLE 35.2 *(continued)*

OPERATIONS	RESULTS
10a. Decision about regulatory operations—to continue or discontinue action, or resume action at a specific time	
10b. Decision about estimative operations to continue to use results from estimative operations or begin a new series of estimative operations	

From: Nursing Development Conference Group. (1979). *Concept Formalization in Nursing: Process and Product* (2nd ed.), D. E. Orem (Ed.). Boston: Little, Brown and Co., pp. 192–193.

self-care deficit; a person who must learn self-care operations associated with a changed state of health and new self-care requisites has a partial deficit.

NURSING SYSTEMS

Persons who can be helped through nursing may be of any age, in various stages of development, in states of good health or poor health, conscious or unconscious. However, each person who requires nursing has a therapeutic self-care demand to be determined and met, and health state-derived or associated-action limitations or incapacities for performance of one or more of the operations of the process of self-care. Nurses, through the operations of nursing practice, identify and particularize existent self-care requisites, calculate the components of their patients' therapeutic self-care demands, identify self-care agency capabilities and limitations, and identify the causes of limitations. Nurses act to regulate the exercise or development of patients' power of self-care agency and ensure that therapeutic self-care demands are known and met. The capabilities and limitations of self-care agency of persons are assessed in relation to the care demand to be met. The nature, causes, and extent of a self-care deficit in relation to an existent (stable or changing) therapeutic self-care demand indicate the amount and kind of nursing required as well as its time and place dimensions.

The components of individuals' therapeutic self-care demands and the development and operability of their powers of self-care agency are conditioned by factors specific to persons as individuals and as members of societal units in time and place locations. Within self-care deficit nursing theory these are referred to as *basic conditioning factors*. Factors specific to individuals include gender, age, developmental state, health state, and health care system factors. Societal unit factors include culture, family-system factors, and socioeconomic factors. Environmental factors and available resources affect persons both as individuals and as members of societal units. Nurses must be knowledgeable about the factors and about how they condition the existence and nature of self-care requisites, methods of meeting requisites, and each identified enabling condition of the power of self-care agency.

Nurses produce systems of care for persons with requirements for nursing. Systems of nursing can be described in terms of nurse role and patient role in knowing and meeting patients' therapeutic self-care demands and in terms of their roles in regulating the development and exercise of patients' powers of self-care agency. The production of nursing is a process based upon the developed powers of nurses to produce nursing for others (nursing agency), the willingness of nurses and nurses' patients to interact and cooperate with each other and to work with one another over time to know and meet stable or changing components of patients' therapeutic self-care demands, and to regulate the development or exercise of patients' powers of self-care agency. Nursing systems are what nurses make when they practice nursing.

CHAPTER 36

Self-Care Deficit Nursing Theory Development Group

This introduction to the subsequent reports of the Development Group focuses on my understanding of the complexity of the never-ending task of theory development and refinement. Development of the self-care deficit theory of nursing encompasses the initial expression of the theory, the creation of insightful conceptual models, formalization of the main conceptual elements of the models, and uncovering the substantive structure, that is, the structural components of the elements. This is the step that leads to identification, description, and explanation of the concrete entities of nursing practice. The pathway of theory formalization and development is not only long but complex, as expressed in the following example.

The group of nursing scholars, the Nursing Development Conference Group, worked to formalize the conceptual elements of the models in the 1960s and 1970s. They drew upon their knowledge of nursing and abilities to work with elements of many sciences and disciplines foundational to understanding nursing—biology, psychology, sociology, the broad field of human behavior, cultural anthropology, the medical sciences, the public health sciences, medical sociology, social philosophy, and education. We explored Sommerhoff's analytical biology, Wiener's work in cybernetics, systems theory as used by behavioral scientists, and various approaches to action theory. The majority of us had essential foundations in logic, epistemology, ethics, and some of us in metaphysics. We were all nurses

This chapter was originally presented via video at the Fifth International Self-Care Deficit Nursing Theory Conference, August 9, 1997, in Leuven, Belgium.

but in a sense we were interdisciplinary with nursing in the foundational sciences and nursing specializations.

As a group we were guided by our developing understanding of nursing as a practical science with theoretically and practically practical components (as described by the philosophers Wallace and Maritain). Eamon O'Doherty, educator, clinical psychologist, occupational psychologist, and human behavioral scientist, helped us clarify our goals, accept nursing as a practical science and a set of applied sciences, understand research specific in the development of practice fields, develop insights about stages of development of the arts and sciences, and clarify the scope and depth of knowledge and technology in forms of education for the occupations and professions.

Basic to all our deliberations was the use of clinical data from nursing cases reported by Group members from their nursing practice endeavors. Some of this early work is narrated in the two editions of *Concept Formalization in Nursing: Process and Product* (NDCG, 1973, 1979).

In 1995 I accepted the need for another formal organized approach to the continuing task of development and refinement of the elements and relationships of self-care deficit nursing theory. At my invitation, the Development Group here today formed itself and took on the task of continuing theory development and refinement. Members meet regularly as a group of the whole and in small work groups. I am grateful to group members for their personal commitments and contributions. It is a pleasure to work with them.

CHAPTER 37

The Formalization of General and Subsidiary Self-Care Requisites and Components of Associated Therapeutic Self-Care Demand for a Particular Health State

PART ONE: FORMALIZED GENERAL AND SUBSIDIARY SELF-CARE REQUISITES OF PERSONS WITH THE PATHOLOGY NAMED BRONCHIAL ASTHMA

The General Requisite

Bring about or maintain adequate pulmonary ventilation by preventing or controlling the pathological processes and their effects, including experienced respiratory difficulty, that characterize attacks of bronchial asthma by engaging in care regimens with some known effectiveness in

1. Reducing swelling and inflammation of the airways of the lungs (smaller bronchioles) that result in their blocking by the production

---

This chapter was originally prepared as part of a consultation with a student at the University of Missouri-Columbia, 1998.

of excess mucus by the mucous membranes of the airways and the leaking of fluid from the blood vessels

2. Preventing or controlling anxiety that may aggravate respiratory difficulty
3. Avoiding, eliminating, or minimizing exposure to allergens, irritants, and other materials and environmental or internal conditions (triggers) that can activate immune cells produced in the body that are associated with inflammation of airway tissues

Subsidiary Self-Care Requisite 1: Accept myself as having periodic attacks of bronchial asthma and learn to understand and fulfill my responsibilities for maintaining or restoring adequate pulmonary ventilation during pending attacks and attacks in process.

Subsidiary Self-Care Requisite 2: Secure and maintain the position of patient in relation to specialized health care professionals (physicians, nurses) who have the knowledge and skills to diagnose the nature and severity of my asthmatic attacks, instruct me in making observations and reporting, prescribe therapeutic measures and regimens, and help me learn to manage myself and my environment and perform care measures to restore and maintain adequate pulmonary ventilation.

Subsidiary Self-Care Requisite 3: Make observations of the occurrence of respiratory difficulties, their nature, the time and sequence of occurrence and their duration, their severity, and the prevailing relevant internal conditions (e.g., respiratory infection) and external conditions (e.g., exposure to extreme cold) at the time of occurrence. On the basis of this information make judgments about the progress and severity of the attack, the preferred regulatory care to be instituted, and the probable outcome if appropriate care is instituted.

Subsidiary Self-Care Requisite 4: Make a decision to and perform the selected regimen of therapeutic care after assembling the medications and equipment required, with understanding of the value of the selected regimen of care in preventing an impending attack or in control of an attack in progress. When respiratory difficulties are severe and may be life threatening immediately place myself under emergency medical care. Family members and associates when informed can assist.

Subsidiary Self-Care Requisite 5:   Make observations of respiratory functioning and the severity and duration of asthmatic symptoms once a therapeutic regimen has been instituted either for prevention or control of an attack in process. Make judgments about the effectiveness of the therapeutic regimen instituted to prevent or to regulate an attack. Report to health care professionals.

PART TWO: THERAPEUTIC SELF-CARE DEMAND COMPONENT

The General Requisites

Constituent activity elements of persons' therapeutic self-care demands express the operations that must be performed to meet formalized and personalized self-care requisites. Health-deviation self-care requisites (such as those for the prevention, regulation, and control of attacks of bronchial asthma) can be formalized only by health care professionals with authoritative knowledge of the nature and structure of the pathological and diagnostic processes involved, and reliable and valid modes of therapy. Once formalized, health-deviation self-care requisites in practice situations must be personalized for individuals by health care professionals on the basis of accurate information about them, what they know about their disease, and what they can and cannot do in their own care.

The following are suggestions about some of the operations involved in meeting each of the five subsidiary self-care requisites named in Part One of this document. Since the general requisite has not been personalized for a specific person, the named operations are viewed as operations of value in meeting each subsidiary requisite. They may offer guides in personalization of the requisites for individuals.

The operations for each requisite are listed separately. For the full expression of each requisite refer to Part One.

Subsidiary Self-Care Requisite 1:   Accept myself as having periodic attacks of bronchial asthma.

Operations to Meet Subsidiary Requisite 1

1. Maintain an awareness that as a person with bronchial asthma I am responsible for acting effectively prior to or during attacks in main-

taining or restoring my pulmonary ventilation, including the securing of professional health care.

2. Reflect upon how I know that I am having an asthmatic attack and isolate in my thoughts my specific experiences and ways I know to represent and describe them: for example tightness of chest, wheezing, coughing, shortness of breath, occurrences when breathing is very difficult.

3. Become able to express what I experience (symptoms), their severity, sequence of occurrence, and duration in order to represent my condition and my experiences to health care professionals. Seek help as needed from physicians and nurses to assist me in learning to describe my symptoms accurately and to make judgments about the severity and meaning of my attacks. Learn the sources of authoritative written materials that will help me in fulfilling my responsibility for care.

4. Learn to work cooperatively with health care professionals and my family to understand and learn to carry out prescribed regimens of therapeutic self-care.

5. Seek and reflect upon information about how my condition of bronchial asthma and its associated care can or should affect my usual routine of self-care and daily living including:

   a. those universal type self-care requisites that need special attention and adjustment to maintain a balance between activity and rest; prevention of hazards to life, health, and well-being; maintaining my normalcy

   b. how to bring about an effective integration of new care elements into my routine systems of self-care and daily living

6. Reflect upon what I now do and what I should do to fulfill my self-care responsibilities associated with bronchial asthma to prevent attacks or control their harmful effects upon me.

Nurse-Compiled Information and Nurses' Prescription With Patient Collaboration

With patient collaboration the nurse ideally collects information sufficient to begin a design for the therapeutic self-care of the patient (including physician input) and a design for a curriculum (an instructional and learning activity design) to help patients become able to fulfill their responsibilities in accord with their developmental state and action potential or to help parents fulfill responsibilities for children.

Subsidiary Self-Care Requisite 2:   Secure and maintain the position of the patient.

The operations to meet this requisite can and should be developed in locales where persons subject to asthmatic attacks reside. Information about available health care should be disseminated on a community-wide basis. This should include how individuals can enter and remain within these systems. From a public health perspective, information about the numbers of persons needing care should be compiled, with attention to their age and mobility, transportation availability, and costs of service.

Nurses providing care to individuals with bronchial asthma need information about

1. Patients' present positions in one or more health care systems
2. Current availability of care: for initial and continuing diagnoses and evaluation of progress with the collection of data from patients' monitoring of attacks, severity of attacks, and their effects on the lives of patients; classifying the severity of patients' attacks; prescribed care regimens for avoidance of triggers; prescribed regimens of care for preventing or controlling attacks; emergency service; and helping patients and families learn to fulfill their care responsibilities
3. Patients' access to care in relation to transportation, costs, their age and mobility, and their independent or dependent status
4. Patients' satisfactions or dissatisfactions with care they are receiving or patients' expressed desires to enter a health care system for help in regulating or controlling their attacks of bronchial asthma

Subsidiary Self-Care Requisite 3:   Make observations of the occurrence of respiratory difficulties.

Operations to Meet Subsidiary Requisite 3

1. Monitor for breathing difficulties
2. Note the time of occurrence of breathing difficulties as well as contact or exposure to external triggers or the presence of internal triggers (cold, engagement in strenuous physical activity, etc.)

3. Note the type(s) of breathing difficulties, their severity, and their progress and duration during each attack of bronchial asthma; note reactions to the attack—the occurrence of degrees of anxiety or outright fear and paralysis for action
4. Make judgments about the nature of the attack, its severity, the prescribed therapeutic self-care regimen to be instituted, the need for help to carry it out, and the need to secure immediate medical care.

Nurses' Activities

The activities depend upon whether the nurses are in physical contact with the patient, have some form of communication, or learn of the patient's activities and experiences following attacks.

Subsidiary Self-Care Requisite 4: Make a decision to and perform the selected regimen of therapeutic self-care.

Operations to Meet Subsidiary Self-Care Requisite 4

1. Reflect upon the judgments made about therapeutic regimens of self-care and make an appraisal of the benefits that can occur from their use. Decide which regimens of care will be instituted, with attention to their preventive value or their value to control impending attacks or attacks in process. Two distinct regimens of self-care should be understood: regimens related to trigger control and regimens directed to control of breathing difficulties.
2. Perform operations to prevent or minimize external environmental triggers. Engage in preventive self-care measures to avoid respiratory infections and self-care to maintain physical, mental, and emotional normalcy.
3. Perform the operations through which prescribed therapeutic self-care regimens to control breathing difficulties are executed, including the assembly of equipment and prescribed medications.
4. Perform operations to control untoward effects of prescribed medications when and if such effects occur.

(Note: For 2 and 3 note differences in time of performance.)

Subsidiary Self-Care Requisite 5:   Make observations of respiratory functioning and the severity and duration of asthmatic symptoms once a therapeutic regimen has been instituted.

Operations to Meet Subsidiary Self-Care Requisite 5

1. Operations to control triggers
    Note changes, if any, in the occurrence of attacks of respiratory difficulty and their severity once controls of known or presumed external environmental triggers are operational. Note changes, if any, in the occurrence of attacks of respiratory difficulty when physical activity is limited to what is of therapeutic value and strenuous physical activity is eliminated. Note effectiveness of operations to control respiratory infections and maintain physical, mental, and emotional health.
2. Operations to control respiratory difficulties
    Note degrees of control of each asthmatic symptom with the use of each therapeutic regimen.

CHAPTER 38

Nursing Practice Models

N ursing, like other human services, requires practice models as one area within its domain of knowledge. Practice models are about actions needed to give the service. They are expositions of the range of types of actions and the articulations of actions and systems of actions of nurses in the designing and the rendering of the human health service of nursing. Practice models have implicit in them the kinds of knowledge that must be applied by nurses in their decision making and in performing the types of actions specified by the practice models.

Model is used in the sense of a pattern or a design for some action to be taken. Nurses take action in nursing practice situations and acquire knowledge needed to make systems of care for specific persons, families, or groups of persons in particular places at this or that time over some duration. Each situation of nursing practice is a concrete reality situation. Practice models, on the other hand, are not concrete. They are abstractions derived from predictable schemes of recurrence of human and environmental events and conditions in nursing care situations. Practice models thus ideally are based upon valid and reliable knowledge of nurses about some range of concrete reality situations of nursing practice. Knowledge necessary for developing practice models for some *range of concrete nursing practice situations* (after Lonergan, 1958) includes the following:

1. Known schemes of recurrence of human and environmental events and properties within situations
2. Validated predictable schemes of variation in the recurring human and environmental events and properties within situations

---

This chapter originated as undated handwritten notes.

3. Validated *means* with some established reliability for (a) acquiring knowledge of, (b) making predictions about, and (c) effecting regulation of human and environmental events and properties with situations. The regulation sought would bring or keep human and environmental events and properties within a range of variations that is compatible with the continuance of life, effective human functioning, and human well-being.

Nurses' initial development, the refinement and continued use of practice models as just described, is necessarily based upon their acceptance of nursing as a practice field. This acceptance, if it has a rational and reasonable basis, includes the understanding that nurses make systems of nursing care for *others* who can benefit from it because of existent or predicted events and conditions that render them in need of nursing, regardless of their needs for other health services. Nurses' development and use of practice models are also related to the state of the art and science of nursing in particular places and at particular times.

Two enduring models used by nurses in their practice are the *task model* and the *medical model*. These models reflect past and to some degree existent orientations of nurses to the domain of nursing knowledge and practice. Neither model in and of itself is a valid nursing practice model. Tasks fit within larger structures of action that nurses should understand and be able to express. Continued acceptance of this medical model by nurses implies their assumption that nursing does not have its own proper object or specialized focus in social groups. This, of course, raises the question of the continued presence of nursing and its significance in society.

Individual nurses and groups of nurses have expressed their understandings of why people need and can benefit from nursing. These expressions by nurses may make explicit, in lieu of the human object, the concern that is proper to nursing and in laying out the domain and boundaries of nursing as a field of knowledge and practice. Nurses' dependence on the task and the medical models of nursing practice have kept nurses *impoverished* with respect to knowledge development about the domain of their own discipline of *nursing*.

GENERAL CHARACTERISTICS

Nursing practice models can be developed at various levels of generality and comprehensiveness. Level of generality is used in the sense of those nursing practice situations for which the model has validity, for example, all nursing practice situations, or only this or that category, or severity of practice situation. Comprehensiveness refers to the inclusion and treatment in the mode of all or some of the human or environmental features of nursing practice situations (see Figure 38.1).

Comprehensiveness refers to the treatment in the mode of all or some of the human or environmental features of nursing practice situations. Development of practice models thus requires on the part of nurse developers a decision about the generalizability of the model and the features of nursing practice situations to be treated by the model. Nursing practice models constitute one product of nurses who engage in the professional work operation of *development*. The other work operations of members of professions performed in order to keep a profession viable in a society are *practice* that is productive of the service, *research, teaching*, and theory development.

Generality of models is understood in terms of the range of appropriateness of the model as a guide for practice in all or some nursing practice situations. Comprehensiveness of practice models is understood in relation to the inclusion and treatment of the features of nursing practice situations. For example, a practice model may be developed around only one feature or

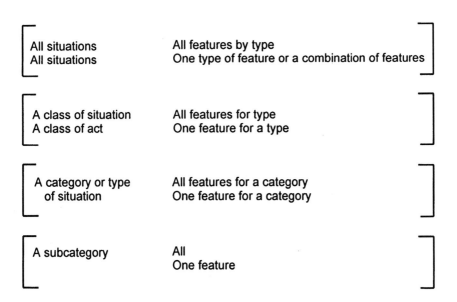

FIGURE 38.1 Features of nursing practice situations.

a set of related features, and yet be useful in all nursing practice situations. Features include not only work operations of nurses in relation to types of nursing cases, but also categories of events and properties, human and environmental.

Since the provision of nursing by nurses to persons in need is a practical endeavor, nursing practice models are designs for practical endeavor that take into account the *doer* of the action, the actor or agent, as well as what the actor does within the situation.

International Perspectives on Orem's Work

S elf-care deficit nursing theory and the work of Dorothea Orem is having a worldwide impact on nursing. A sampling is presented in this section.

The theory has been found to be helpful to nurses in Australia, Belgium, Canada, Germany, Holland, Japan, Norway, Spain, Sweden, Thailand, and Uruguay, to name some of the countries that we know about. In chapters 39, 40, and 41, nurses from Mexico, Germany, and Thailand share information about the impact of self-care deficit nursing theory on nursing in their countries. As indicated in these papers, although some translations exist, major difficulty in using the theory in non–English-speaking countries is the lack of adequate translations of Orem's writings.

CHAPTER 39

The Contribution of Self-Care Deficit Theory to Nursing in Mexico

Esther C. Gallegos

Without survey or interview data, but having watched and heard several groups of Mexican colleagues conduct research and discuss Orem's theory, we assert that Orem's Self-Care Deficit Nursing Theory (SCDNT) has had an enormous influence on nursing education, research, and practice in our country.

Possibly the first to learn about the Self-Care Deficit Theory were the instructors at nursing schools that were affiliated with the Mexican Federation of Nursing Schools (Federación Mexicana de Escuelas y Facultades de Enfermería, FEMAFEE). This association of educational institutions has taught workshops on nursing theory, including SCDNT, throughout the country since the 1980s. It appears that the theory was introduced to academics when self-care nursing theory literature reached leaders in the nursing field. In addition, chapters in books such as the one by Marinar-Tomey (1994), available in Spanish, also helped to disseminate this theory, although in a limited manner.

Another mechanism that has had an influence in spreading the theory to a greater number of nurses has been through Master in Nursing students from several Mexican states, whose curricula include courses on nursing theory. Orem's book (1993), translated to Spanish, is utilized in these courses, thus helping to spread knowledge about the theory. Master's programs have also promoted theory-based research and proposals.

Nursing services in social security institutions (Instituto Mexicano del Seguro Social, IMSS), as well as private hospitals, have also utilized this theory as a basis for designing nursing care. These efforts are attributable to the enthusiasm nurses show for discovering interventions that prove their professional independence, given that historically, nursing care in hospitals has essentially consisted of responding to medical orders in terms of treatment and diagnostics.

The conference titled "Theoretical Self-Care Model," held on October 11, 1995, was a milestone event in the acceptance of the theory within the Mexican nursing industry. Orem herself participated in this conference, along with distinguished members of the Orem Society, who shared their experiences in a two-day workshop following the conference. During the workshop, participants were able to study different applications of the theory in nursing education, research, and practice in the United States and Canada. Three hundred eighty Mexican nurses attended the Orem conference; ninety-four of them participated in the workshop. Most found answers to their questions about theory application.

More recently, we have heard of at least two nursing schools (located in the states of Chihuahua and Veracruz) that want to restructure their curricula based on Self-Care Deficit Theory, although we know of others that are already working under this framework, such as Instituto Politécnico Nacional in Mexico City.

The main difficulties nurses have faced in applying the theory can be summarized as follows: few instruments that would make concepts operational in nursing research and care, few accessible references that address how to use the theory to organize curricula or nursing syllabi at the undergraduate level, and the absence of texts in Spanish.

CHAPTER 40

Self-Care Deficit Nursing Theory in Germany

Gerd Bekel

The discussion about the application of nursing theories in nursing practice did not start in Germany until after 1982. Since nursing science was not integrated into nursing education, the discussion was essentially directed toward the practice use of theories. The scientific use of nursing theories was not the subject of professional discussion before that time. The central ideas of different nursing theories, their definitions of what nursing is and should be were only presented in textbooks. The rather superficial discussion of nursing theories had to do with the lack of valid translations of the theories. Translations did exist in the form of working papers for only very few theories. These were predominantly used for seminars and training courses for nurses but unfortunately were not integrated systematically into education programs at that time.

FIRST STEPS

The growing discussion about nursing theories in Germany was influenced by the development of nursing in Switzerland. In 1991 the first publication focusing on self-care deficit nursing theory appeared in the literature (Ricka & Schmidli-Bless, 1991). This was just before the debate concerning the development of nursing as an academic profession reached its peak in Germany. This occurred between 1991 and 1995. The result of this debate led to the development of the first academic courses for nursing at universities and schools of applied science.

During this period, the publications appeared introducing the self-care deficit nursing theory as a basic concept for nursing practice. Because of the lack of reasonable translations from international nursing literature, a large number of these articles were written at an introductory or explanatory level (Botschafter & Moers, 1991). Articles published later reported on the use of self-care deficit nursing theory in a variety of nursing practice settings (Strunk & Osterbrink, 1995). Research papers, concerning developmental work regarding self-care of particular patient populations or research results related to self-care can not be found for this period.

UTILIZATION OF SELF-CARE DEFICIT NURSING THEORY IN NURSING EDUCATION

Little is known about the use of self-care deficit nursing theory in nursing education. Nevertheless there have been reports since the late eighties that self-care deficit nursing theory was recognized as valuable in nursing education. The majority of nursing schools after 1985 used an Activities of Daily Living based nursing model (ADL), originally developed in England. The first German translation of this nursing model was published in 1987 (Roper, 1987).

The concepts of self-care deficit nursing theory as a structure for teaching were used only by individuals who had the ability to use the original editions of *Nursing: Concepts of Practice*. However, in 1989, the University of Osnabrueck offered courses in which studying the basic concepts of self-care deficit nursing theory was included. Dr. Georges C. Evers from Catholic University of Leuven introduced self-care deficit nursing theory from a research and practice perspective in courses for nursing teachers. His experience in using the theory in the Netherlands and Belgium has had an important impact on further use of the theory in multiple nursing curricula.

In 1991 at the Institut für Weiterbildung in der Krankenpflege (IWK) in Delmenhorst, the self-care deficit nursing theory was integrated into the education of nursing teachers. Gerd Bekel offered special seminars for using the theory in practice settings of hospitals and nursing homes. The activities at Osnabrueck and Delmenhorst, were certainly the first attempts to integrate the self-care deficit nursing theory systematically in nursing education and nursing practice in Germany.

With students from these courses in Delmenhorst, work groups were established in 1993 using the self-care deficit nursing theory in the study of nursing cases. The intention of working group members was to describe which self-care operations should be done by patients and to give direction for the calculation of the therapeutic self-care demand for particular patient population by analyzing certain nursing cases. This was done in particular for patients suffering with incontinence and for patients with psychiatric diseases. In the summer of 1994 the first national conference on self-care deficit nursing theory was held at the IWK in Delmenhorst. Members of the work groups presented their developmental work in nursing practice and education. Dr. Violetta Berbiglia, from the University of Texas in San Antonio, presented at the First National Conference on self-care deficit nursing theory in Germany. At the second Conference on self-care deficit nursing theory in December 1994, further development of group work was presented.

In September 1994, encouraged by the results in using the theory in teaching and work groups, staff members at IWK started the development of a curriculum for the education of nursing consultants. The theoretical basis and the core concepts for this program were completely based on self-care deficit nursing theory. It was the first time that written documents indicated that the self-care deficit nursing theory was systematically included in a nursing curriculum.

Emphasis was put on the fact that the nursing diagnostic procedure based on self-care deficit nursing theory should be at the center of nursing consultation with patient and family members. Although the theory today is used in a variety of nursing schools, at the present time no further reports exist about how the theory is used in nursing curricula.

In 1999, Elisabeth Holoch and colleagues published a textbook for pediatric nursing based on self-care deficit nursing theory (Holoch et al., 1999). It is one of the first nursing textbooks in Germany based on a nursing theory. The German translation of the fifth edition of *Nursing: Concepts of Practice* was first published in 1997 (Orem, 1997).

UTILIZATION OF SELF-CARE DEFICIT NURSING THEORY IN NURSING PRACTICE

The application of self-care deficit nursing theory in nursing practice began in Germany in approximately 1995. This process has been facilitated by the increasing development of nursing programs at the university level. Several hospitals developed projects to apply the theory to nursing practice. In 1995, a hospital in Hanover introduced the concepts of self-care deficit nursing theory in a geriatric rehabilitation department. The aim of this project was to align entire nursing care planning and documentation on the basis of self-care deficit nursing theory. Further projects followed in 1996 in Bremen. In St. Remberti, a nursing home, extensive diagnostic instruments for nursing care planning related to exploration of self-care agency and dependent-care agency were developed. Parallel to this work, in 1996 nurses in two hospitals in Bremen started to use self-care deficit nursing theory for direction in their practice. Members of a work group at the Diakonissen Hospital in Bremen chose self-care deficit nursing theory among several nursing theories as the basis for the nursing department. At the end of 1996 the Central Hospital Links der Weser in Bremen started a training program for nurses based on self-care deficit nursing theory. Later, concepts were developed using self-care ideas for nursing practice. In 1997 further projects followed in the Community Hospital in Schorndorf and in the General Hospital in Harburg. The University Hospital in Ulm, the pediatric hospital Olgahospital in Stuttgart, and the City Hospital in Munich-Schwabing, one of the largest hospitals in Munich, began to use self-care deficit nursing theory in developmental nursing projects. Further projects were begun in 2001 at hospitals in Neumuenster and Quaken-brueck. Today there are approximately 15 institutions using self-care deficit nursing theory systematically for nursing practice—that is, their nursing philosophy and care planning are totally based on self-care oriented models.

STRUCTURE OF DEVELOPMENTAL PRACTICE PROJECTS

The overall goals for the implementation process of self-care deficit nursing theory are:

1. Facilitating continuity of nursing processes related to patient treatment
2. Facilitating continuity of interdisciplinary treatment processes of patients
3. Developing and utilizing nursing-specific language related to a nursing theory

Concept Design

The implementation of self-care deficit nursing theory in various nursing practice fields is based on a four-step concept.

Step 1:   Identification of problems and structures of nursing in the health-care institution; theoretical introduction of the concepts of self-care deficit nursing theory

Step 2:   Formulation and analysis of nursing relevant patient situations in various nursing fields; development of systematic descriptions of patient problems related to the health-care situation and the therapeutic self-care demand associated with the situation

Step 3:   Development of instruments for nursing diagnostic procedures

Step 4:   Development of nursing therapeutic procedures specific to relevant nursing practice situations

Each project lasts for one year (steps 1 to 4). Depending on the goals of the individual facility the project involves three to five wards with approximately ten to fifteen registered nurses. That means that in each institution almost sixty registered nurses will be involved in project work.

UTILIZATION OF SELF-CARE DEFICIT NURSING THEORY IN NURSING ADMINISTRATION

In 1991 an extensive discussion began in Germany related to cost reduction and reorganization of the health care system. Never before did nursing have to face such changes in the procedures for financial calculation and payment of nursing service. An instrument was introduced to make it possible to determine the exact staffing requirements. Unfortunately it turned out that this instrument was not valid, and several years later the government discontinued this program.

However, many hospitals are still using this instrument for internal purposes of staffing calculation for nursing units. In addition to this in June 2001 the government passed an initiative to introduce the Diagnostic Related Groups (DRG) as the basis for financing health care in the future. Particularly in the above-mentioned hospitals, the nursing management staffs have started initiatives to use self-care deficit nursing theory-based developmental work (care plans, etc.) for nursing management purposes. As a result of the tremendous and extensive changes in the health care system and the impact on nursing, the nursing managers in those hospitals using self-care deficit nursing theory as their basis for practice founded the German Network of Self-Care Deficit Nursing Theory in April 2001. The main purpose of the network is to share results of practical and theoretical work in using self-care deficit nursing theory.

To date, results of the work done in institutions relating to calculating nursing demand based on self-care deficits of patients show the potential of the self-care deficit nursing theory-based diagnostic process. It is obvious that care plans that focus primarily on the proper object of nursing will show the relationship between nursing-relevant patient problems and Diagnostic Related Groups. This will be supported by results from research. Some self-care deficit nursing theory-based research projects on self-care in patients with dialysis and patients with leg ulcer and asthma already give insight on how self-care concepts will influence financing nursing intervention.

CHAPTER 41

An Integrative Review and Meta-Analysis of Self-Care Research in Thailand: 1988–1999 [Supported by Faculty of Medicine, Ramathibodi Hospital]

Somchit Hanucharurnkul, Jariya Wittaya-sooporn, Yuwadee Luecha, and Wantana Maneesriwongul

Self-care has been one of the key domain concepts in nursing since 1959, with the development of Orem's self-care model. Recently, self-care has become increasingly evident in health care, making even more sense in the face of the world economic crisis and the need for health care reform in Thailand. Self-care is an attempt to promote optimal health, prevent illness, detect symptoms at an early date, and manage both acute and chronic conditions of illness. Thus, self-care decreases the dependence of an individual on others. Even with rapid progress in medicine and technology, self-care is necessary. If people can mobilize their own resources and actively participate in their own health care, they may exceed life expectancies and significantly improve their quality of life.

In Thailand, The National Health Care Reform Committee included self-care as one of the key elements in primary care that is integrated, continuous, and holistic in nature (Simenton, Matthews-Simonton, & Creighton, 1978). In order to promote self-care among individuals, families, and communities, graduate nursing students in various universities have been applying Orem's General Theory of Nursing in clinical practice and conducting extensive research studies related to self-care over the past ten years. There are currently more than 200 master's theses on this topic. These activities have contributed to greater understanding of self-care phenomena. However, to build knowledge that will have an impact on nursing practice and to further advance self-care nursing science, a systematic and integrative review of accumulated research findings is needed. Thus, the purpose of this study is to describe ten years of self-care research in Thailand and to present the effectiveness of self-care promotion intervention on patient outcomes in various populations.

RELEVANT LITERATURE

Review of research and meta-analysis are increasingly more important in advancing knowledge development and facilitating evidence- or research-based practice. The number of nursing studies is rapidly increasing. However, most of the nursing research review and meta-analyses were conducted in the United States to determine the effectiveness of the specific intervention. For example: meta-analysis of the effects of psychoeducational interventions on length of post-surgical hospital stay (Devine & Cook, 1983), meta-analysis of critical outcome variables in non-nutritive sucking in preterm infants (Schwartz, Moody, Yarandi, Anderson, et al., 1987), meta-analysis of diabetic patient education (Brown, 1988, 1990, 1992), meta-analysis of relaxation training on clinical symptoms (Hyman, Feldman, Harris, Levin, Malloy, et al., 1989), meta-analysis of effects of heparin flush and saline flush (Goode, Titler, Rakel, et al., 1991), meta-analysis on strategies for teaching patients (Theis & Johnson, 1995), integrative review and meta-analysis of ten years of oncology nursing research (Smith & Stullenbarger, 1995).

In Thailand, meta-analyses were found mostly in the education field (Wiratchai & Wongwanich, 1999). In nursing, there is one report of meta-analysis of the effect of surgical preparation on biopsychosocial adjustment in women (Unhasut, Rabeub, Sinthu, et al., 1996). Two other studies described the characteristics and results of the studies in diabetic patients (Menettip, 1997) and cervical cancer patients (Aksiriwaranon, 1998).

Self-Care Research in Thailand

Self-care research in Thailand, based on Orem's general theory of nursing, includes descriptive, experimental, and qualitative participatory action research. Study samples have included healthy, acute, and chronically ill persons.

In descriptive research, there are studies that describe self-care practices ranging from simple or routine care in daily life measures (Hoornboon-herm, 1999a, 1999b, 1999c; Singhala, 1999; Sombutlah, 1999) to the highly complex skills of managing a chronic illness (Wattradul, 1994). These studies do not meet the criteria for meta-analysis because they describe only one variable. The largest number of studies tested the relationships between basic conditioning factors of age, gender, education, socioeconomic status, health state, knowledge, and social support with self-care or dependent care, that is, agency, efficacy, behaviors, deficit, and burden; or have tested the relationship between self-care and outcomes, that is, glycosylate hemoglobin and fasting blood sugar in diabetic patients, quality of life in cancer patients (Hanucharurnkul, 1988; Nuaklong, 1991; Takviriyanun, 1991; Vudhisethakrit, 1999). These descriptive correlation studies have contributed to confirming or refuting the theoretical proposition of self-care deficit theory, which states that self-care or dependent care is conditioned by age, developmental state, life experience, social cultural orientation, health and available resources (Orem, 1995). However, the findings cannot be conclusive without systematic review and meta-analysis.

The self-care concept is historically rooted in nursing and many nurse leaders accept that promoting the ability of individuals to care for themselves or dependent members of the family is the important and unique function of the profession. However, studies in Thailand indicate that chronically ill patients and their families report that they did not receive adequate information and guidance from nurses in caring for themselves (Hongtrakul, 1989; Uckanit, 1991) or dependent members (Gasemgitvatana, 1994). These studies have limited generalizability because they were conducted mostly in large tertiary-care settings; furthermore, they reflect the philosophy of more acute, episodic, curative-centered care approaches, rather than holistic, continuous care. Promoting individuals' self-care requires reformulating the health care service system as well as increasing health care professional knowledge, attitude, and skills.

Since nursing is a practice discipline in which the aim of research is to build nursing science to improve the health of people, developing and testing the effectiveness of nursing interventions is crucial. Nursing investigators who designed intervention programs based on Orem's nursing system usually tested the effectiveness of self-care promotion programs. The outcome of the interventions included self-care or dependent-care agency, efficacy, behavior, deficit or burden; health, for example, symptom experiences, complications, metabolic control; quality of life or well-being; satisfaction with care; and length of hospital stay. The most common methods that investigators use are (1) providing information by various strategies, (2) promoting patient participation in self-care, or (3) family participation in caring for the patients. Most of the studies yielded a positive outcome. However, the impact of these programs on clinical practice is limited.

Some investigators tend to believe that, since self-care is necessary to maintain life, health, and well-being of individuals, it is more appropriate to explore how to promote and sustain self-care efforts of the person than it is to test the effectiveness of self-care promotion programs using experimental design. In this design, in which the control group receives no treatment, researchers see a trend to violate human rights by withholding the desirable treatment (Gasemgitvatana, 1993). Therefore, participatory action research (PAR) was used to develop models to promote self-care among various populations, especially for chronically ill patients such as those with diabetes (Hanucharurnkul, Keratiyutawong, & Archananupapr, 1997; Phonploy, 1995; Tantayotai, 1997), HIV/AIDS (Nantachaipan, 1996), or cancer (Chotanakarn, 1996; Jirajarat, 1996). Results of these studies provide more insight and deeper understanding of self-care agency and how to enhance self-care agency in patients with chronic illness. Furthermore, this method of research increased nursing competence among the investigators.

Another line of self-care research is based on the notion that self-care has been perceived narrowly as an individual following professional advice (Sritanyarat, 1996). Two studies of self-care processes in diabetic and hypertensive patients were conducted using grounded theory and symbolic interaction as a conceptual framework (Panpakdee, 1999; Sritanyarat, 1996). Three other studies used ethnographic methodology to describe self-care by HIV/AIDS patients (Sangchart, 1997; Songsang, 1997) and elderly persons (Naka, 1999). Discoveries from these studies provide a comprehensive understanding of self-care that incorporates social and cultural perspectives. Also, self-care alternatives are evident. Results of the studies can be used for establishing a basis in helping patients to meet their self-care requirements within their social and cultural context.

In conclusion, self-care has been extensively studied in Thailand within the last ten years, especially by master of nursing science students. Integrative review and meta-analysis are necessary in order to summarize the findings and to set the direction for further study. The project reported here describes the synthesis of ten years of self-care research in Thailand, using integrative review and meta-analysis. The project was directed toward five goals:

1. To describe the status of self-care research in Thailand from 1988 to 1999
2. To summarize the magnitude of the effect size of related factors on self-care
3. To assess the effectiveness of self-care promotion intervention on outcomes in various populations
4. To set the direction for further study
5. To present self-care process derived from qualitative studies

METHODS

The project was implemented by a 16-member team consisting of four graduate faculty members, ten doctoral, and two master's nursing students. Three graduate faculty members teach in the area of adult nursing, and pediatrics, and two are familiar with Orem's general theory of nursing. One teaches research method and statistics and has experience in meta-analysis.

Sampling Procedures

Computer searches at The National Research Council of Thailand were used to locate master's theses and doctoral dissertations from all universities in Thailand that offered graduate programs from 1988 to 1999, using the heading *self-care, as related to health and illness*. In addition, the names of master's and doctoral graduates from all faculties of nursing, departments of nursing, and faculties of public health were requested, with the aim of finding topics of their master's thesis or doctoral dissertations that were related to self-care in health and illness. For non-master's theses or doctoral theses, hand searches were used to locate the studies at The Library of the National Research Council of Thailand, and at the research database from the Faculty of Nursing, Mahidol University. When searches were completed, potential studies were evaluated to assure that the studies were conducted between 1988 and 1999 and that the topics were related to self-care in health and illness.

One hundred and eighty studies were found, but only 123 met the criteria for meta-analysis. Five were qualitative studies and 52 were descriptive studies on health behavior or described only self-care behavior.

Coding Procedures

Studies were coded according to the coding form, which was composed of four characteristics as follows:

1. General characteristics, including research topic, name of research discipline, year reported, and type of publication
2. Substantive characteristics, including information about the studied subjects, such as age, gender, educational level, unit of study (e.g., individual, family, or groups), characteristics of intervention (type, length of intervention, and follow-up)
3. Methodological characteristics, including type of research design, method of sampling, sample size, and group assignment
4. Quality of the study, including research design method of sampling, quality of the instrument, statistics used for data analysis

Information from each study was identified and entered on the coding form by the ten doctoral nursing students and the two master's nursing students who completed their theses and were waiting for thesis defense. Six hours of special lectures on meta-analysis were provided for these students before performing data coding. Inter-rater reliability checks were performed at the completion of five studies, which were independently and periodically coded by each student with a project director. After completion of all study coding, it was checked by the project director for completeness. Any disagreement identified would be discussed until agreement was achieved.

Data Analysis

For the descriptive studies, which describe the relationship between basic conditioning factors and self-care, the formula shown in Figure 41.1 was used to convert simple correlation (r), chi-square (X^2), and t value to the effect size index (Cohen, 1977). See Figure 41.1.

Effect sizes for each variable pertinent to this research were calculated for each study using the above formulae. Similar variables were combined; self-care agency, self-care behavior, self-care efficacy, self-care deficit, and self-care burden were combined to self-care agency (the negative value of deficit and burden were changed to positive value). Glycosylated hemoglobin and fasting blood sugar were combined to glucoregulation.

For the magnitude of effect size, Cohen (1977) has provided guidelines for interpretation as follows: an effect size 0.2 is considered small, 0.5 is moderate, and 0.8 and above is large. These guidelines are used in this meta-analysis.

Results

Of the 123 studies selected there were 67 (54.47%) descriptive studies and 56 (45.53%) experimental studies, including participatory action research. Since the five participatory action research studies included quantitative data of pre- and posttest, the meta-analysis could be performed. The studies were predominantly master's thesis (86.33%) with purposive sample (69.78%) of chronic illness (76.78%). Orem's general theory of nursing was used mostly as a conceptual framework alone (76.78%) or in combination with others (10.79%).

Individuals were the unit studied, with few focusing on families as caregivers. The subjects were predominantly adults with chronic illness, and the elderly were not clearly identifiable. Gender combinations were studied, and educational level, socioeconomic status, and sociocultural orientation of the subjects were also reported. Self-care in health promotion, disease prevention, and early detection were addressed less often than in chronic illness.

To convert simple correlation (r), chi-square (X^2) and t value to the effect size index:

$$d = 2r \sqrt{1 - r^2}$$

d = effect size
r = simple correlation

For chi-square statistics, convert to r using the following formula:

$$r = \sqrt{\frac{x^2}{n}}$$

n = sample size, use only for 2 x 2 frequency tables (df = 1)

For converting t to r, use the following formula:

$$r = \sqrt{\frac{t^2}{t^2 + df}}$$

Then convert r to effect size, using the previous formula.

For intervention program studies, the formula for calculating effect size estimate, as suggested by Glass, was used:

$$d = \frac{X_e - X_c}{S_c}$$

where d is the effect size
X_e is the mean of the experimental group
X_c is the mean of the control group
S_c is the standard deviation of the group

Average effect size (weighted mean) was determined by using the following formula:

$$d_{average} = \sum_{i=1}^{k} n_i d_i \left/ \sum_{i=1}^{k} n_i \right/ \sum_{i=1}^{k} n_i$$

where d = effect size for each independent study, n = the number of subjects in each study, and k = number of studies

FIGURE 41.1 Formulae.

Relationship Between Basic Conditioning Factors and Self-Care Agency

In meta-analysis of 67 descriptive studies, all simple correlations, chi-square, and t value were converted to effect size of various basic conditioning factors on self-care agency. As shown in Table 41.1, weighted mean effect size across the study for health state is large (1.15), for education and knowledge is moderate (0.68 and 0.59, respectively), and for income, social support, duration of illness, and age is small. It is noted that weighted mean effect size of age and duration of illness on self-care are both positive and negative, yielding the weighted mean effect size across studies at small size.

The Effectiveness of Self-Care Promotion Intervention

There were 56 self-care promotion interventions in various populations but predominantly in patients with chronic illness. (76.78%), particularly diabetic patients (35.71%). Sample size was mostly between 30 and 60 subjects. Purposive or convenience sampling was predominant. The number of studies in each population group was as follows: diabetes—20, cancer—12, HIV/AIDS—4, chronic obstructive pulmonary disease—4, thalassemia—3, surgery and pregnancy—7.

To present the weighted mean effect size of self-care promotion intervention, outcome variables with at least three studies were selected. Table 41.2 shows the weighted mean effect size of each outcome variable. Weighted mean effect size of *self-care agency* is large in diabetic patients, HIV/AIDS patients, pregnant women, and thalassemia patients, whereas it is moderate in patients with cancer and chronic obstructive pulmonary disease. For *quality of life*, weighted mean effect size is large in HIV/AIDS patients and moderate in cancer patients. In diabetic patients, the

TABLE 41.1 Mean, SD, and Range of Effect Size of Basic Conditioning Factors on Self-Care Agency

	Number of studies	d	SD	Range	
Age	24	0.19	0.39	−0.72	−0.77
Education	28	0.68	0.34	0.45	−0.99
Income	26	0.48	0.26	0.06	−1.29
Social Support	14	0.40	0.31	0.16	−1.62
Heath State	8	1.15	0.63	0.52	−2.44
Duration of Illness	18	0.22	0.30	−0.19	−1.02
Knowledge	10	0.59	0.39	0.07	−1.27

TABLE 41.2   Effects of Outcome Variables According to Disease Group

Disease group	Outcome variables	No. of study variables	Weighted mean effect size (d)	SD	Range
Diabetes	SCA	16	1.66	0.77	0.32–3.47
	Knowledge	10	1.80	0.57	0.96–3.00
	Glucoregulation	13	0.61	0.26	0.13–1.39
	Disease control	5	1.27	0.35	0.73–1.79
Cancer	SCA	6	0.60	0.29	0.05–1.76
	Quality of life	9	0.64	0.07	0.27–1.15
HIV/AIDS	SCA	4	1.90	0.13	0.90–2.47
	Quality of life	4	1.05	0.33	0.41–1.68
Pregnancy	SCA	6	1.28	0.76	0.14–2.31
	Knowledge	3	0.87	0.54	0.64–2.56
Thalassemia	SCA	3	1.53	0.31	1.02–1.96
COPD	SCA	3	0.77	0.33	0.44–1.10
Surgery	Pain	5	0.64	0.55	0.10–2.14
	Complication	6	0.74	0.71	0.04–2.50
	Satisfaction	5	0.87	0.47	0.43–1.92
	Length of stay	4	0.37	0.17	0.25–0.82

intervention produced moderate effect size on glucoregulation and large effect size on disease control. In surgical patients, weighted mean effect size of satisfaction is large, complication and pain are moderate, and length of stay is small. When the mean length of hospital stay (LOS) was compared between the control group (M = 6.18) and the experimental group (M = 5.03), it was found that mean LOS in the experimental group was 1.15 days less than the control group.

Five participatory action research studies were aimed at the development of self-care agency, improvement of quality of life, and disease control among the chronically ill, HIV/AIDS, diabetic, and cancer patients. Final results yielded the practice model, which includes patients' effort to perform self-care and helping methods provided by the nurse investigators. The results also identified various basic conditioning factors that explain the rationale for taking or not taking various self-care actions.

The model reflected that, in order to perform self-care behavior, patients must use their time, effort, and resources in taking whatever action they judge to be appropriate, even though it is neither pleasurable nor appealing to them. For example, they have to take chemotherapy even though it causes nausea and vomiting. In addition, patients tried to discover, by trial and error, self-care strategies to relieve their symptoms, learning from other patients who had previously experienced the symptoms, or seeking information from brochures they received from the hospital.

The core helping methods provided by the nurse investigators in these five studies were (1) managing symptoms, (2) coordinating care, (3) providing counseling to patients and families, both by telephone and personal interaction, (4) providing information regarding type of treatment and its outcome, (5) involving families in patient care, (6) reinforcing continuing treatment and self-care, and (7) mobilizing resources to assist patients and families. There are some specific methods of helping for each group of patients. For example, for cancer patients, they included promoting a positive attitude toward the disease's treatment, and correcting the myths of cancer. Helping diabetic patients in negotiation with the physician regarding their treatment is important. These methods of helping provided more concrete actions in extension of Orem's helping methods, and were provided through the nurse–patient relationship or interpersonal system, according to Orem's perspective, intertwining to increase mutual efficacy.

Participatory action research also provided the data related to basic conditioning factors that influence self-care behavior in this group of chronically ill patients. These basic conditioning factors were both personal and environmental in nature. The personal factors included socioeconomic status and occupation, health state (especially symptomatic experience), perception and belief about their disease, and hope. The environmental factors were social support, health care service, and resources. Disease and treatment strongly influence self-care behaviors and effort. These factors explain why the patients performed or did not perform such self-care behavior or the way they performed such behaviors.

DISCUSSION

Graduate education in nursing has been a major source of self-care research in Thailand over the last decade: master's thesis (86.33%) and doctoral dissertation (8.63%). The studies were descriptive, experimental, participatory action research, and purely qualitative in nature, with purposive or convenience samples of fairly small size. Intervention programs to promote self-care were titled differently as educative-supportive, health education, patient participation in self-care, counseling, and planned teaching. However, the strategies used were very similar and usually combined various methods of helping, as suggested by Orem in the theory of nursing system (Orem, 1995). These methods of helping are teaching, guiding, supporting, and providing an environment for self-care. Other methods may be added, such as counseling, group meetings, and mutual goal setting. Thus, many replications of the studies were found, especially testing the effectiveness of self-care promotion programs but in various chronically ill and surgical patients.

Self-Care and Related Factors

Descriptive correlational study provided evidence in support of Orem's proposition that the individual's ability to engage in self-care or dependent care is conditioned by age, developmental state, health state, sociocultural orientation, family system, pattern of living and environmental factors (Orem, 1995). Health state produced positive large effect size on self-care agency; education and knowledge produced positive moderate effect size; while income and social support yielded positive small effect size. For age and duration of illness, the effect sizes on self-care agency were both positive and negative. For age, it indicated that self-care agency increases from children to adults and declines with aging. This state of development of self-care agency is the foundation of self-care when an individual has a chronic illness. For the duration of the illness, the patients might need some time to develop their self-care agency; however, self-care agency could decline with the length of illness because of health deterioration.

Qualitative studies provide a basis for understanding why basic conditioning factors influence patients' ability to perform or not perform some therapeutic self-care demands, or the way people meet their self-care requisites. For example, a diabetic patient who was working as a hairdresser could not eat on time because of her job demands. Qualitative studies in patients with chronic illness have also provided deep understanding of self-care as a process by which patients struggle to care for themselves in order to live normally. This kind of knowledge is very useful in helping patients to meet their self-care requisites.

Effectiveness of Self-Care Promotion Intervention

The current emphasis on the use of outcomes for the evaluation of health care effectiveness is crucial. Jennings, Staggers, and Brosch (Cohen, 1988) established a meaningful framework for viewing the various dimensions of outcomes. The dimensions included patient-focused outcomes with both diagnostic specific indicators and holistic indicators, provider-focused outcomes in both professional and significant others, and organization-focused outcomes. Most of the outcomes of self-care promotion intervention included in this analysis are patient-focused. These outcomes are diagnostic specific, such as glycosylated or fasting blood sugar in diabetic patients, or pain and complications in surgical patients. The outcomes for holistic indicators are self-care agency, knowledge, quality of life, and patient satisfaction. Only four studies in surgical patients included organization-focused outcomes, that is, the length of hospital stay, and one study in diabetic patients included cost in reduction of medication used.

The weighted mean effect size across all studies in each patient group in this analysis suggests that self-care promotion intervention yields a moderate to large positive effect size on various outcomes. This reflects consistency with clinical findings in that cancer patients who are receiving treatment and patients with chronic obstructive pulmonary disease usually encounter many symptoms that limit their ability to care for themselves while self-care requisites are complicated. Thus, self-care promotion intervention may not be enough, since the patients still need help from others. Also, the weighted mean effect size for quality of life in HIV/AIDS patients (M = 1.05, SD = 0.33) is higher than in cancer patients (M = 0.64, SD = 0.33), which may be caused by the fact that most of the study subjects were HIV-infected without serious symptoms.

In surgical patients, the first study to test the effectiveness of promoting patients' participation in self-care on postoperative recovery and satisfaction with care was conducted by Hanucharurnkul and Vinya-nguag (Jennings, Staggers, & Brosch, 1999), in adult surgical patients with pyelolithotomy and nephrolithotomy. This was replicated in five other studies on surgical patients such as gynecological patients, orthopedic patients, patients undergoing spinal cord surgery, or with the same group of surgical patients but in other settings. The intervention and the outcome were almost the same. The findings suggest that patient participation in self-care yields a large positive effect size on patient satisfaction, a moderate positive effect size on reduction of pain and complication, and a small positive effect size on length of hospital stay. The intervention can reduce cost by reducing the length of hospital stay by 1.15 days.

The magnitude of the effect size of self-care promotion intervention over the last decade did not change from 1988 to 1999. This reflects the minimal impact of self-care research in clinical practice. However, the studies were conducted in various population groups and there were a small number of studies in each group, except in diabetic patients. Furthermore, the measurement of self-care is different in each study. Thus, the meta-analysis cannot be done comprehensively. Also, the relationship between outcome effect of self-care promotion intervention and study characteristics cannot be determined.

CONCLUSION

In spite of many limitations in this integrative review and meta-analysis, growing confidence in the effectiveness of self-care promotion intervention is warranted and supported by consistency of findings in various studied groups. Also, basic conditioning factors should be taken into account in order to help clients develop their self-care agency.

Contribution of Graduate Students and Faculties to Nursing Knowledge in Self-Care

The majority of research on self-care in Thailand were master's theses. This finding is not surprising, since an essential goal of advanced nursing education is creation and dissemination of nursing knowledge (Wilson & Raines, 1999), and every master's program in nursing has thesis requirements. Faculty advisors spend a great amount of time providing supervision to the students. Thus, both graduate students in nursing and faculty advisors make valuable contribution to the advancement of self-care knowledge. Educators must continue to improve research-related courses and activities. Curriculum planners should be aware of barriers to research such as students' lack of writing skill (especially for those universities that require theses to be written in English), or lack of understanding of the importance of research in practice. Evidence-based practice is necessary to improve quality of care. Since evidence-based practice is the integration of "individual clinical expertise with the best available external clinical evidence from systematic research" (Rosswurn & Larrabee, 1999), advance practice nurses with graduate education who possess knowledge and skills in conducting and/or utilizing research are necessary in practice.

Future Directions of Research on Self-Care

The review of the 123 descriptive and experimental studies, including participatory action research in self-care over the last decade, provides the bases for future study as follows:

1. Quantitative studies of the relationship between basic conditioning factors and self-care agency globally do not provide or extend existing knowledge. However, studies should explore which and how each basic conditioning factor operates in specific groups of patients. Also, qualitative study may provide more understanding of the ways persons are meeting their self-care requisites.
2. Intervention outcome of self-care should include not only patient-focused outcome indicators but also provider-focused outcome and organization-focused outcome, such as burden of family caregiver or health care professional, and cost of the care.
3. Identification should be made of group units of analysis for study as well as individuals, with an increase in the number of studies in family and community care.
4. Expand settings of study to include home and hospice temples.
5. Increase the number of studies of age-specific population, particularly the elderly, older adult, adolescents, and children, also focusing on specific health problems.

6. Increase the number of gender-specific interventions in male and female groups with specific problems such as chronic illness.
7. Increase the study of the effectiveness of specific interventions that patients or families usually perform by themselves for health promotion or symptom management in chronic illness and the specific outcome for each intervention.
8. Expand studies to include health system research to develop appropriate systems in promotion of self-care in various settings.

Implication for Nursing Practice

Nursing practice should provide the system for research-based practice by creating the position of Advanced Practice Nurse in specialty areas, according to clients' needs. These Advanced Practice Nurses need skills and resources to appraise, synthesize, and diffuse the best evidence of systematic research into practice.

The authors would like to express sincere appreciation to the fifth class of doctoral nursing students, Apiradee Plodnaimeung and Thantawan Natethong, for their time and effort in coding the data.

References

Aksiriwaranon, W. (1998). *A survey of nursing research related to cervical carcinoma in Thailand.* Unpublished Master' s Thesis in Science (Nursing), Mahidol University, Bangkok, Thailand.

Allport, G. W. (1960). *Personality and social encounter.* Boston: Beacon.

Alumnae Association of The Johns Hopkins Hospital School of Nursing. (1967). *Response to change in health services: Papers from the seventy-fifth anniversary program.* Baltimore: Author.

American Nurses' Association first position on education for nursing. (1965). *American Journal of Nursing, 65*(12), 106–111.

Aquinas T. (1974). *Summa theologiae* (Vol. 36, T. Gilby, Trans.). Cambridge, MA: McGraw-Hill.

Aristotle (1919). *The ethics of Aristotle.* New York: Carlton House.

Arnold, M. B. (1960). Emotion and motivation. In *Emotion and personality: Psychological aspects* (Vol. I). New York: Columbia University Press.

Arnold, M. B. (1960). *Emotion and personality: Neurological and physiological aspects* (Vol. II). New York: Columbia University Press.

Ashby, W. R. (1964). *An introduction to cybernetics.* London: Chapman & Hall.

Backscheider, J. (1969). Rules pertaining to technologies. Unpublished paper.

Backscheider, J. (1973). Dynamics of concept development. In Nursing Development Conference Group (Ed.), *Concept formalization in nursing: Process and product.* Boston: Little, Brown.

Barnard, C. (1962). *The functions of the executive.* Cambridge, MA: Harvard University Press.

Blocker, C. E., Plummer, R. H., & Richardson, R. C. (1965). *The two-year college: A social synthesis.* Englewood Cliffs, NJ: Prentice-Hall.

Botschafter, P., & Moors, M. (1991). Pflegemodell in der Praxis—8. Folge: Dorothea Orem. Die Selbstfursorge-Defizit-Konzeption der Pflege. *Die Schwester Der Pfleger, 30*(8), 701–707.

Brown, E. L. (1948). *Nursing for the future.* New York: Russell Sage.

Brown, S. A. (1988). Effects of educational interventions in diabetes care: A meta-analysis of findings. *Nursing Research, 37*(15), 223–230.

Brubacher, J. S., & Rudy, W. (1958). *Higher education in transition.* New York: Harper & Row.

Chotanakarn, P. (1996). *Development of self-care agency model in breast cancer patient receiving chemotherapy.* Unpublished Master's Thesis in Science (Nursing), Mahidol University, Bangkok, Thailand.

355

Cleland, V. (1972). Nurse clinicians and nurse specialists: An overview. In *Three challenges to the nursing profession: Selected papers from the 1972 ANA convention.* New York: American Nurses' Association.

Cohen, J. (1977). *Statistical power analysis for behavioral science.* New York: Harcourt Brace.

Cohen, J. (1988). *Statistical power analysis for the behavioral science.* Hillsdale, NJ: Lawrence Erlbaum Associates.

Commission on Professional and Hospital Activities (1966, June). *Professional activity study: Discharge analysis B.* (hospital files).

Dependent-care practices of women with children aged 0–5. (1999). Paper presented at the The 6th International Self- Care Deficit Nursing Theory Conference, Bangkok, Thailand.

Devine, C. E., & Cook, D. T. (1983). A meta-analytic analysis of effects of psychoeducational interventions on length of postsurgical hospital stay. *Nursing Research, 32*(5), 267–273.

Dickoff, J., & James, P. (1968). On theory development in nursing: A theory of theories. *Nursing Research, 47*(3), 197–203.

Doherty, E. P. (1965, March 16). *Human behavior: Lecture transcript.* Washington, DC: The Catholic University of America.

Faculty Participants (1979). *The faculty scholar: One adventure in thinking.* Hattiesburg, MS: University of Southern Mississippi School of Nursing.

Gasemgitvatana, S. (1994). *A casual model of caregiver role stress on wives of chronically ill patients.* Unpublished Doctoral Dissertation in Nursing Science, Mahidol University, Bangkok, Thailand.

Georgetown University School of Nursing (1976). *Organization of nursing faculty responsibilities.* Washington, DC: Author.

Gerstl, J. E. (1967). Education and the sociology of work. In D. A. Hansen & J. E. Gerstl (Eds.), *On education: Sociological perspectives.* New York: Wiley.

Glass, G. V. (1981). *Meta-analysis in social research.* California: Sage Publications.

Goode, C. J., Titler, M., & Rakel, B. (1991). A meta-analysis of effects of heparin flush and saline flush: Quality and cost implication. *Nursing Research, 40,* 324–330.

Grzegorzlinski, E. (1965, September). Medical education in developing countries. *The Journal of Medical Education, 40*(9).

Hanucharurnkul, S. (1988). *Social support, self-care, and quality of life in cancer patients receiving radiotherapy in Thailand.* Unpublished Doctoral Dissertation, Wayne State University, Michigan.

Hanucharurnkul, S., Keratiyutawong, P., & Archananuparp, S. (1997). Self-care promotion program for diabetes. *Thai Journal of Nursing Research, 1*(1), 115–137.

Hanucharurnkul, S., & Vinya-Nguag, P. (1991). Effects of promoting patients, participation in self-care on postoperative recovery and satisfaction with care. *Nursing Science Quarterly, 4*(1), 14–20.

Hare, R. (1970). *The principles of scientific thinking.* Chicago: University of Chicago Press.

Henderson, V. (1955). *Harmer's: A textbook of principles and practices of nursing* (5th ed.). New York: Macmillan.

Holoch, E., Gehrke, U., Knigge-Demal, B., & Zoller, E. (1999). *Lehrbuch Kinderkrankenpflege.* Bern: Huber Verlag.

Hongtrakul, J. (1989). *Relationships among selected basic conditioning factors, social support, and self-care agency in essential hypertensive patients.* Unpublished Master' s Thesis in Science (Nursing), Mahidol University, Bangkok, Thailand.

Horn, B. J., & Swain, M. A. (1977). *Development of criterion measures of nursing care.* Springfield, VA: National Technical Information Service.

Hornboonherm, P. (1999). *Dependent-care practices of women with school age children.* Paper presented at the the 6th International Self-Care Deficit Nursing Theory Conference, Bangkok, Thailand.

Hyman, R. B., Feldman, H. R., Harris, R. B., Levin, R. F., & Malloy, G. B. (1989). The effects of relaxation training on clinical symptoms: A meta-analysis. *Nursing Research, 38*(4), 216–220.

Jennings, B. M., Staggers, N., & Brosch, L. R. (1999). A classification scheme for outcome indicators. *Image: Journal of Nursing Scholarship, 31*(4), 381–388.

Jirajarat, M. (1996). *Development of self-care agency model in colorectal and anal cancer patients receiving treatments in outpatient clinic.* Unpublished Master' s Thesis in Science (Nursing), Mahidol University, Bangkok, Thailand.

King, A. R., & Brownell, J. A. (1966). *The curriculum and the disciplines of knowledge: A theory of curriculum practice.* New York: Harper & Row.

Kneller, U. F. (1966). *Educational anthropology: An introduction.* New York: Wiley.

Kotarbinski, T. (1965). *Praxiology: An introduction to the sciences of efficient action* (O. Wojtasiewicz, Trans.). New York: Pergamon.

Lonergan, B. J. F. (1958). *Insight. A study of human understanding.* London and New York: Darton, Longman and Todd, Philosophical Library.

Lonergan, B. J. F. (1967). *Insight.* New York: Philosophical Library.

Lonergan, B. J. F. (1972). *Method in theology.* New York: Herder and Herder.

Lonergan, B. J. F. (1978). *Insight: A study of human understanding* (Rev. student ed.). New York: Harper & Row.

Macmurray, J. (1957). *The self as agent.* London: Faber & Faber.

Macmurray, J. (1961). *Persons in relation.* New York: Harper and Brothers.

Maritain, J. (1940). *Science and wisdom* (B. Hall, Trans.). London: Centenary Press.

Maritain, J. (1959). *The degrees of knowledge* (G. B. Phelan, Trans.). New York: Scribner.

McEwan, L. (1986). *A retrospective study to identify the import of SCDT framework upon the process of diagnosis, prescription and design of care for R.* Columbia, MS: Harry S Truman Memorial Veterans Hospital.

McGrath, E. J. (1962). The ideal education for the professional man. In N. B. Henry (Ed.), *Education for the professions: The sixty-first yearbook of the National Society for the Study of Education, part II.* Chicago: University of Chicago Press.

Menettip, S. (1997). *A survey of nursing research related diabetic patients in Thailand.* Unpublished Master' s Thesis in Science (Nursing), Mahidol University, Bangkok.

Merritt, R. (1988, August). State health reports. *Nation's Health: The Official Newspaper of the American Public Health Association.*

Moyer, R., & Beach, K. (1967). *Developing vocational instruction.* Palo Alto, CA: Fearon.

Mueller, S. (1974, Fall). Higher education or higher skilling. *Daedalus: Journal of the American Academy of Art and Sciences,* pp. 150–151.

Naka, K. (1999). *Life-style and self-care of the elderly in a rural Thai village in Southern Thailand.* Unpublished Doctoral Dissertation in Nursing Science, Mahidol University, Bangkok, Thailand.

Nantachaipan, P. (1996). *Development of self-care agency model in persons with HIV infection/AIDS.* Unpublished Master's Thesis in Science (Nursing), Mahidol University, Bangkok, Thailand

National League for Nursing (1972). *Policies and procedures of accreditation for programs in nursing education associate degree programs, baccalaureate and higher degree programs, diploma programs, practical nursing programs.* National League for Nursing: Division of Accreditation, National League for Nursing, and Division of Accreditation (Eds.). New York: Author.

Niemeyer, M. F. (1951). *The one and the many in the social order according to Saint Thomas Aquinas.* Washington, DC: The Catholic University of America Press.

Nuaklong, W. (1991). *Self-care agency and quality of life in cervical cancer patients during and post receiving radiotherapy.* Unpublished Master's Thesis in Science (Nursing), Mahidol University, Bangkok, Thailand.

Nursing Development Conference Group (1973). *Concept formalization in nursing: Process and product.* Boston: Little, Brown.

Nursing Development Conference Group (1979). *Concept formalization in nursing: Process and product* (D. Orem, Ed.). Boston: Little, Brown.

O'Doherty, E. P. (1965, March 16). *Human behavior: Lecture transcript.* Washington, DC: The Catholic University of America.

Orem, D. E. (1956). *Hospital nursing service. An analysis.* Indianapolis: Division of Hospital and Institutional Services.

Orem, D. E. (1959). *Guides for developing curricula for the education of practical nurses.* Washington, DC: Government Printing Office.

Orem, D. E. (1968a, March 7–May 2). In-service education and nursing practice. In D. D. Petrowski & M. T. Partheymuller (Eds.), *Forces affecting nursing practice: The proceedings of the Continuing Education Series.* Washington, DC: The Catholic University of America Press.

Orem, D. E. (1968b). *Foundations of nursing and its practice.* Unpublished manuscript.

Orem, D. E. (1969). Levels of nursing education and practice. *Alumnae Magazine Johns Hopkins School of Nursing, 68*(1), 2–6.

Orem, D. E. (1971). *Nursing: Concepts of practice.* New York: McGraw-Hill.

Orem, D. E. (1980). *Nursing: Concepts of practice* (2nd ed.). New York: McGraw-Hill.

Orem, D. E. (1985). *Nursing: Concepts of practice* (3rd ed). New York: McGraw-Hill.

Orem, D. E. (1988). The form of nursing science. *Nursing Science Quarterly, 1*(2), 75–79.

Orem, D. E. (1990). A nursing practice theory in three parts 1956–1989. In M. E. Parker (Ed.), *Nursing theories in practice* (pp. 47–60). New York: WLN.

Orem, D. E. (1991). *Nursing: Concepts of practice* (4th ed.). St. Louis, MO: Mosby Yearbook.

Orem, D.E. (1993). *Modelo de Orem. Conceptos de enfermeria en lapractica.* (M. T. Luis, Trad.) Barcelona, Espana: Ediciones Cientificas y Tecnicas. (Trabajo original publicado en 1991).

Orem, D. E. (1995). *Nursing: Concepts of practice* (5th ed.). St. Louis, MO: Mosby.

Orem, D. E. (1997). *Strukturkonzepte der Pflegraxix.* (Translated by G. Bekel). Wiesgaden: Ullstein-Mosby.

Orem, D. E. (2001). *Nursing: Concepts of practice* (6th ed.). St. Louis, MO: Mosby.

Orem, D. E., & Taylor, S. O. (1986). Orems general theory of nursing. In P. Winstead-Fry (Ed.), *Case studies in nursing theory* (pp. 37–71). New York: National League for Nursing.

Panpakdee, O. (1999). *Self-care process of the patients with essential hypertension.* Unpublished Doctoral Dissertation in Nursing Science, Mahidol University, Bangkok, Thailand.

Parsons, T. (1951). *The social system.* New York: Free Press.

Parsons, T. (1964). *The structure of social action.* New York: McGraw-Hill.

Preface to the Issue "Adulthood." (1976, Spring). *Daedalus: Journal of the American Academy of Art and Sciences,* pp. v–viii.

Phonploy, W. (1995). *Self-care promotion for blood sugar controlling of non-insulin dependent diabetes mellitus.* Unpublished Master's Thesis in Adult Nursing, Prince of Songkla University, Songkla, Thailand.

Ricka, R., & Sclimidli-Bless, C. (1991). Pflegensches Fachwissen nach dem Modell der Selbstpflege von Dorothea Orem—1. Teil: Die Schlusselkonzepte. *Pflege, 4*(1), 65–72.

Robb, I. H. (1893). *Papers and discussions from International Congress of Charities, Correction and Philanthropy.* Chicago: Republished (1949) New York: McGraw-Hill.

Robb, I. H. (1907). *Educational standards for nurses.* Chicago: E. C. Koecker.

Robinson, V. (1986). Relationship of theory-based nursing and defined populations in using Orem's self-care deficit theory of nursing in practice, education, and research. *School of Nursing, University of Missouri, Conference.* Columbia, MO: Curators of the University of Missouri, November.

Rogers, J. (1944). *In-service staff education for the professional groups in the nursing department of a hospital: A selected annotated bibliography.* New York: National League for Nursing Education.

Roper, N. (1987). *Die Elemente der Krankenpflege.* Basel Recom: Verlag.

Rosswurm, M. A., & Larrabee, J. H. (1999). A model for change to evidence-based practice. *Image: Journal of Nursing Scholarship, 31*(4), 317–322.

Sangchart, B. (1997). *Culture of self-care among persons with HIV infection and AIDS: A study in the Northeast, Thailand.* Unpublished Doctoral Dissertation in Nursing Science, Mahidol University, Bangkok, Thailand.

Schwartz, R., Moody, L., Yarandi, H., & Anderson, G. C. (1987). A meta-analysis of critical outcome variables in Nonnutritive sucking in preterm infants. *Nursing Research, 36*(5), 292–295.

Self-care practices of children. (1999). Paper presented at the The 6th International Self-Care Deficit Nursing Theory Conference, Bangkok, Thailand.

Self-care: The art and science of nursing. (2nd ed.) (1993). Bangkok, Thailand: V. J. Printing.

Simonton, O. C., Matthews-Simonton, S., & Creighton, J. (1978). *Getting well again.* California: J. P. Tarcher, Inc.

Singhala, K. (1999). *Self-care behavior of youths in rural areas of Mahasarakham Province.* Paper presented at the The 6th International Self-Care Deficit Nursing Theory Conference, Bangkok, Thailand.

Smith, M. C., & Stullenbarger, E. (1995). An integrative review and meta-analysis of oncology nursing research. *Cancer Nursing, 18*(3), 167–179.

Sombutlah, S. (1999). *Self-care behavior of menopausal women: A case study in urban and rural areas of Mahasarakham Province.* Paper presented at the The 6th International Self- Care Deficit Nursing Theory Conference, Bangkok, Thailand.

Songsang, S. (1997). *Self-care of AIDS in a Thai culture context at a temple in Southern Thailand.* Unpublished Master's Thesis in Adult Nursing, Prince of Songkla University, Songkla, Thailand.

Sorokin, P. A. (1957). *Social and cultural dynamics.* Boston: Extending Horizons Books.

Sritanyarat, W. (1996). *A grounded theory study of self- care processes among Thai adults with diabetes.* University of Texas at Austin, Austin.

Strunk, H., & Osterbrink, J. (1995). Pflegetheorie nach Dorothea Orem. Von der Pflegephilosophie zur Aufgabenbeschreibung—angewandt in einer Schmerzklinik. *Die Schwester Der Pfleger, 34*(12), 1057–1063.

Studies of educational interventions and outcomes in diabetic adults: A meta-analysis revisited. (1990). *Nursing Research, 39*(16), 189–215.

Takviriyanun, N. (1991). *Self-care agency and quality of life in head & neck cancer patients while receiving and after completion of radiotherapy.* Unpublished Master's Thesis in Science (Nursing), Mahidol University, Bangkok, Thailand.

Tantayotai, W. (1997). *Development of self-care agency model in insulin-dependent diabetic patients.* Unpublished Doctoral Dissertation in Nursing Science, Mahidol University, Bangkok, Thailand.

Theis, S. L., & Johnson, J. H. (1995). Strategies for teaching patients: A meta-analysis. *Clinical Nurse Specialist, 9*(2), 100–105.

Uckanit, W. (1991). *Self-esteem and self-care practice in patients with chronic obstructive pulmonary disease.* Unpublished Master's Thesis in Science (Nursing), Mahidol University, Bangkok, Thailand.

Unhasut, K., Rabeub, P., & Sinthu, S. (1996). Meta-analysis of effect of surgical preparation on biopsychosocial adjustment in women. *Journal of Nursing, 14*, 32–47.

Van Eron, M. (1985). Clinical application of self-care deficit theory. In J. Riehl-Sisca (Ed.), *The science and art of self-care* (pp. 208–274). Norwalk, CT: Appleton-Century-Crofts.

Vickers, G. (1957). Control, stability, and choice. In L. von Bertalanffy & A. Rapaport (Eds.), *Yearbook of the Society for General Systems Research.* Bedford, MA: Society for General Systems Research.

von Bertalanffy, L. (1967). *Robots, men, and minds: Psychology in the modern world.* New York: Braziller.

Vudhisethakrit, P. (1999). *Basic conditioning factors, self-care deficit and spontaneous abortion.* Paper presented at the The 6th International Self-Care Deficit Nursing Theory Conference, Bangkok, Thailand.

Wall Street Journal, December 2, 1966.

Wallace, W. A. (1979). *From a realist point of view. Essays on the philosophy of science.* Washington, DC: University Press of America.

Wattradul, D. (1994). *Promotion HIV/AIDS patients participation in self-care.* Unpublished Master's Thesis in Science (Nursing), Mahidol University, Bangkok, Thailand.

Wilson, A. H., & Raines, K. H. (1999). Contributions of graduate students to nursing knowledge in women's health. *Image: Journal of Nursing Scholarship, 31*(4), 403.

Winstead-Fry, P. (Ed.). (1986). *Case studies in nursing theory.* New York: National League for Nursing.

Index

Printed in the United States
74626LV00003B/1-72